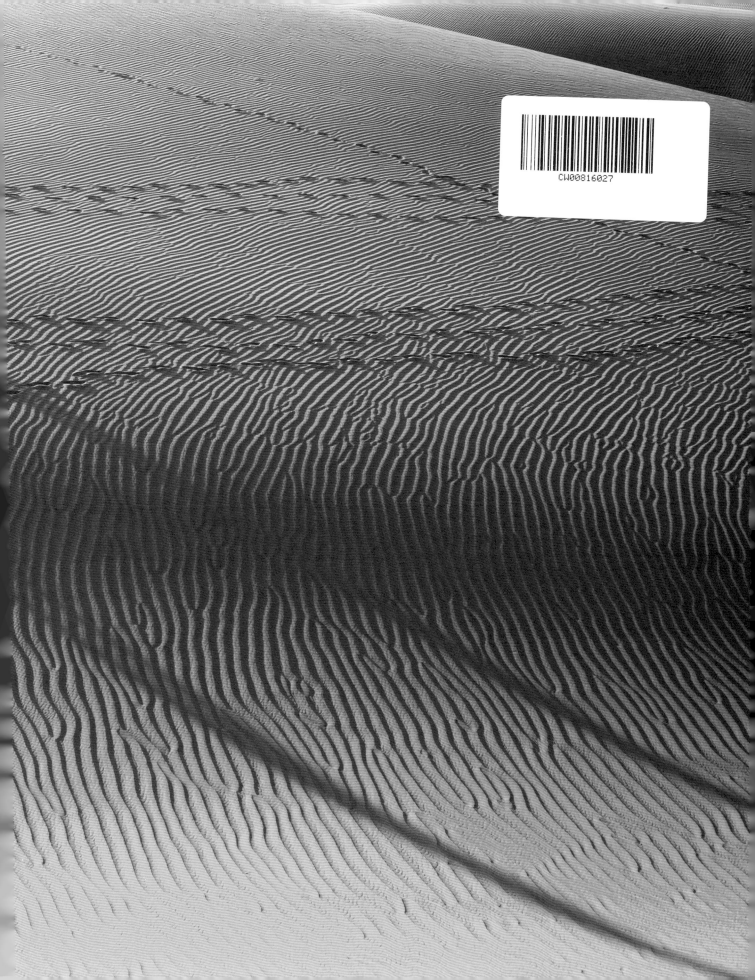

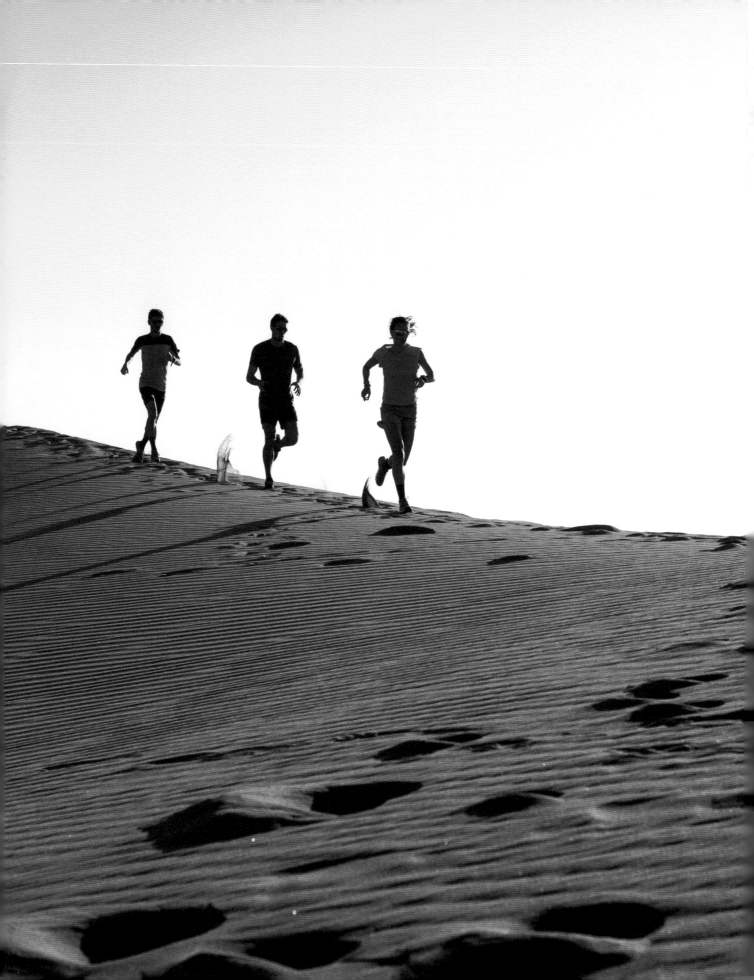

On the Run

Running Across the Globe

gestalten

Contents

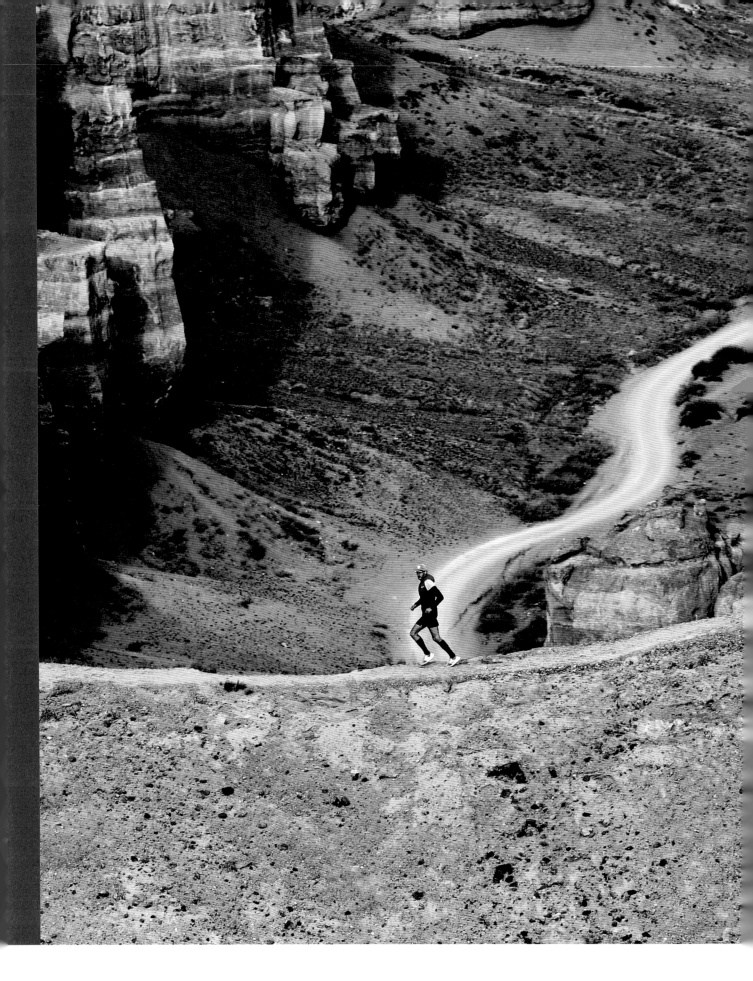

On Your Marks

Why do humans run? At one stage we simply had no choice. Our ancient ancestors evolved to run as a necessity for successful hunting and self-preservation. In fact, much of how the human body looks and functions is the result of our species becoming better runners.

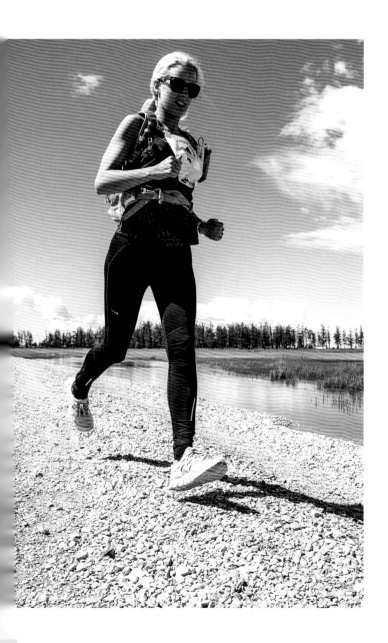

We no longer have to hunt for food, yet we desire running more than ever. Today we run for fun and fitness. What was once purely essential to survival now brings joy. Every year, millions participate in official races around the world, and many more put on their running shoes simply for the sake of putting their bodies in motion. We run vast distances, sometimes in places too harsh for vegetation to flourish, and can justify it in a million ways. Running quantifies new frontiers of athletic achievement—100 meters in under 10 seconds, the four-minute mile, the sub-two-hour marathon—but mostly we run to push our personal frontiers.

In his book *What I Talk About When I Talk About Running* (2007), Japanese author Haruki Murakami wrote: "Exerting yourself to the fullest within your individual limits: that's the essence of running, and a metaphor for life." In this exertion, as the body floods the brain with feel-good chemicals to the point of euphoria—what is called a "runner's high"—we feel a unity of mind and matter. It may be the closest most of us come to a conscious, legal, non-religious transcendental experience. For some, gaining access to this metaphysical realm makes running a form of therapy. For others, it's more of an escape, an antidote to screens and algorithms, and the noise and restlessness of the modern world. The wonderful thing about running, of course, is that it can be both, and it is accessible at almost any time.

Running is, first and foremost, a competition against oneself. We compete against our own limitations, doubts, and fears. Every step is a small victory that gets us into the habit of winning and every run offers the potential to reach beyond the limits of sport— to make a political statement, to express oneself, or to empower marginalized communities and subcultures. When considered in this light, all of a sudden running doesn't feel like an individual sport, but when it is just you, alone with your thoughts or in the absence of the working of your mind, that's where the transcendence happens, the meditation of running, of learning from our body and our body learning from us—just the way it's always been. ∎

Running: A Very Human History

About 2 million years ago, when we were somewhere on the path of development from apes to humans, our species underwent a momentous physical transformation: we evolved to run.

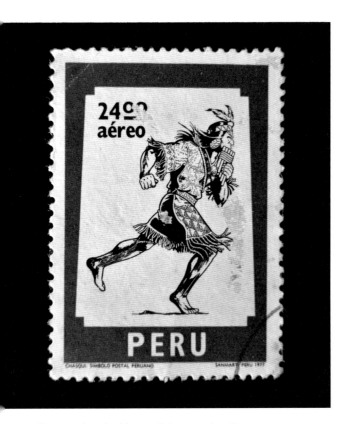

Above: an Inca *chaski*—one of a large number of messenger-runners whose network formed a kind of verbal postal system across the empire—immortalised on a Peruvian stamp. Opposite, top: a stone relief shows Ramses running to reaffirm his 30-year rule. Opposite, bottom: a Neolithic rock drawing at Tadrart Acacus, Libya, depicts humans hunting—an example of how ancient civilizations captured the concept of running in their art.

The prevailing theory for this evolutionary step forward is that we developed the ability to run to survive. Just as fish developed fins and gills, our bodies self-optimized to hunt and avoid being hunted. Our skulls were reconfigured for better balance when moving at speed and to prevent overheating. Our buttocks grew to increase stability and power, while the shock-absorbing ligament in our spines became far more pronounced. We blossomed, becoming upright and vibrant, as if having been unpacked from a box after millions of years. In short, we not only evolved to walk, but also to run. These physiological changes made early humans exceptional endurance runners, which meant that while our prey was faster over short distances, we had the stamina to give chase until an animal was exhausted. Life is indeed a marathon, not a sprint. As the German biologist and record-breaking runner Bernd Heinrich noted in his book *Why We Run* (2002), the smarts, stamina, and desire to win that developed during this period were integral to human ascent in the food chain.

Over the years, running itself evolved, too, becoming more ceremonious, sporting, and social. There is evidence of running for sport in ancient Egypt, about 3000 BCE, where pharaohs demonstrated their fitness to inspire confidence in their authority. In Ireland, from about 1600 BCE, footraces were part of funeral festivities performed to commemorate the dead. Mostly, running was connected to sports like mob football, the chaotic predecessor of today's beautiful game.

From about 1438, the Inca, like the Greeks before them, recognized the value of runners as messengers. The Inca empire was connected by a massive road system of about 40,000 kilometers (25,000 miles), and in order to communicate important military or trading information they set up a network of sprinters, or *chaskis*, as a sort of human telephone—long before Alexander Graham Bell's patent in 1876. *Chaskis* would run between special stations

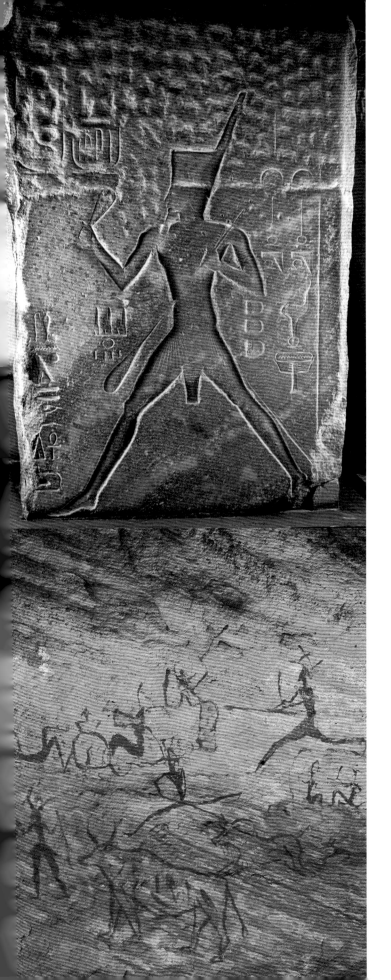

placed up to 15 kilometers (9 miles) apart and pass on messages for another runner to relay to the next station. In this way, precious information could travel up to 240 kilometers (150 miles) in a single day. To be named as a *chaski* was a great honor bestowed only on the fastest athletes, but the role also came with great responsibility—those who failed or delivered misinformation could face execution.

The most renowned messenger, of course, was the Greek Pheidippides who, in 490 BCE, ran a 480-kilometer (300-mile) round trip from Athens to recruit the Spartan army for a decisive battle in the village of Marathon. He then ran 40 kilometers (25 miles) to Marathon; upon arriving back in Athens to report the Greek victory, he collapsed and, with his dying breath, declared, *"Nike! Nenikekiam!"* ("Victory! We are victorious!"). Pheidippides's trek from Athens to the site of the battle is the inspiration for what is today the world's most famous race: the marathon.

Greek storytelling also most certifiably leads us to the roots of competitive running, to the inaugural ancient Olympics, in 776 BCE. The spectacle featured only one event, the *stadion*, a 180-meter (200-yard) sprint performed naked and barefoot. It wasn't until 13 Games later that another sport was added: the double-*stadion*. In 1896, the marathon debuted alongside five other running events at the first modern Olympic Games in Athens.

As athletics garnered more news coverage in the twentieth century, star athletes themselves became more prominent, raising awareness of important issues such as racism, discrimination, and civil rights. One would be hard-pressed to think of a more defiant sporting moment than when African-American sprinter Jesse Owens won four gold medals at the 1936 Olympics in Berlin, thereby undermining the Nazis' campaign of racial superiority.

And yet, as late as the 1960s, women were still excluded from many running events around the world. In 1966, Roberta "Bobbi" Gibb applied to run the Boston Marathon but received a rejection claiming that women were not capable of running long distances. Gibb ran the race anyway and became the first ▶

Just as fish developed fins and gills, our bodies self-optimized to hunt and avoid being hunted. Our skulls were reconfigured for better balance when moving at speed and to prevent overheating.

As athletics garnered more news coverage in the twentieth century, star athletes themselves became more prominent, raising awareness of important issues such as racism, discrimination, and civil rights.

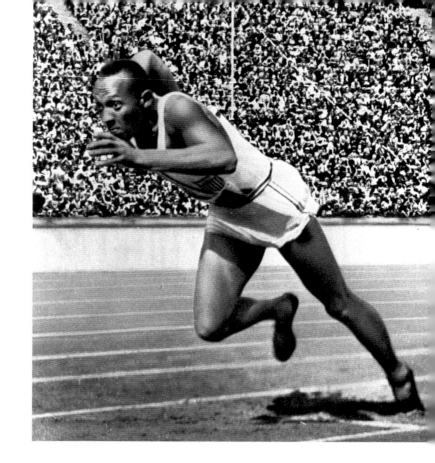

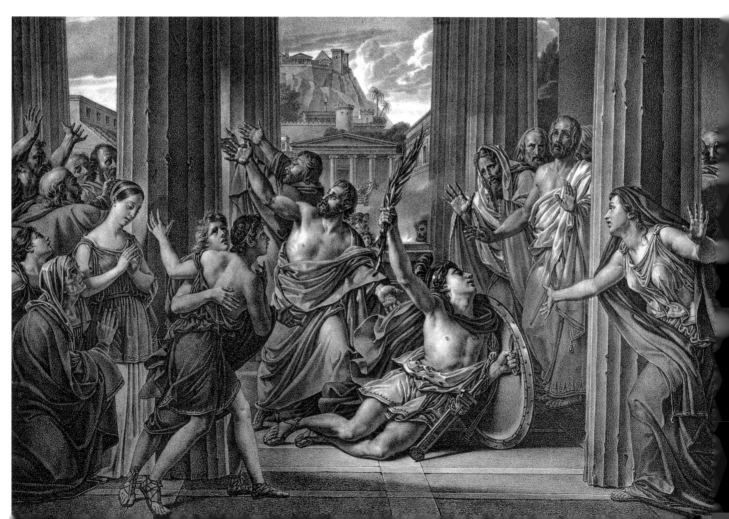

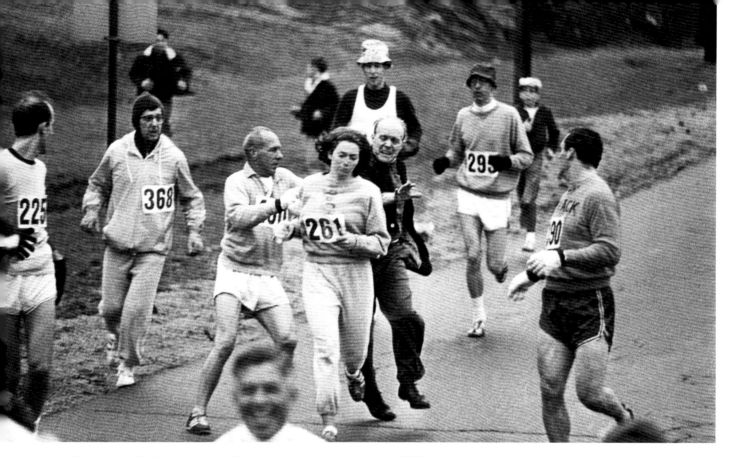

Above: a race official attempts to stop Kathrine Switzer from taking part in the 1967 Boston Marathon.
Opposite, top: American athlete Jesse Owens at the start of his 200-meter victory at the 1936 Berlin Olympics.
Opposite, bottom: a depiction of Pheidippides delivering his news of the Greek victory at Marathon.

▶ woman to complete the course, albeit unregistered. She ran again the next year, as did another woman, Kathrine Switzer, who had managed to register officially. However, Switzer's race was not stress-free: there were repeated angry interventions from race organizers, who claimed her registration was a mistake. It took another five years before the Amateur Athletic Union would officially sanction a women's marathon division. In many countries today, up to a third of marathon runners are women.

Competitive and professional running have continued in a variety of roles over the centuries, including the operation of treadmills for use in raising water or grinding grain. The British even managed to introduce the concept into corporal punishment for prisoners in the early nineteenth century. When the Irish poet and playwright Oscar Wilde was sentenced to two years' hard labor for the crime of homosexuality in 1895, he faced grueling six-hour stints on the treadmill.

Despite Wilde's experience, running flourished as a literary subject in the twentieth century and writers increasingly used it as a metaphor for everything from class division to existentialism. British author Alan Sillitoe's *The Loneliness of the Long-Distance Runner* (1959), perhaps the most famous story ever written about running, except

for *Forrest Gump,* is an example of the sport's profound allegory. In one passage, Sillitoe likens running to an awakening, both of himself and of life: "Sometimes I think that I've never been so free as during that couple of hours when I'm trotting up the path out of the gates and turning by that bare-faced, big-bellied oak tree at the lane end. Everything's dead, but good, because it's dead before coming alive, not dead after being alive."

The determination of these runners is echoed in William J. Bowerman's book *Jogging* (1967), which inspired an entire generation to hit the road in the name of health. It sold more than a million copies and presented running as an antidote to Americans' increasingly sedentary suburban lifestyles. The publication of *Jogging*—peppered as it is with inspirational quotes popular with Instagram influencers, such as "Everything you need is already inside"—was a seminal step in democratizing the sport for the everyday citizen. What began as counterculture to the TV-dinner generation quickly went mainstream. As one jogger told the *New York Times* in 1968, "At first you think everyone is staring at you—and they are. After a while you enjoy jogging so much you don't give a damn." Bowerman, a track-and-field coach at the University of Oregon and a co-founder of Nike, ▶

▶ worked obsessively to design the perfect shoe for his athletes, and the marriage of performance and fas the hion promoted by companies such as Nike was born. Among the Oregon athletes was long-distance runner Steve Prefontaine. He was the consummate poster boy for the sport and crowds filled bleachers to watch him perform. His stardom arguably did for running what David Beckham did for soccer in the U.S. When he died in 1975 in a car accident at just 24 years old, Prefontaine held every American track record between 2,000 and 10,000 meters.

Alongside seminal literary works, the postwar period also produced a pantheon of running greats. In 1952, Emil Zátopek of Czechoslovakia became the only athlete to claim gold in every long-distance event (5,000 meter, 10,000 meter, marathon) at a single Olympic Games. Astonishingly, having already won two medals, he decided at the last minute to compete in the marathon—his first. Eight years later, at the 1960 Games in Rome, Ethiopa's Abebe Bikila won an Olympic gold medal after running the marathon barefoot. The era's probably most famous runner, the Brit Roger Bannister, wasn't a runner at all. A medical student who was only able to train when his studies permitted it, he entered sports lore in 1954 by becoming the first person to run a sub-four-minute mile. And yet Bannister's record stood for just 46 days. The next year, three runners ran a sub-four-minute mile in the same race. "My mind took over. It raced well ahead of my body," Bannister recalled about his historic feat—proof that running is as much about clearing mental hurdles as physical ones.

Marathons and sprints became marquee events at the Olympics, which were broadcast on television for the first time in 1960. By the 1964 Games in Tokyo, the Olympics reached living rooms worldwide. Around the same time, amateur running exploded. Cities began hosting marathons to cater to hobby runners looking to emulate what they saw on TV.

For the less ambitious, there was the half-marathon. Five- and 10-kilometer races also no longer took place only on tracks but also on streets, trails, and beaches.

Meanwhile, as in other disciplines, possibilities in running began to expand for athletes with disabilities. In 1984, the wheelchair marathon was included for the first time at the Paralympic Games, which had themselves debuted in 1960. Arguably the event's most successful athlete is Germany's Heinrich Köberle, who has won four gold Paralympic medals. Outside the marathon, the Russian-born American Tatyana McFadden, who is paralyzed from the waist down and competes in a wheelchair, has scooped seven Paralympic golds, four of which were secured at the 2016 Games in Rio de Janeiro, where athletes competed in nine different running events within 10 disability categories, from the blind to amputees and those of short stature.

Below: running barefoot, Ethiopian Abebe Bikila passes the tomb of the Marathon Warriors in Rome, on his way to victory in the marathon event at the 1960 Summer Olympics. Opposite, from top: Roger Bannister on completing his sub-four-minute mile; an early example of Nike athletic shoes featuring William J. Bowerman's 'waffle sole' design; a taxi passenger follows the 1964 Tokyo Olympic Games on a screen in the back of the vehicle.

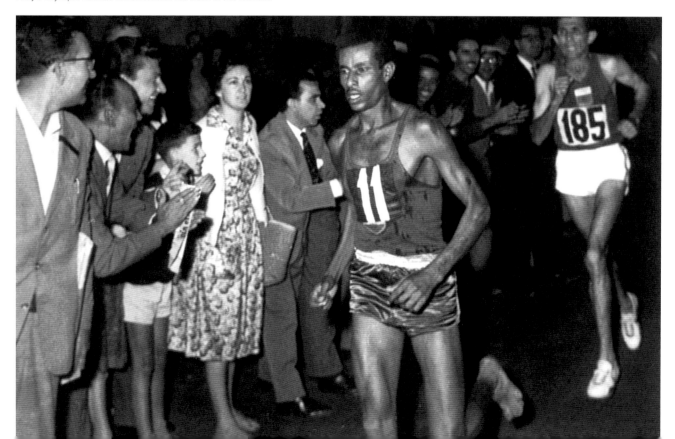

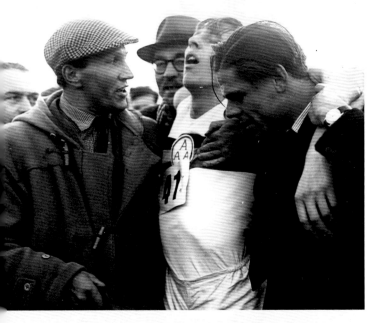

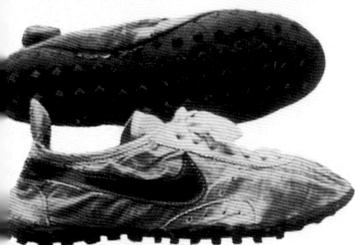

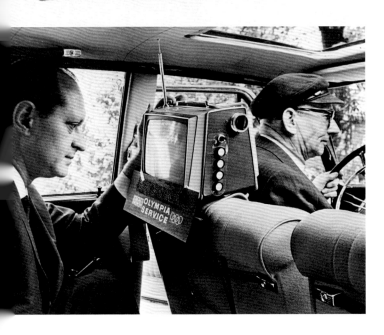

Today it is estimated that there are more than 800 marathon events and more than 2 million people run a half-marathon annually in the U. S. alone. We wear the sport on our sleeves, and on our wrists, and may also soon on our faces via virtual-reality headsets.

Today it is estimated that there are more than 800 marathon events and more than 2 million people run a half-marathon annually in the U. S. alone. We wear the sport on our sleeves, and on our wrists, and may also soon on our faces via virtual-reality headsets. Our obsession is fueled by apps such as Strava that feed our desire for community, mastery, competition, reward, and status. Through this "gamification," we are driven to compete with ourselves and others. At their core, these apps perhaps tap into the very reason we run today.

As we demand more from ourselves, we also demand more from our runs, as evidenced by the popularity of ever-ambitious races such as the 217-kilometer (135-mile) Badwater 135 ultramarathon through Death Valley, or the 617-kilometer (383-mile) 6633 Arctic Ultra, whose finish line is beyond the point where trees can survive. Likewise, we demand more of our athletes. Runners such as Justin Gallegos, who has cerebral palsy, have smashed the definition of what it means to be able-bodied, and in Kenyan runner Eliud Kipchoge we have the perfect example of an athlete pushing the limits of the human body. In 2019, 12-time marathon winner Kipchoge became the first person in record history to run a marathon distance in under two hours—arguably the greatest sporting achievement of all time.

Even the notion of running as an individual sport is being challenged, thanks to the proliferation of running crews, which combine sport with the arts, fashion, and activism. Sprouting up in cities, towns, slums, and favelas in every corner of the world, from European capitals to Soweto, Shanghai and Rio de Janeiro, running crews encourage people of different backgrounds and abilities to take up the sport. Each with their own running philosophy, they are unified by the motto that you are not alone—quite fitting for an activity that has literally shaped us, and through which we, as social animals, can understand who we are and how we got here. ∎

Distances and Terrains: A Beginner's Guide

It used to be that when you told someone you were going for a run, they could easily imagine what that meant—what you wore, how you moved, and roughly where and for how long. Running today demands a little more specificity.

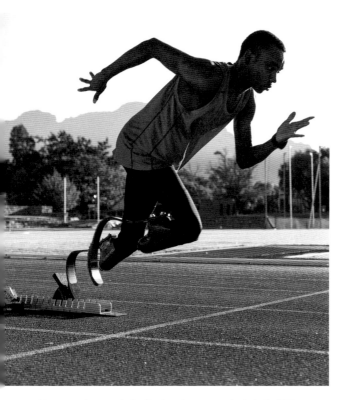

Above: track events in the Paralympic program include the 100-meter, 200-meter, and 400-meter sprints; middle-distance runs of 800 meters and 1,500 meters; and long-distance runs of 5,000 meters. There is also a universal relay (4 × 100 meters). Opposite: while track races are confined to, usually, eight competitors per heat, road races have participants in their thousands. Almost every country in the world now hosts a major long-distance race, whether it's a half-marathon, marathon, or ultramarathon.

There are more than a dozen ways to do it, and countless different events to train for and compete in. The former fringes of the sport are going mainstream, and with more gateways than ever, an increasing number of people are starting to take it seriously. What used to be an excuse to get off the couch is now a lifestyle fueled by apps, adventure, and competition. Navigating this expansive landscape as a newcomer can be exhausting not only for the legs but also the brain. What follows is a brief introduction to distances and terrains to help you find your way.

Track

The footrace is probably the world's oldest sporting contest—so old that we've likely been doing it since before we had the tools to record the activity. Ancient Greek sources suggest that organized track racing was first seen at the inaugural Olympic Games in 776 BCE. It was a 180-meter sprint on a dirt path, performed nude, and remained the only Olympic event for more than 50 years. Today, the Games feature 12 track events, and you will see all-weather running tracks everywhere, from high-school playing fields to 80,000-seat stadiums.

Track events are essentially divided into three groups: nonstop sprints, pretty much nonstop sprints, and sprints with obstacles. In 100-meter, 200-meter, and 400-meter races, the goal is to reach your top speed as fast as possible and maintain it until you cross the finish line. These events are all about explosive power, which you can improve by working on your fast-twitch muscle fibers through exercises such as powerlifting and squats.

Middle-distance track races—800 meters, 1,500 meters—leave a little more room for strategy and pacing. Should you start steady and gun it at the end? Or flash out of the gates and hang on for dear life as the finish line, and your competition, nears? There

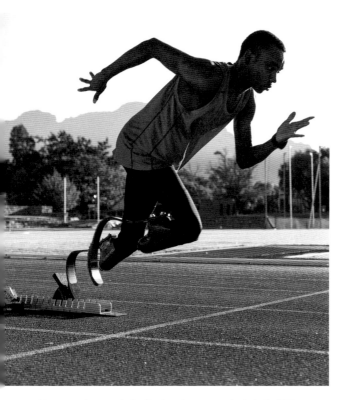

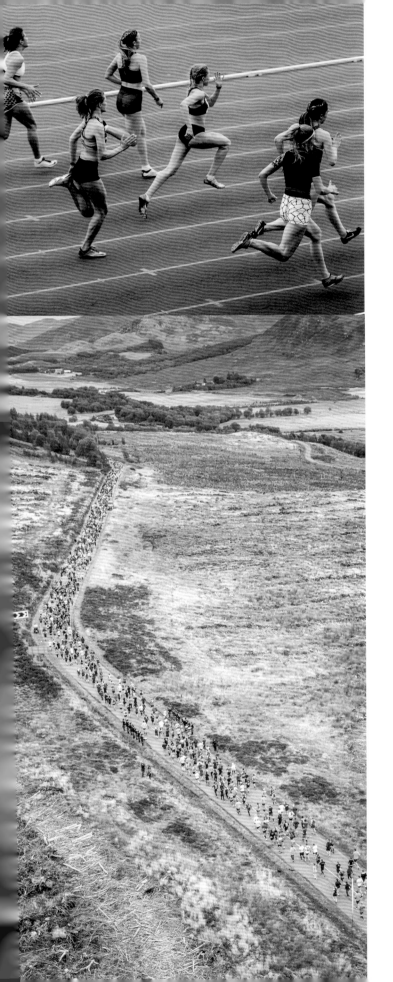

is no absolute consensus, but most competitive runners prefer to save their best for last. Running the second half of the race faster than the first is known as a negative split.

Long distances on the track—5,000, 10,000 meters—are all about going as fast as possible without burning out before the home stretch. These distances have produced some of the sport's best all-around athletes, including Kenenisa Bekele, Haile Gebrselassie, and Paavo Nurmi. If you're hoping to get to their level you'll need to employ longer, slower exercises in your workouts, which will help to develop your slow-twitch muscle fibers and boost stamina and oxygen capacity. Combine these with weekly interval-training sessions to simultaneously stimulate your fast-twitch fibers.

Not every track offers a clear path, as is the case with hurdles and steeplechase. Hurdles are 100-meter (women), 110-meter (men), or 400-meter sprints that require runners to jump over horizontal bars between 68 and 107 centimeters (27 and 42 inches) high. The strategy is simple: run fast and don't fall. Meanwhile, the steeplechase (a horse race adapted for human competition) demands a little more pacing—and has less room for error. The standard steeplechase is a 3,000-meter run complete with 28 grounded barriers. For additional difficulty, there are also seven water jumps.

Road

The world's most famous long-distance race is the 42.2-kilometer (26.2-mile) marathon. In 2018, about 1.3 million people participated in races worldwide, most of which were typically run on road. If you ask someone what Boston is famous for, a respectable number will say the marathon before naming the Celtics or Red Sox. Berlin is the place to see records broken, and the New York marathon might ▶

The footrace is probably the world's oldest sporting contest— so old that we've likely been doing it since before we had the tools to record the activity. Ancient Greek sources suggest that organized track racing was first seen at the inaugural Olympic Games in 776 BCE.

The world's most famous long-distance race is the 42.2-kilometer (26.2-mile) marathon. In 2018, about 1.3 million people participated in races worldwide, most of which were typically run on road.

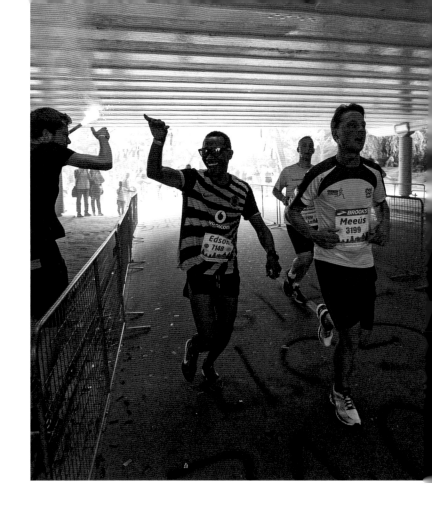

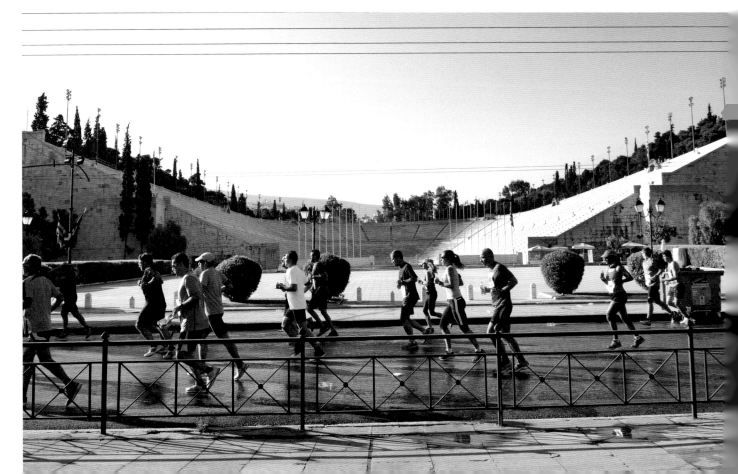

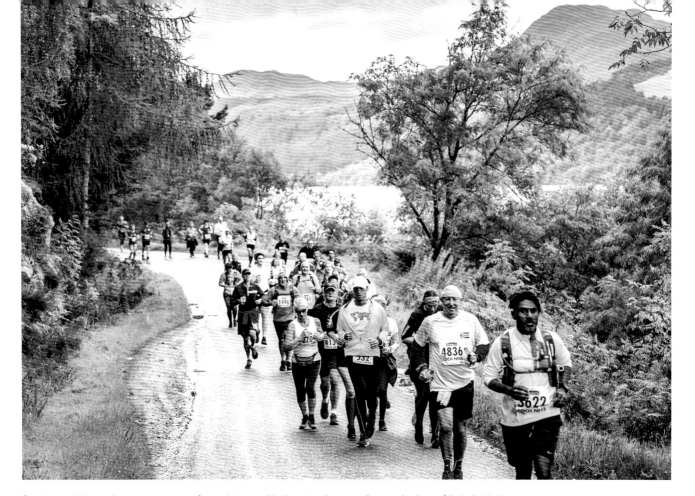

Participants in long-distance events are often as interested in the natural surroundings and culture of their destination country as they are in challenging their bodies. For this reason, many such events offer extended visits with added sightseeing options for those taking part in the running event. Savanna safaris, urban tours, scaling volcanoes, environmental volunteering, and camping at Mount Everest base camp are just some of the exciting extras on offer.

▶ just be the best way to see all five boroughs. Along with three other cities—London, Tokyo, Chicago— these races comprise what is called the World Marathon Majors. Competitors who have run in all are known as Six Star Finishers.

There's an adage that anyone can run a marathon. It just takes 12 to 20 weeks of training and masochistic tendencies. For many finishers, it will be the toughest physical challenge of their lives. So how did marathons become the sporting event *du jour*? A few decades ago, most runners ran to achieve a good time. Today, they run to *have* a good time. It's about the experience, not the performance, as evidenced by a decline in finishing times over the past 15 years, while enthusiasm has reached a fever pitch. Instagram is flooded by images of Garmins on wrists, medals around necks, and race-day outfits during every marathon season. Attending a race can feel akin to being at a music festival. Today's marathon field consists mostly of hobby runners looking to check an item off their bucket list.

More approachable perhaps is the half-marathon, the world's fastest-growing long-distance race for more than a decade. In 2018, more than 2.1 million runners finished a half. Most part-time runners can be half-marathon-ready with eight to twelve weeks of training. The 2000 Broloppet half-marathon was one of the largest running events ever held, compelling more than 90,000 people to run the Øresund Bridge between Denmark and Sweden.

Meanwhile, more ambitious runners have moved on to a new thrill: the ultramarathon. Usually defined as any race longer than 42.2 kilometers (26.2 miles), many ultramarathons cover hundreds or thousands of kilometers. British endurance athlete Mimi Anderson, for example, ran a staggering 3,568 kilometers (2,217 miles) across the U. S. in 2017. Notable ultramarathons include the Spartathlon in Greece, the U. K.'s London to Brighton run, and South Africa's Two Oceans. Distance isn't the only challenge. In many races, runners also have to face extreme heat or cold, exhaustion, navigation, and boredom. While you could pull off a marathon with a few months ▶

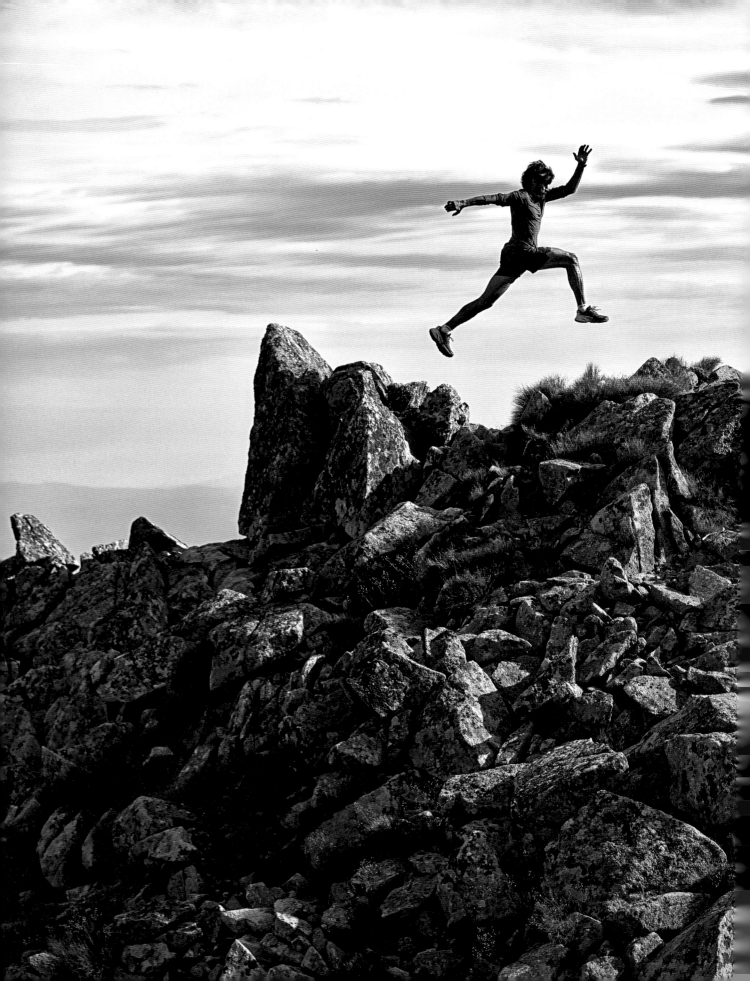

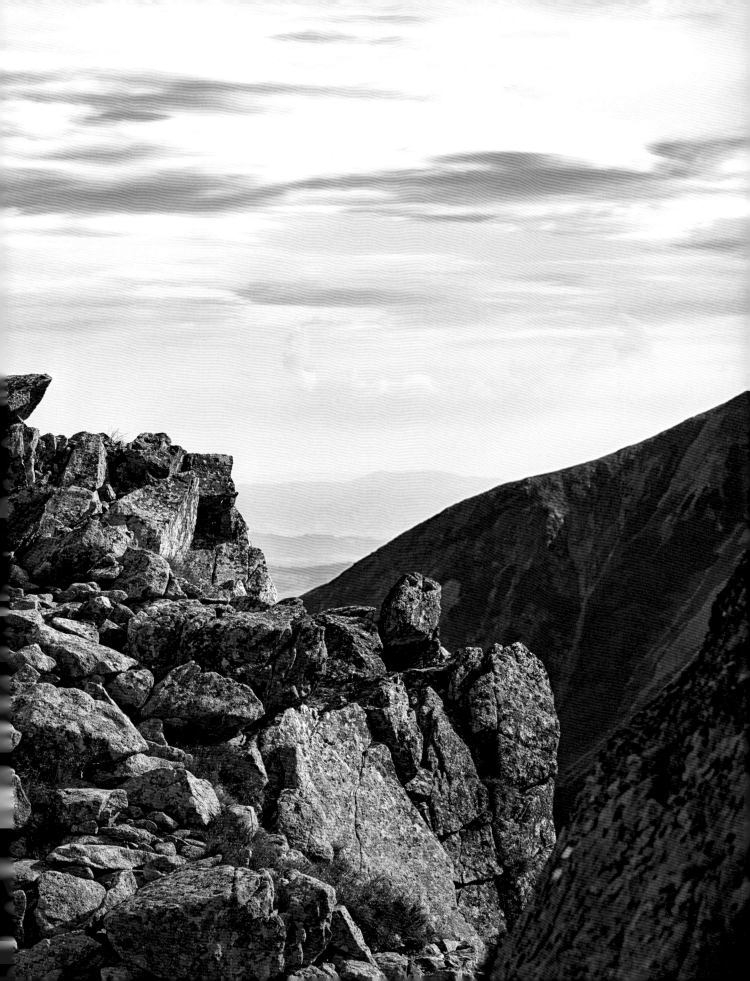

▶ of training, preparing your body for an ultra is a very different beast and something more akin to taking on a part-time job.

Off-road

Runners are increasingly looking for a sense of adventure and to reconnect with our ancestral roots. It is no longer enough to put one's head down and plug away. Off-road runs satisfy a yearning for the great outdoors and encourage us to look up and take in our surroundings. We put our feet on gravel, grass, rocks, sand, or ice, and our eyes look toward the horizon.

Trails are by far the most popular way to navigate nature. There are more than 1,800 trail races around the world, covering simple forest footpaths to treacherous treks through glacial peaks. Trail running has seen a meteoric rise in popularity over the past decade as we increasingly seek to reconnect with nature. No terrain is off-limits—hills, mountains, plateaus, canyons, valleys, and peninsulas are all fair game as long as the path goes up, down, and around. Many races cover ultramarathon distances and have aid stations along the way for runners to fuel up on snacks and drinks. A set of ethics known as "leave no trace" obliges runners to tread lightly and carefully on the ground they cover.

In more demanding off-road races, runners will often carry the "10 Essentials," which should include a compass or GPS, headlamp, food, water, and a first-aid kit. Some extreme races—such as the annual Badwater 135 ultramarathon, which kicks off below sea level in Death Valley, the hottest place on Earth, and finishes at an elevation of 2,548 meters (8,359 feet)—require more equipment than you might take on the average vacation. Grueling physical punishment aside, running in nature is actually very much like taking a trip—you plan, pack, travel, see something new, briefly disconnect from the world, and hate going to work the next day. You count down the days until next time, and you can't stop telling your friends about it.

Trail running combines a host of outdoor-running genres, including fell running, skyrunning, fastpacking, and swimrunning. Fell running is like trail running, except more extreme: it has rougher trails, steeper inclines and declines, and a governing body that

Across the globe, there are huge swathes of land that have remained untouched for many thousands of years. There is no better way to connect with nature than to run one of the many off-road events that happen worldwide. Whether you find yourself coursing up and down the undulating hills of rural England, scaling mountains in the Swiss Alps, swimming the icy waters of Scandinavia, or pulling your own sled across the Arctic, you cannot fail to feel at one with the Earth.

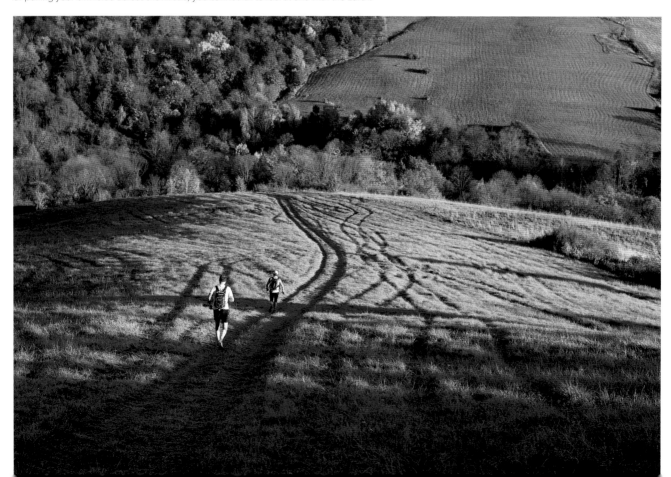

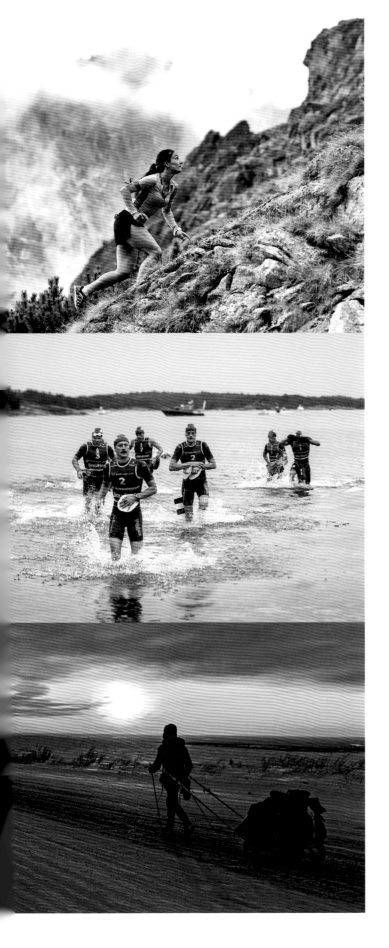

Off-road runs satisfy a yearning for the great outdoors and encourage us to look up and take in our surroundings. We put our feet on gravel, grass, rocks, sand, or ice, and our eyes look toward the horizon.

oversees up to 500 races in the U. K. annually. The sport's roots date all the way back to the eleventh century, when the Scottish King Malcolm III initiated a fell race to find the best messenger. The majority of fell races tend to take place in the U. K.; other parts of the world might call it mountain or hill running.

Skyrunning is any mountain run that takes place above 2,000 meters (6,561 feet) with an incline that exceeds 30 percent. There are official SkyMarathons and Ultra SkyMarathons, and a federation that enforces rules, recruits new runners, and conducts scientific research. At the more extreme end there are races that incorporate ridge running and oxygen deficiency. The Tromsø Skyrace, for example, straddles the Norwegian mountains above the Arctic Circle and takes runners through 4,800 meters (15,750 feet) of vertical gain over a 57-kilometer (35-mile) course.

Fastpacking means carrying enough essentials on your back to survive a couple days and nights on the trails, while swimrunning involves running a trail with intervals of swimming in between. The latter sport originated with the ÖTILLÖ Swimrun, which challenges participants to island-hop the Stockholm archipelago from Sandhamn to Utö. The course includes 21 runs and 20 swims.

It seems that humans will never stop finding new ways to challenge themselves. Today, running continues to take on new forms and configurations. Why not combine a marathon with a 180-kilometer (112-mile) bike ride and a 3.9-kilometer (2.4-mile) swim, in what is known as an Ironman? Some races go even further: Can you run while being electrocuted? In soaked, freezing clothes? How's your traction on a grease-slicked quarterpipe? But no matter how many obstacles, or how many miles, and regardless of everything around you, running will always be as simple as putting one foot in front of the other. ∎

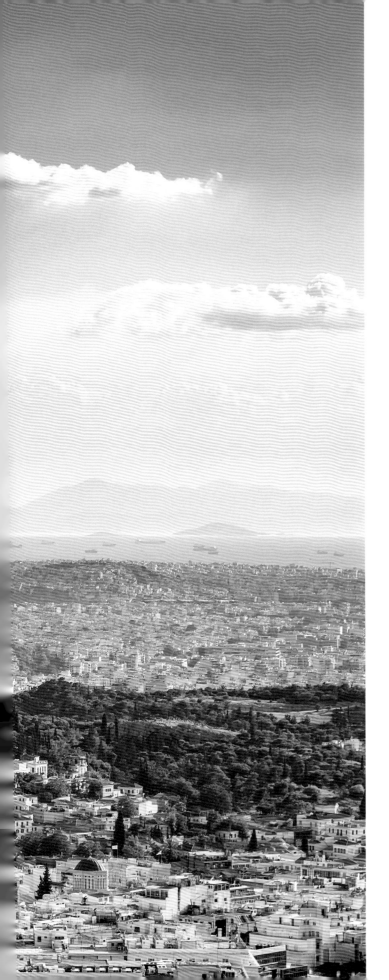

ATHENS MARATHON— THE AUTHENTIC

For marathon runners, this is the birthplace of the sport. The race itself—the Authentic— is tough, largely uphill, but covers the ancient steps of the first marathon, finishing in the stone Panathenaic Stadium. It's a world-famous race that, once run, can never be forgotten.

Even for non-runners, the route from Marathon to Athens has a special and significant place in the history books. It is the path Pheidippides, a soldier and messenger, is said to have taken to bring news of victory in the Battle of Marathon to the Athenians in 490 BCE. More than 2,000 years later, this legend inspired the men's marathon race created for the 1896 Olympic Games—the first modern Games. Greek athlete Spyridon Louis won the gold medal at this event, becoming a national hero. The 42.2-kilometer (26.2-mile) race itself has become famous in its own right, as the original and "authentic" marathon.

The route is hilly and unpretty, and the organization imperfect, but every runner must at some point run from Marathon to Athens. And thousands do, every year—from elite and professional athletes to first-timers, alongside the power walkers ▶

21

The route from Marathon to Athens has a special and significant place in the history books. The 42.2-kilometer (26.2-mile) race itself has become famous in its own right, as the original and "authentic" marathon.

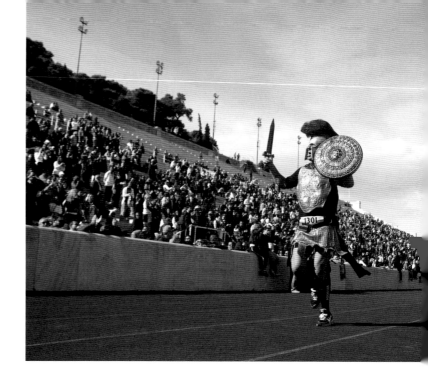

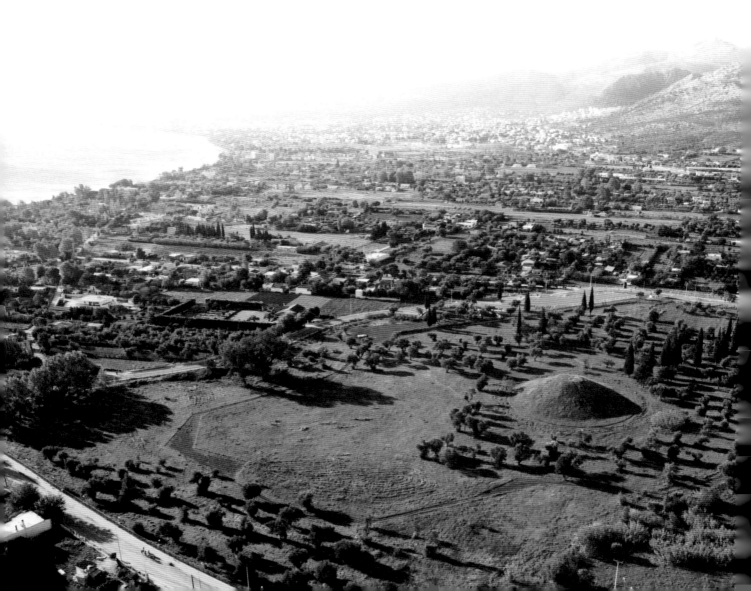

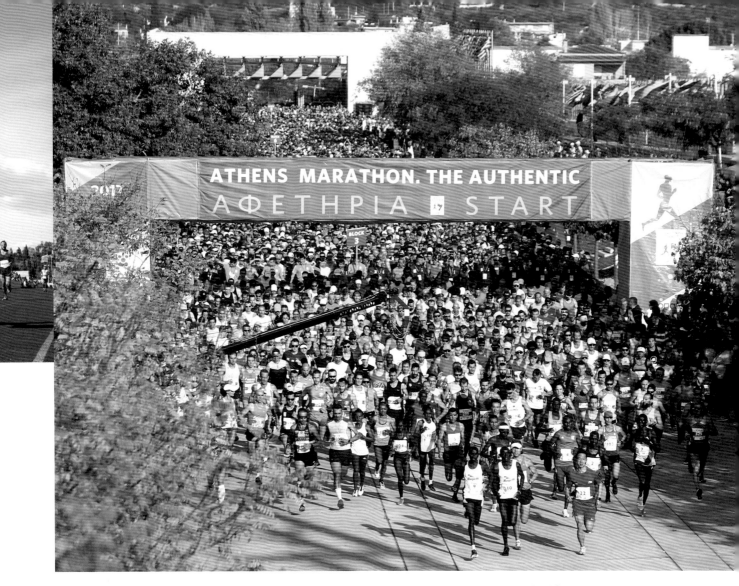

Above: the starting line at Marathon. As many as 40,000 athletes cross this line to embark on the race across mainland Greece. Some claim it has the toughest uphill climb of any major marathon—a 21-kilometer (13-mile) stretch from about 10 kilometers (6 miles).

▶ completing the same course and runners completing the shorter, city-center courses.

The athletes follow a particularly demanding route, with the central half of the race distinguished by steep inclines and undulating terrain, which only begins to flatten out in the last 5–6 kilometers (3–4 miles) of the course, with the finish line only visible for the last couple of meters. All finish under the arch at the historic Panathenaic Stadium, which is not only an ancient monument, but a part of modern Olympic history, too, having hosted the opening and closing ceremonies of the first revived Games in 1896. This is the finish line of finish lines.

Athens is not just a sporting event, a hard race, or a particularly tough road marathon. In the eyes of the event organizers, the race has broader significance, with distance running, especially in this historic location, seen as a model for cooperation, solidarity, resilience, and fellow feeling. Initiatives such as the 2018 Runners' Forest, which replanted woodland along the course following the Greek wildfires of that year, exemplify this broader social mission. ■

Length: 10 or 42.2 km (6.2 or 26.2 mi)

Location: Athens, Greece

Date: November

Type: road/city

Temperature Ø: 12–18 °C (59–64 °F)

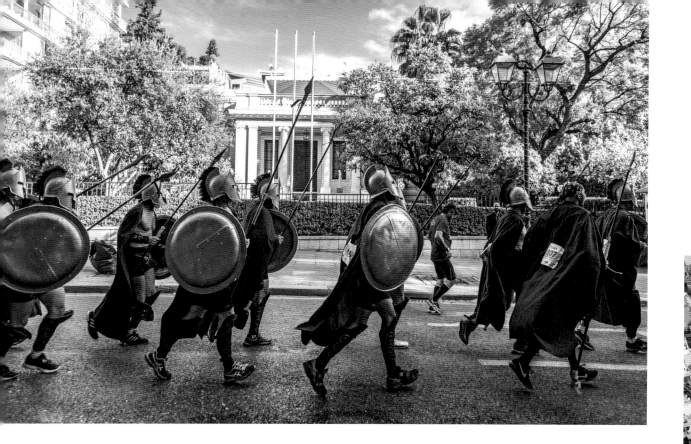

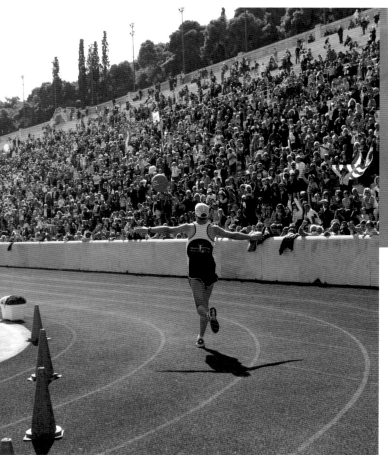

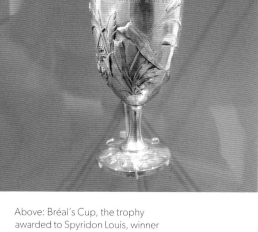

Above: Bréal's Cup, the trophy awarded to Spyridon Louis, winner of the first marathon held in the modern Olympic Games, 1896. The Authentic doubles as the country's national event, with some participants proudly dressing as soldiers in honor of Pheidippides. Opposite: the Panathenaic Stadium.

All finish under the arch at the historic Panathenaic Stadium, which is not only an ancient monument, but a part of modern Olympic history, too, having hosted the opening and closing ceremonies of the first revived Games in 1896.

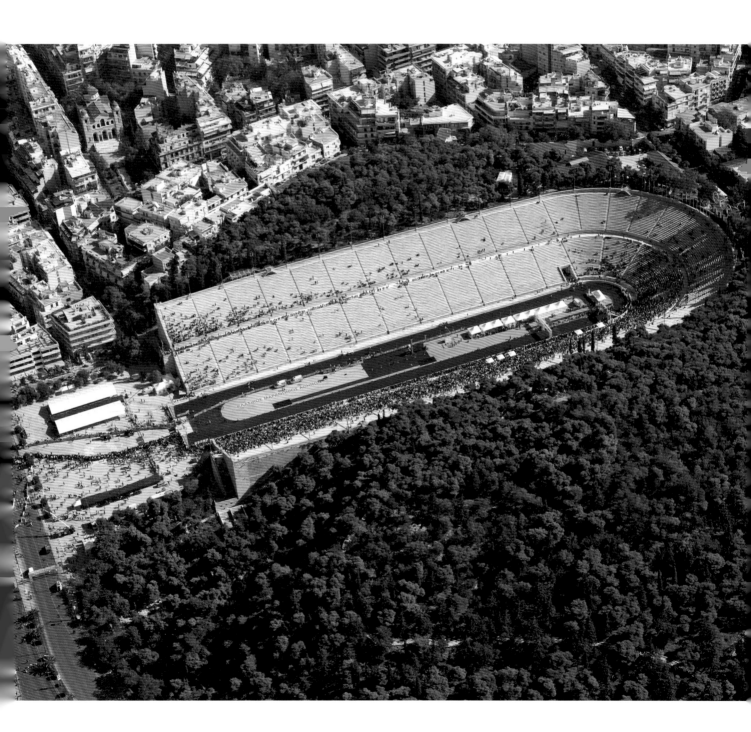

ENDURE24

A must in U. K. ultra racing, this event combines a festival-style approach—music, firepits, and tepees and tents line the route—with intense endurance running. The ants on the ground are trying hard to complete as many laps as possible in the time allowed. It's a great one for teams and beginners trying longer distances, as the atmosphere is one of the best in British running.

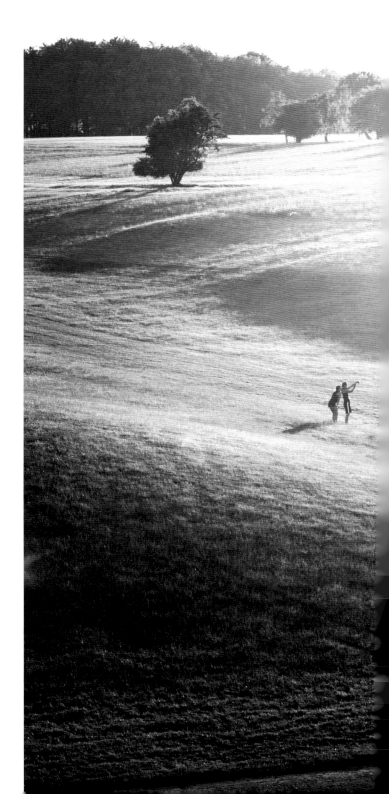

Endure24 is a 24-hour solo or team relay race run on 8-kilometer (5-mile) trail loops, with entrants racing the clock rather than the distance: the aim is to get as far as you can in the time. It's held in both Reading and Leeds, and virtually anyone of any level of experience can take part—even walking is allowed, meaning that this is a uniquely beginner-friendly event.

Of course, this kind of challenge also attracts experienced athletes, and the solo race in particular lives up to its "Epic, Brutal, Relentless" tagline. The course record for solo entrants at the Reading event is 225 kilometers (140 miles) among male competitors, and 193 kilometers (120 miles) among women. Achieving 20 laps, or 160 kilometers (100 miles), at either of the two courses is recognized by admittance to the Endure24 100 mile Club, and only a small proportion of the 300 (Reading) or 800 (Leeds) entrants ▶

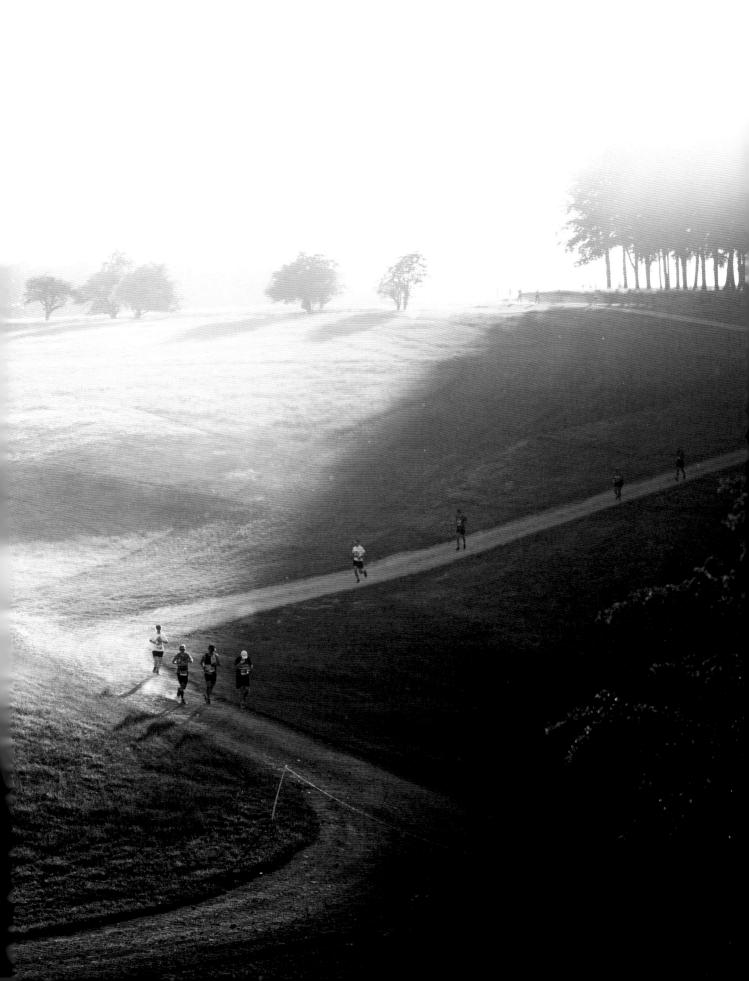

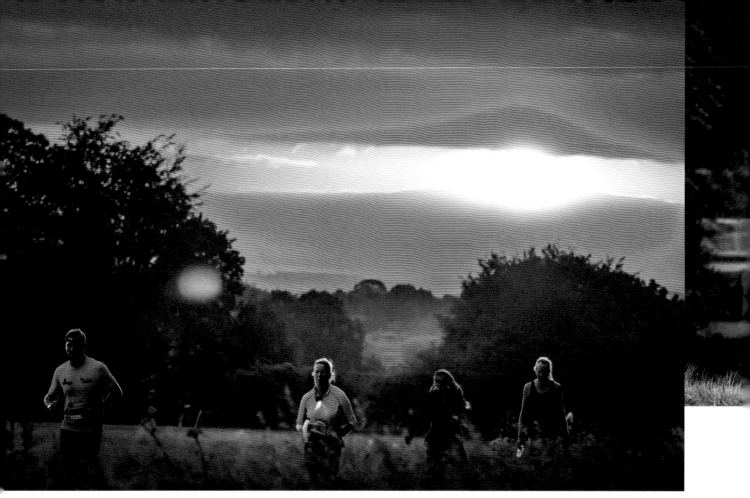

Participants in the Endure24, whether in Leeds or in Reading, benefit from some of the prettiest English countryside—shady woodland glades, open pastures, gentle slopes, and tree-lined avenues dotted with the odd stately home or folly await them.

▶ reach this milestone. These solo runners have their own dedicated campsite and are allowed a support crew to provide supplies and support (but no pacing).

Meanwhile, the possibility of running in teams of up to 12 people (XXL Fun Teams), the lack of pressure, and the unique festival-style set-up at these paired events—not to mention the well-groomed surroundings (the races take place on private estates)—mean that these events have a well-deserved reputation for an enjoyable and supportive atmosphere, perhaps the best in the U. K. On site, the food that's on offer is one of the most appealing spreads in the sport. With retail outlets, bars, entertainment, and even massage therapists available in the race village, it's no wonder the event has earned the title of "the Glastonbury of running."

The route itself appears flat and easy on lap one. By lap five, runners will be nearing a marathon distance, and all of a sudden the road begins to look hilly. As the day turns to night, runners continue to make their way along the forested trails, and on gravel roads, and grass and dirt tracks. In darkness the atmosphere gets serious, with racers often checking the leader board while the course is lit with lanterns and fairy lights (racers themselves are required to wear head torches). Endure24 is known for its hyper-enthusiastic volunteers, however, and the supportive ambience drives many runners to achieve personal bests, with even novices running farther than they imagined they could.

The brilliance of this event is that supporters, family, first-time runners, and extreme ultra athletes all take part together. How often do the non-runners get up close and personal with 24-hour athletes achieving such astonishing feats? ∎

Length: varies

Location: Reading/Leeds, U. K.

Date: June and July

Type: trail

Temperature Ø: 10–20 °C (50–68 °F)

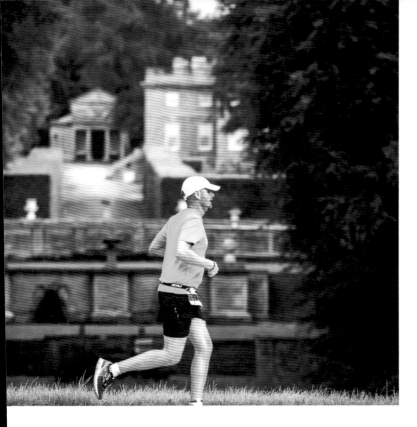

Endure24 is a 24-hour solo or team relay race run on 8-kilometer (5-mile) trail loops, with entrants racing the clock rather than the distance: the aim is to get as far as you can in the time.

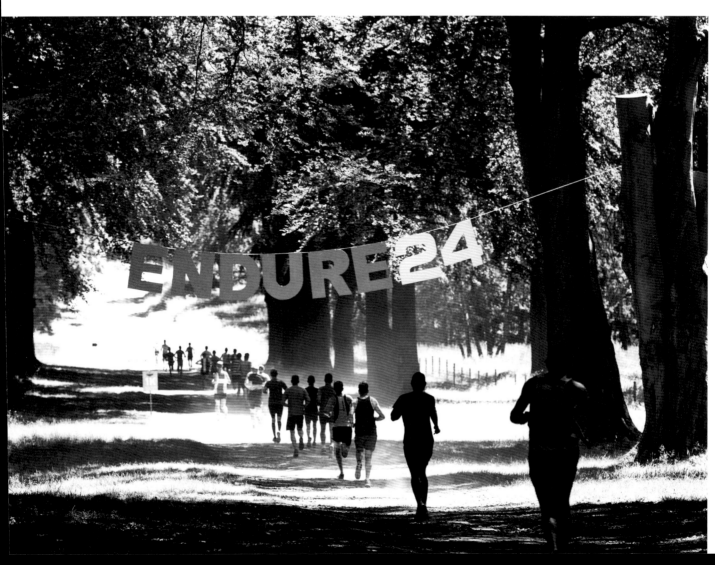

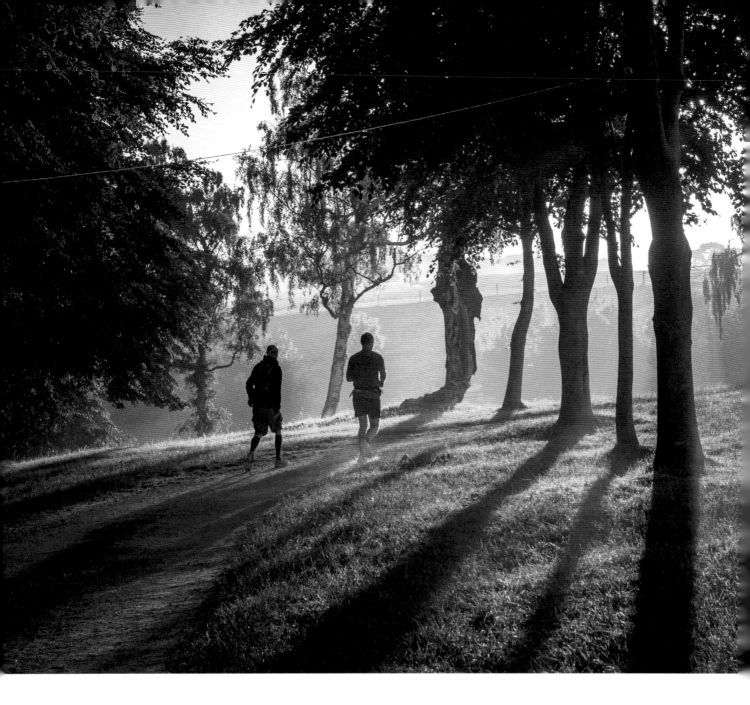

Endure24 is known for its hyper-enthusiastic volunteers, and the supportive ambience drives many runners to achieve personal bests, with even novices running farther than they imagined they could.

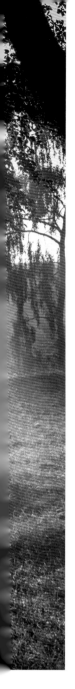

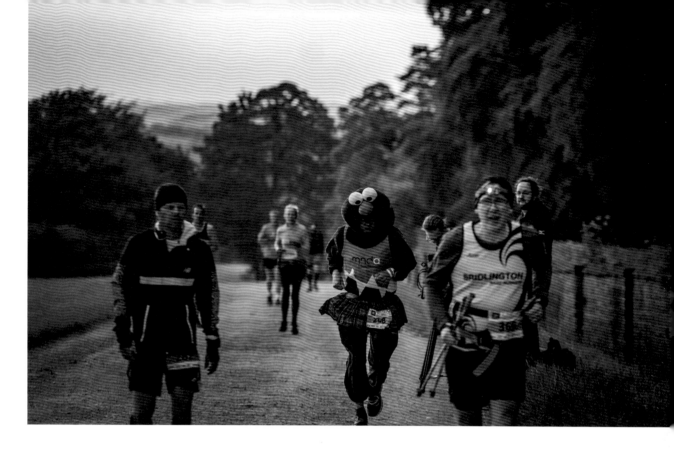

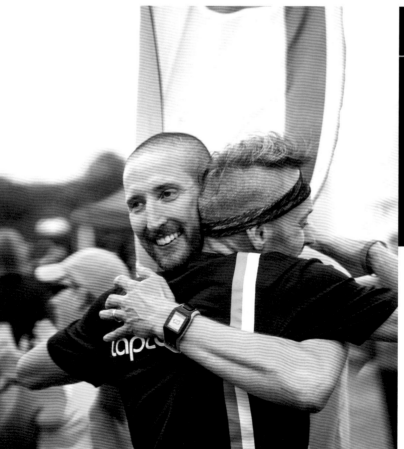

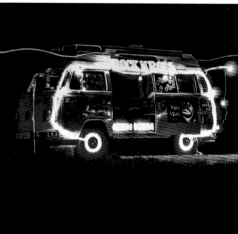

With the race taking place around the clock, participants jog through beautiful sunsets and on into the night, leaving their teams and family members to occupy themselves in the "race village" that sets up in both locations.

ENDURANCE-LIFE NORTHUM-BERLAND

Northumberland's exposed coastline is a place to find peace in your soul and sand in your shoes. With only a handful of runners racing the longest distance at this event, it's a great one for learning the trade of mind over matter. You may finish, but the elements will win—wind, rain, and sun. The views help.

The Northumberland coastline boasts some of the most dramatic, historic scenery in the U. K. The full ultra Endurancelife event is the best way to experience, and indeed endure, a long-distance run amid the rugged beauty of this stretch of coast.

There are few sights in the country to compare with Bamburgh Castle in its exposed, bayside setting. Its Norman keep dates back to the eleventh century, with settlements recorded here as far back as the sixth—the enormous rocky escarpment on which it sits made it an ideal defensive position for the Celtic Britons, and adds to its drama today. The arched entrance to the castle marks the starting line for the Endurancelife event; a small group of shivering runners usually assembles here before the starting gun, listening to the safety announcements and preparing to face the weather. ▶

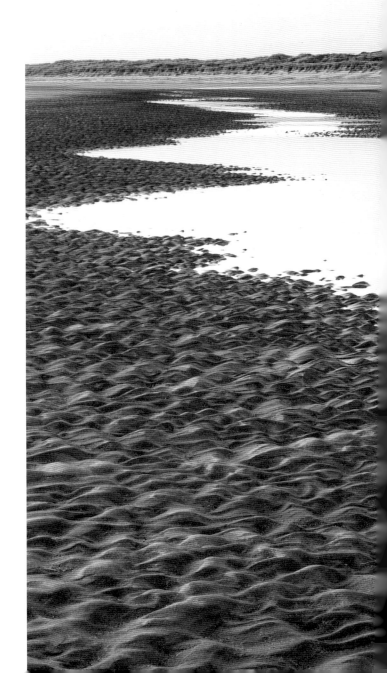

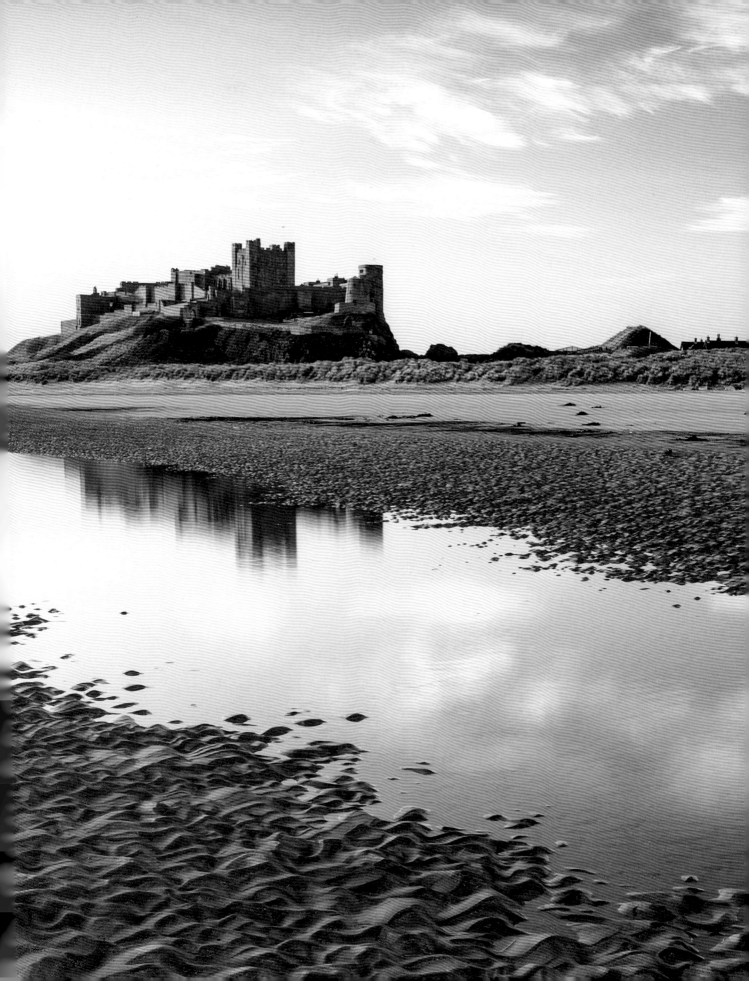

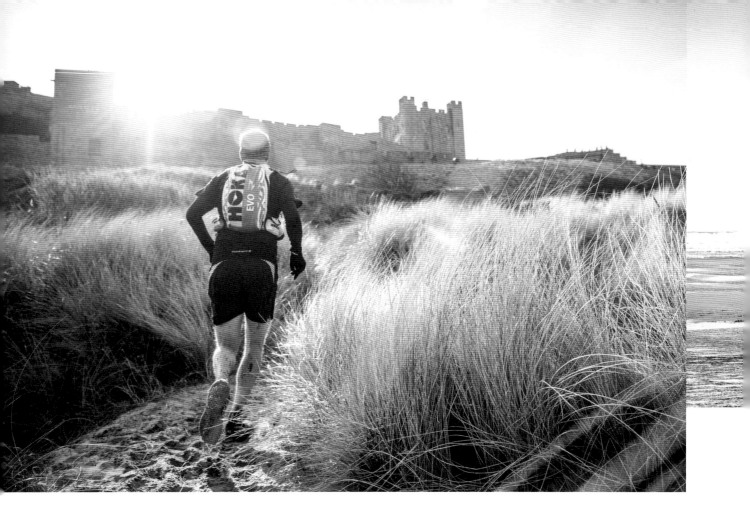

Above: Bamburgh Castle. Opposite, bottom: the ruins of Dunstanburgh Castle. The coast at Bamburgh is known for is wide sandy beaches and grassy dunes—it looks benign, but the winds blowing in from the North Sea can be punishing.

▶ This is a race for those who love the outdoors in all its forms. You never know what Mother Nature will throw at you. From the sky, the sun or rain (or both) may come. Underfoot, the sandy beaches, rolling dunes, scree, and rock. Prepare to feel sand in your shoes, wind in your face, and the love of nature, however grudging, in your heart.

As runners make their way south from Bamburgh, keeping the sea on their left, a host of conservation sites reveal themselves, including two National Nature Reserves. Historic monuments and scenic lookout spots are also in abundance; ultra runners will spot the ruins of fourteenth-century Dunstanburgh Castle as they approach the southernmost point of the course. The best bit? Runners on this longest route reach a point just north of the town of Craster, before turning back toward Bamburgh; depending on how close you are to the front, you'll see every runner that's behind you on the way back north.

The race doesn't have tens of thousands of entrants; you can enjoy your thoughts alone as you pant up and down the hills of the barren coast. It's beautiful running and, although you'll likely be trudging it out with very few runners around to urge you on, the well-stocked aid stations and race crew are never far away. A classic clipboard- and pen-wielding official will check you in and out of each checkpoint with a smile.

The Endurancelife coastal trail series is a well-established and much-loved series of events around the coast of Britain, including of the Gower Peninsula, Dorset, and the North York Moors. Northumberland has been on the calendar for many years for a reason. It's one of the best. ∎

Length: 10, 21.1, 42.2, or 52 km (6.2, 13.1, 26.2, or 32.3 mi)

Location: Bamburgh Castle, U. K.

Date: February

Type: trail/coastal

Temperature Ø: 8 °C (46.4 °F)

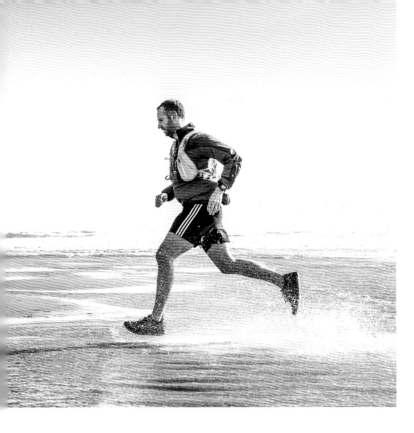

This is a race for those who love the outdoors in all its forms. You never know what Mother Nature will throw at you. From the sky, the sun or rain (or both) may come. Underfoot, the sandy beaches, rolling dunes, scree, and rock.

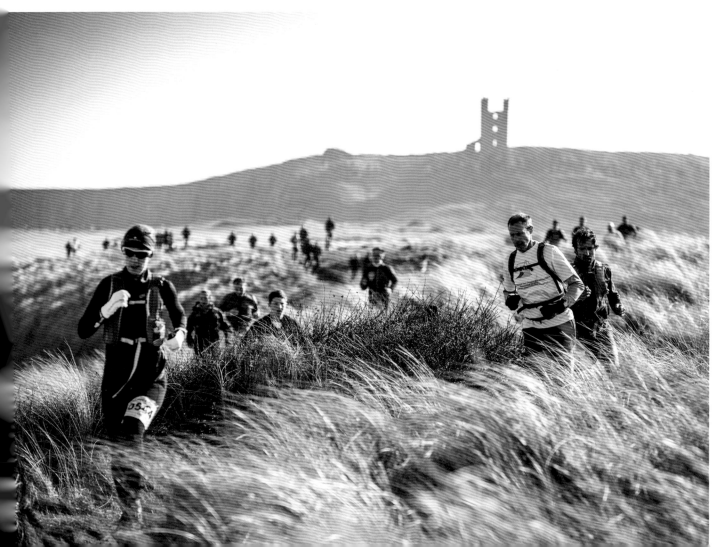

The race doesn't have tens of thousands of entrants; you can enjoy your thoughts alone as you pant up and down the hills of the barren coast. It's beautiful running.

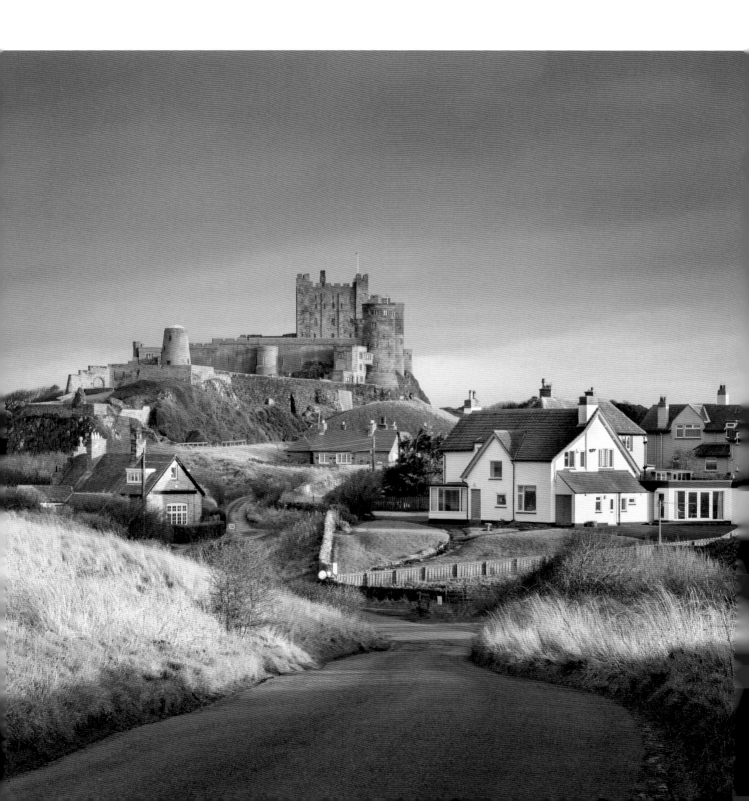

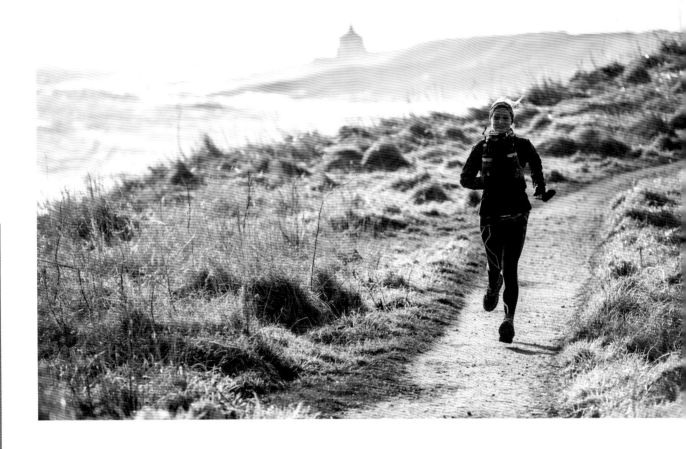

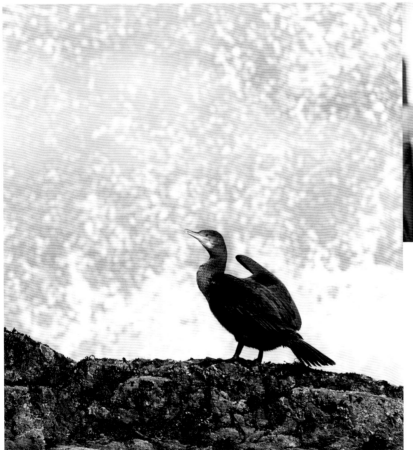

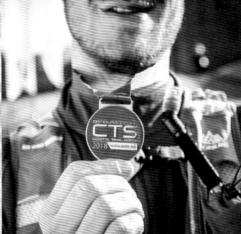

Above: those who complete an Endurancelife Coastal Trail Series event receive a medal for their efforts, stamped with the year and location—one of eight (and counting) hosting runs like this in the U. K. Opposite: the picturesque village of Bamburgh, with its castle rising up behind it.

Pavement Pounding: Vibrant Runs in the Heart of the City

It's not all about the marathons. City running is an opportunity to hit the streets while exploring a new country. Some of the best routes are found in unexpected places—say hello to Pristina, Kosovo—and combine challenging running with unique gastronomic, architectural, and cultural experiences.

Hanoi city center

Escaping the busiest streets, this route through central Hanoi will take you around the beautiful West Lake.

Start outside the Quán Thánh Temple and run clockwise around the lake. You'll pass the beautiful Trấn Quốc Pagoda—the oldest in the city—as well as bustling street markets. This one will be a warm and humid run, so make sure you stay hydrated. If you find yourself in need of an energy kick, be sure to sample the famous Vietnamese coffee. Mopeds are the main mode of transport here, so don't be surprised at the amount of horn-beeping!

If you're running a marathon distance, be sure to look out for the Marathon Café and have your photo taken for the wall!

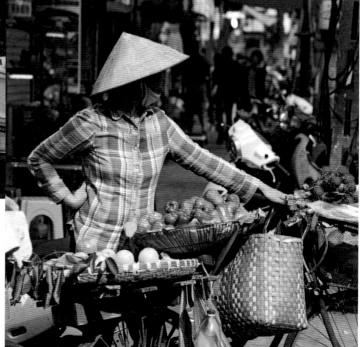

Hanoi has a number of dedicated running paths, particularly around its numerous lakes. Take a run around Hoàn Kiếm Lake, in the center of Hanoi, then dive into the historic center, where the narrow streets are bustling with activity.

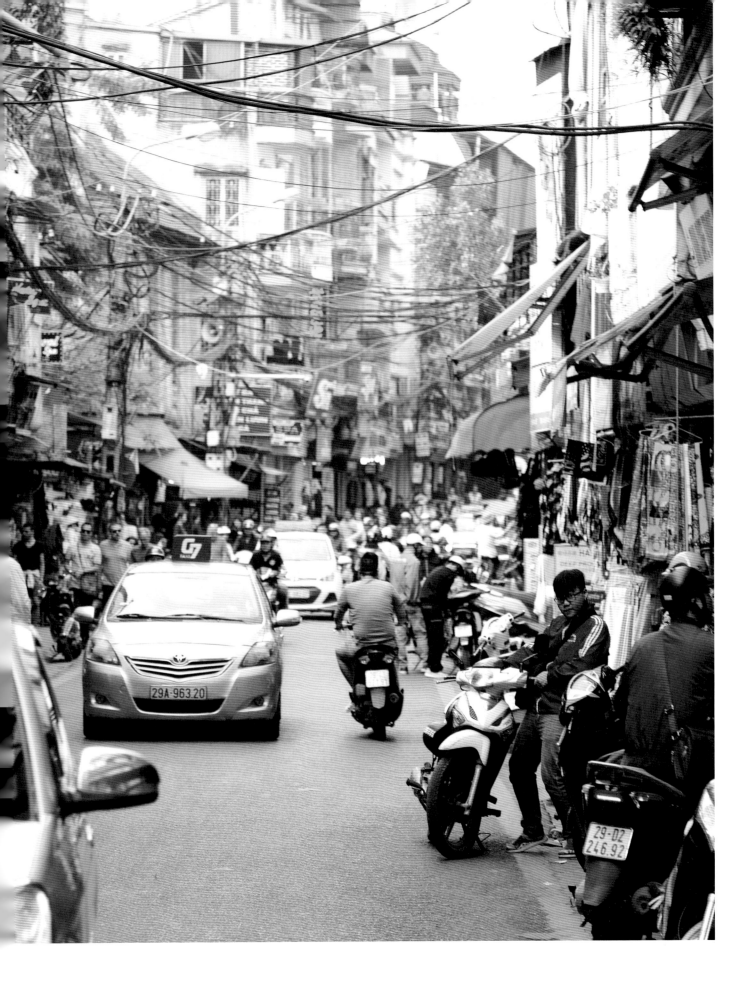

Monaco

The location of one of the most exhilarating races in motorsport, the tiny, twisting streets of Monaco are full of hills, tight squeezes, bridges, and tunnels, plus the famously glitzy oceanfront marina, home to the most super of the super-yachts. There aren't many places where you can run a Formula One circuit—an entire country, in fact—and be back in time to stop off for some luxurious breakfast in a seafront brasserie or restaurant.

Run any distance you like. Monaco may be small, but it comes with several impressive and challenging mini-loops, such as up to the Prince's Palace of Monaco on the hill and back to the small high street and quirky shops. You can even run along the pontoons to see the boats up close. Ask nicely and you may be allowed a peek inside.

This gorgeous and luxurious microstate on the French Riviera is not only ideal for running, but a short walk will take you to the French coastline. For a getaway in summer, this is the place—perfect for training and indulging in the best food.

Pristina

Kosovo and its capital, Pristina, are not often on the must-see lists of world travelers. This is a shame, however, as the café culture, stunning countryside, and incredibly hospitable citizens make this a truly special destination.

Run from the center of town northeast, heading out of the city center. Your starting point, the Newborn Monument, marks Kosovo's declaration of independence from Serbia and was unveiled in 2008, making this the youngest country in Europe (among those states who recognize it). Once out of the center and past the National Library of Kosovo—a somewhat divisive, if intriguing presence— you'll be on the trails around the city.

It's bleak here in the winter, but gorgeous in summer, so time your trip right in order to enjoy the farmlands and rural paths and tracks of the city's outskirts. There's accommodation to suit all budgets and traditional dishes include stuffed peppers and kebabs made of beef, lamb, or chicken.

Add Pristina to your bucket list—you're likely to revisit.

Below: an aerial view reveals the scope of Pristina, Kosovo. Opposite, top: the principality of Monaco rises above Port Hercule. Opposite, bottom: a lone runner strides past the Petronas Towers in Kuala Lumpur.

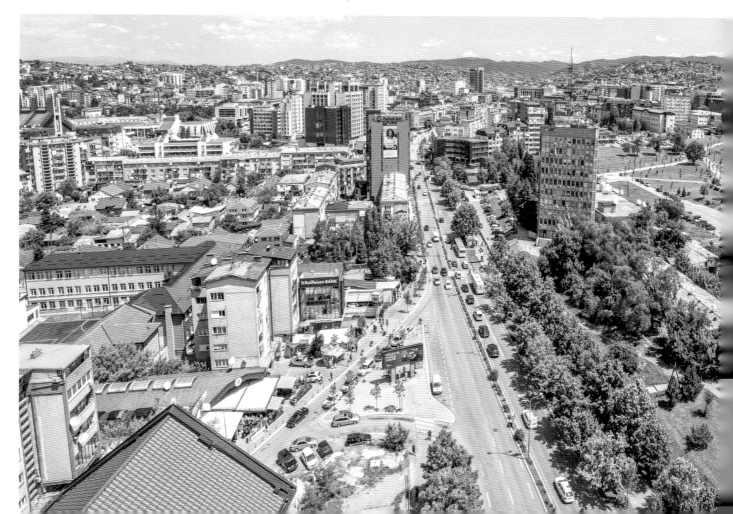

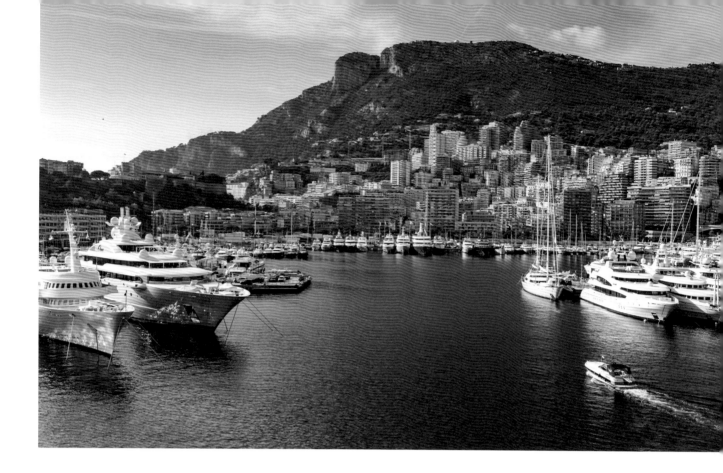

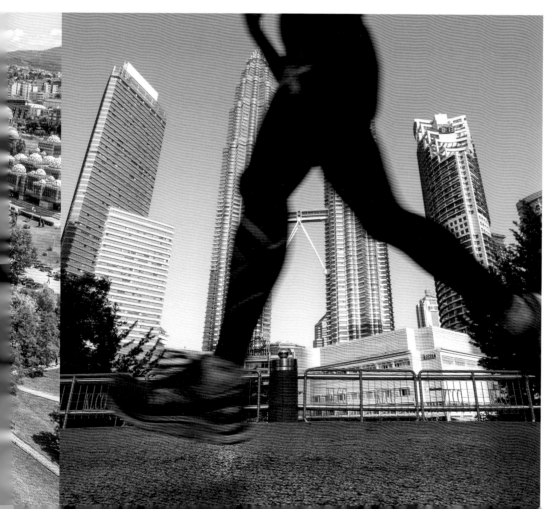

San Francisco

Located in the northern part of California, between the San Francisco Bay and Pacific Ocean, San Francisco is one of the most visited cities in the world. Our route will allow you to tick off all the San Fran bucket-list items in one go!

Starting at Fisherman's Wharf, spot the seals basking on the pontoon and then head south to Powell Street—a great place for cable-car spotting. From there, move west among the Victorian-style townhouses to meet the Painted Ladies (the postcard-perfect painted Edwardian and Victorian houses for which San Francisco is famous). Veering north you'll then run to the Golden Gate Bridge; if you're lucky the fog will have lifted and you will see it in all its glory! Finally, run east back to Fisherman's Wharf, where you can spot Alcatraz Island and grab a much-deserved bite to eat!

This 16.1-kilometer (10-mile) circuit is ideal for those runners wanting to explore, but any running route here will blow you away. With flat elevation around the bay, it's perfect for all abilities.

Kuala Lumpur

KL, as locals know it, is the largest city in Malaysia and home to 1.8 million people.

The KLCC Park, at the foot of the famous Petronas Towers, is where you'll likely be running. On a surfaced running track, you'll make your way through this lush space alongside other addicts and around a lake, waterfalls, fountains, and reflecting pools, with the two 452-meter (1,483-foot) skyscrapers as your backdrop. Alternatively, head to the KL Forest Eco Park or, for marathon addicts, join the annual, city-wide race, held in October.

In the evening, head up to one of the city's many swanky rooftop bars or pools and look out over the twinkling lights while you sip your drink of choice and the sun sets behind the two spectacular towers.

If you're wanting to explore a little more, you can run the 15-kilometer (9.3-mile) stretch from the Petronas Towers to the Batu Caves, which ends with a challenging run up 272 multicolored steps.

Below: a San Franciscan takes an early-morning jog near the Golden Gate Bridge. Opposite: Titiwangsa Lake Gardens, in Kuala Lumpur, is a popular recreational park for joggers—also in the center of the city.

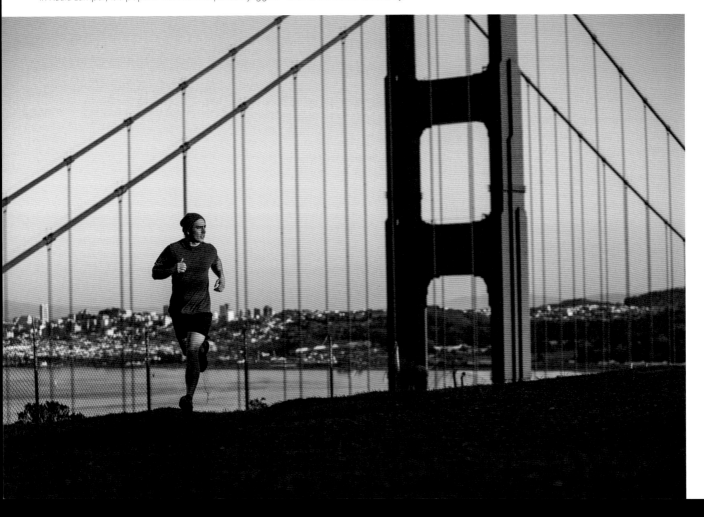

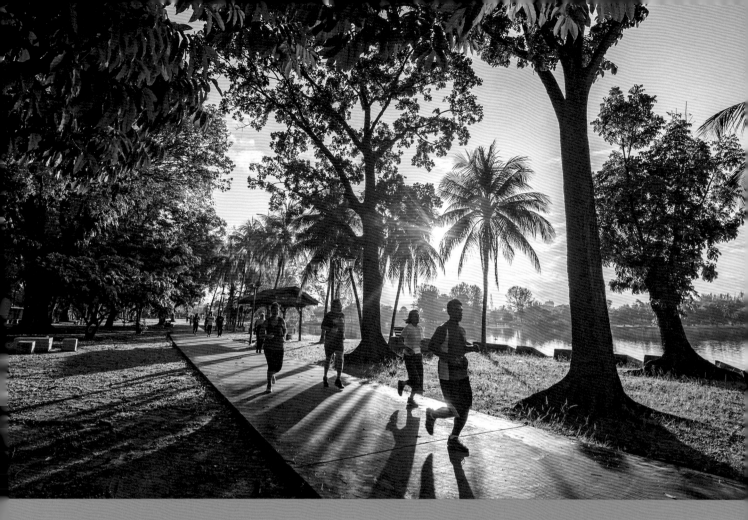

City Runs: The Basics

Hanoi city center
Vietnam
Route:
around West Lake
Distance:
17 km (10.6 mi)

Monaco
Route:
varies
Distance:
varies

Pristina
Kosovo
Route:
varies
Distance:
varies

San Francisco
California, U. S.
Route:
Fisherman's Wharf–Powell Street–
Golden Gate Bridge
Distance:
16.1 km (10 mi)

Kuala Lumpur
Malaysia
Route:
KLCC Park;
KL Forest Eco Park;
or Petronas Towers–Batu Caves
Distance:
varies

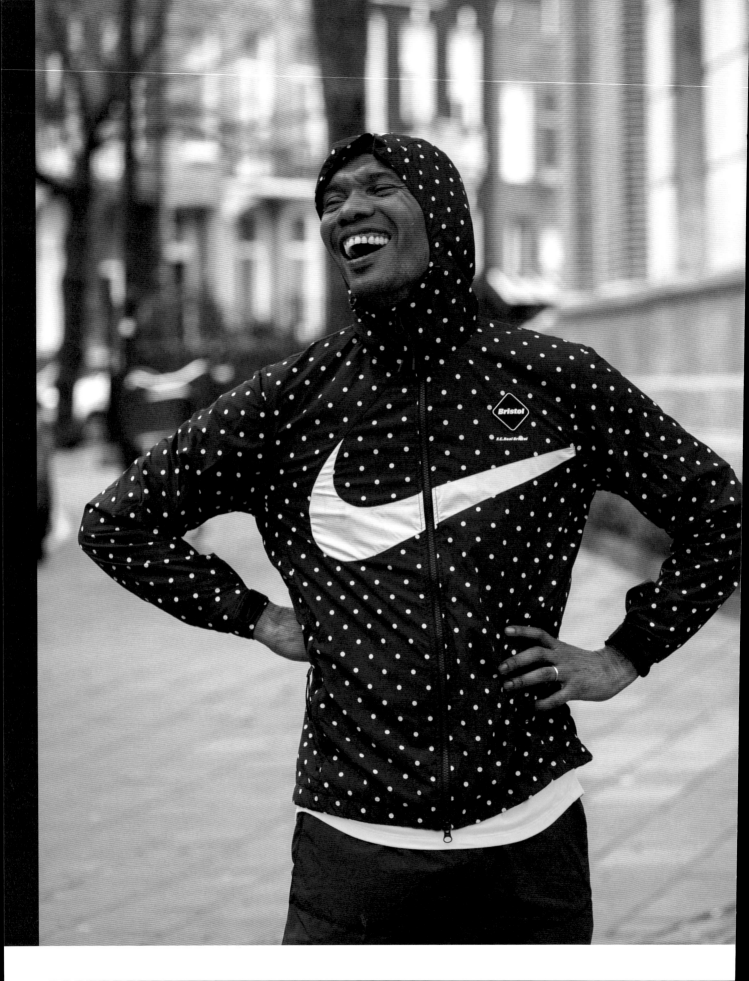

Running Till You Drop with Streetwear Pioneer Edson Sabajo

In 2010, Edson Sabajo created the Patta Running Team for people who wanted to run without cramping their style (or their vices).

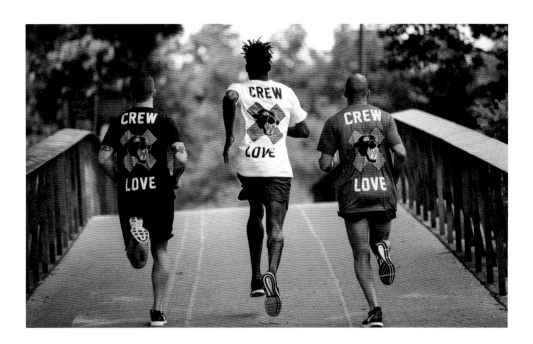

"I smoke and I drink," Edson Sabajo says in a 2017 video about his running philosophy. "And I'm 45. If I can do it, y'all motherf*ckers can do it too." Sabajo is the founder of the Amsterdam-based Patta Running Team, a diverse crew of multi-hyphenates—tattoo artist-DJs, designer-photographers, writer-activists—who also happen to run. Some are fellow *Mokummers* (a colloquial term for natives of Amsterdam), many are not. Seeing them converse before or after a session, you might mistake them for enthusiasts on a smoke break at a sneaker drop.

Sabajo can be credited for bringing sneaker drops to the Netherlands. Starting in the 1990s, he would fly to New York and stuff duffel bags full of styles you couldn't find in Europe. Back in Amsterdam, he flipped them for a profit among a small crew of local sneakerheads—part of a subculture that was just beginning to take off outside the U. S. This was long before reselling shoes was a viable business, when deals were sealed with a handshake instead of a click, and the term "hypebeast" for a trend-obsessed fashion addict hadn't been coined. In 2004, Sabajo and his longtime friend, Guillaume "Gee" Schmidt, opened a store in the red-light district and gave the side hustle a name: Patta, which means "shoe" in their ancestral home of Suriname.

Within a few years, Patta had partnerships with many of the brands Sabajo scouted on his sneaker safaris, including Nike. Sabajo also started to take running more seriously. "I was playing football for a long time but at one point my feet didn't do what my head was telling them, so I stopped and started running," he says. In 2010, a collaborator from Nike asked Sabajo if he wanted to create a running team. "I said, a'ight, but we wanna to do it our way," he says. His way meant Eric B. & Rakim and gold rings instead of "Eye of the Tiger" and Jolly Rancher colorways. Sabajo saw the opportunity as a way for the sport to attract people who didn't adhere to running's straight-edge ethos. Fit non-athletes. Anti-jocks. Artists, skaters, boxers, rappers. Hustlers like Sabajo and Schmidt. "Running isn't just for people who want to change their whole lifestyle," Sabajo says. "Running was and is for everybody."

Urban running crews are now in vogue, but when the Patta gang rocked up to races a decade ago, they looked like aliens. "In the beginning, when we were running some athlete venture ▶

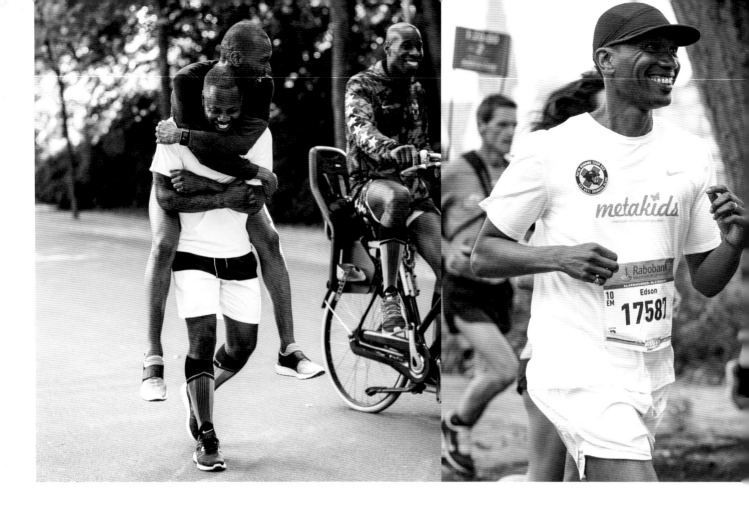

▶ thing, we all came decked out in some hyped gear and people looked at us like, 'What the hell they be doing here?'" Sabajo says. "But for us, we just want to run, and if we can look fly innit? Oh, hell yes." Patta is without doubt the best-dressed crew at every running event, often clad head to toe in gear made bespoke for the occasion. Style remains integral to the running team's identity. Music and parties are also part of Patta's catalogue of necessary running accessories: hip-hop before the race and Hennessy after. One never gets the impression that this is all a charade. "There is no scientific formula for that," says Sabajo. "First and foremost, we are fans of the stuff we're doing. If you like all these things, why not combine them instead of segregate them? Keep it simple. If you don't like something, don't force it. You're not bigger or better if you do. Be you and do you."

As far as Sabajo is concerned, the idea that you shouldn't turn your passion into a career is terrible advice. His life's work is simply his life. Running is his way of meditating on the job. "I use running as a tool to clear my head and be mentally and physically ready to enjoy life," he says. "At the end of the day, you feel like a winner every time. You can't tell me different." Today, more than 100 people run with Patta. They come from all backgrounds and creative vocations. Some are looking for a distraction from their everyday life, others to enrich it. One of the crew's recent initiatives involved training a group of young people to run a half-marathon along the dunes and beaches of the Dutch coast. "We feel it's necessary to give the youth tools to work with," explains Sabajo. "We're trying to create a legacy, so we're taking people with us on this journey."

That journey has taken the Patta Running Team global, from Moscow to Hong Kong, as part of a run-party-repeat tour called Bridge the Gap. Created by the captains of New York's Bridge Runners and London's Run Dem Crew, Bridge the Gap invites running crews from around the world to crash a host crew's hometown and couches. On Sunday morning, sometimes hungover, they run a half- or full marathon together. Most of the crews are sponsored by brands such as Nike, Puma, or Adidas, who hook them up with bibs for the race. "I think Run Dem Crew and Bridge Runners, when they founded Bridge the Gap, they set the tone and pace for urban running worldwide," says Sabajo. "And luckily we were a part of that." Marquee stops on the tour include Berlin, Belgrade, Paris, Copenhagen, Bali, Seoul, Tokyo, Tel Aviv, and Johannesburg. "Show me where you drink, show me where you eat, show me your routes," Sabajo says, "and I will show you mine."

Ultimately, people run with Patta for the same reason they choose to do anything: because it's fun. "I'm always surprised that they wanna join my dumbass ideas, but I love 'em for that," Sabajo says. Also, long-distance running can be a nightmare. It's not always easy to motivate yourself. Sabajo's remedy? Crew love. "That winner mentality with your people," he says. "It looks like a one-man sport, but actually you're doing it with a team." Unite and conquer. ∎

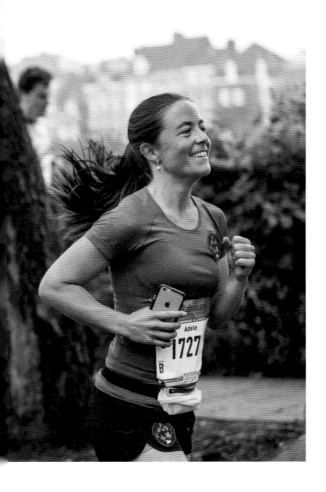

"In the beginning, when we were running some athlete venture thing, we all came decked out in some hyped gear and people looked at us like, 'What the hell they be doing here?' But for us, we just want to run, and if we can look fly innit? Oh, hell yes."

Right and opposite, far left: it's clear from the many photos of Sabajo's crew that a love of life and camaraderie are high on the agenda for Patta team members. Above: Edson joins other runners for the "10 English mile" (16 km) event in Maastricht.

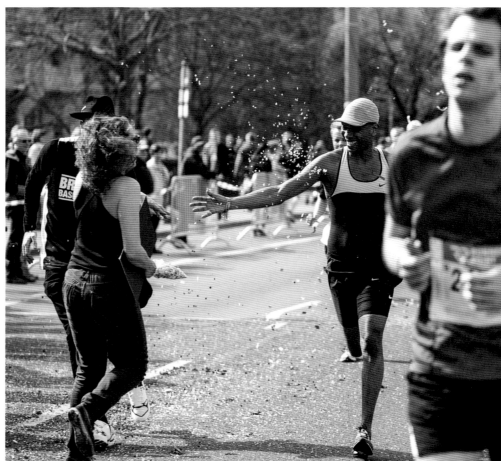

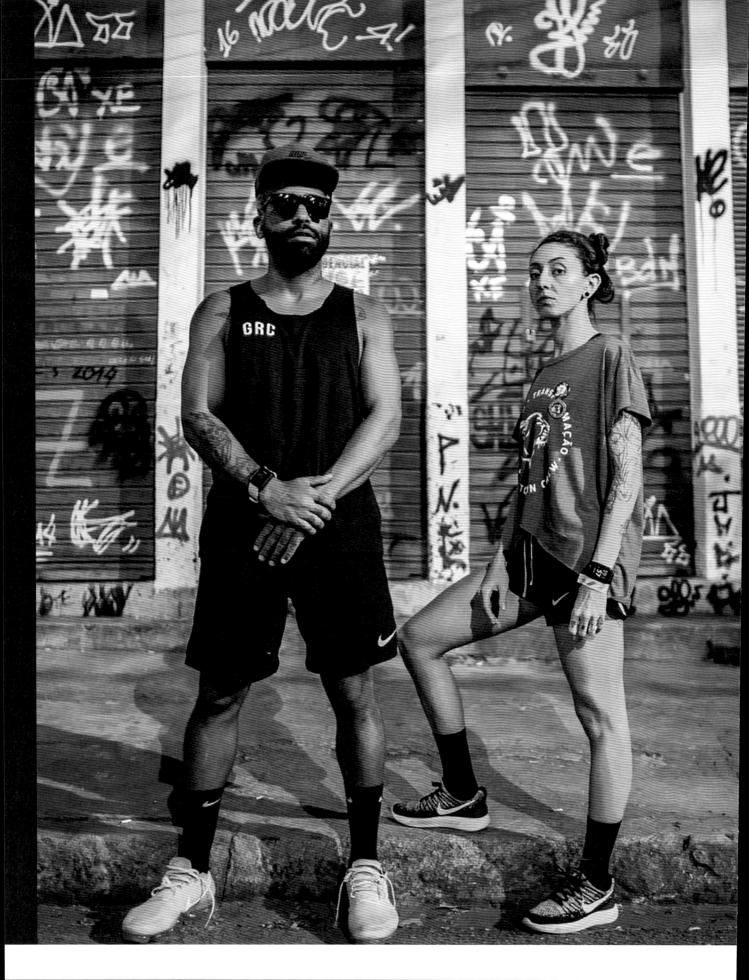

Reclaiming the Streets with Júnior Negão and Gisele Nascimento

Few people would recommend running through the favelas of Rio de Janeiro after dark, but Ghetto Run Crew is here to change that.

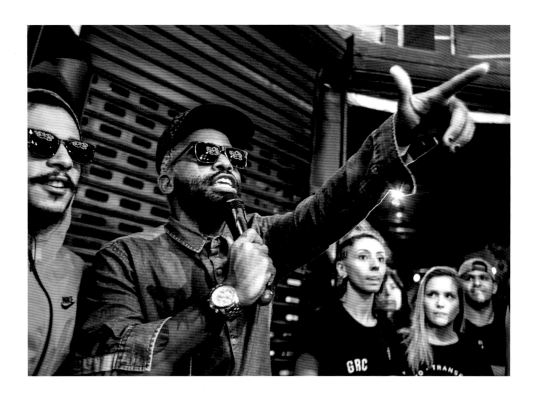

Cops can get testy when black-clad youths run through the Rio favelas after dark. All the more reason, then, for Júnior Negão and his crew to occupy the streets. "We are not a club, we are a crew, a cultural resistance," announces Negão, who founded Ghetto Run Crew in Rio de Janeiro after a late-night run with his wife, Gisele Nascimento, in 2013. Today, many of the crew's runs kick off at midnight. "Running at night was a way of engaging with other cultural activities that only really happened after dark, such as samba, skateboarding, and graffiti," Negão explains. The crew suffered a lot of repression at first, principally because the police felt it was not acceptable to go running in the favelas at night. With persistence and determination, however, they have managed to create a movement.

Negão never imagined himself as a runner. "When you live at the top of mountains or hills, in the places where the favelas are, running is a normal part of life … but I decided to use it as a tool for social empowerment." Favela residents are looked down upon by the rest of society and face a constant struggle to survive. Women have it particularly tough. "My mother, my wife, so many others, who despite being real-life winners, are still undervalued," says Negão. "The idea with Ghetto Run was to bring these women together and, through running, provide them with the means to strengthen themselves as individuals." Running became a gateway to confidence, the kind of confidence that transcends sport. "You can overcome any challenge in any area of your life," explains Nascimento as she talks about what she's learned from running. "Whether as a professional, as a mother, or as a daughter, I learn to be a better human being. And that does not depend on anyone else. It depends only on you."

Independence is the lifeblood of Brazil's creative communities, but it is a freedom that many worry is under threat as President Jair Bolsonaro's attempts to shape the country according to ▶

> *"We are a counterculture because we allow other body types, other lifestyles, to participate in traditional running cultures. We don't use running as competition, but as a tool for cultural representation."*

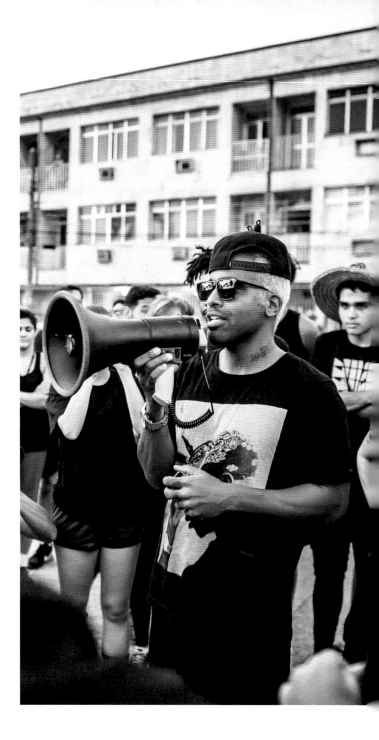

▶ Conservative values. On the day of his inauguration in January 2019, Bolsonaro dissolved Brazil's Ministry of Culture, and it was later announced that public funding for the arts would be limited to government-sanctioned projects. As Nascimento explains: "We live in a society that plots to assassinate the culture, ancestry, and artistic creativity of the people. The Ghetto Run Crew has become what it is today without any government looking out for us, without providing us with documents, space to work, or investment. So we do it our way—down to earth, with planning, one step at a time."

Negão calls this process "citizen solutions," which often originate in the favelas and have produced some of Brazil's most celebrated subcultures that are integral to the country's creative capital. Negão grew up in a favela in Rio's North Zone, where most Ghetto Run Crew meetups take place. He sees it as a privilege to represent the cultures that contribute to the city's cultural economy. "It's not just about us rising," says Negão. "It's about bringing our community, our society, with us on this journey. I never wanted to be a leader. I created the Ghetto Run Crew to help other movements tell a story."

And with 15 other storytellers in the Ghetto Run Crew, and an extended family that runs into the hundreds (including rappers, skateboarders, graffiti artists, dancers, DJs, and poets), they have created a powerful space in which their stories can be told. "We are a counterculture because we allow other body types, other lifestyles, to participate in traditional running cultures," says Negão. "We don't use running as competition, but as a tool for cultural representation."

Part of Negão's mission is to increase Afro-Brazilians' visibility in running, which he says isn't immune from racism. "How many black people have changed, are changing, and will change running?

How many have built, are building, and will build strong bridges with their passion, and yet don't have space in our memories? If the world's best runner was white and called Rick Springfield instead of Eliud Kipchoge, you can guarantee the story would be different." Ultimately, young people need to see that art, sport, and social engagement can earn them respect in the world. Creating such role models, and giving them a platform, is what Ghetto Run Crew is building toward. "The world has Jesse Owens, Tommie Smith, John Carlos, Aída dos Santos, Colin Kaepernick, Charlie Dark, and many others who prove the value of black power," Negão says. "One day, we will also be on that list." ∎

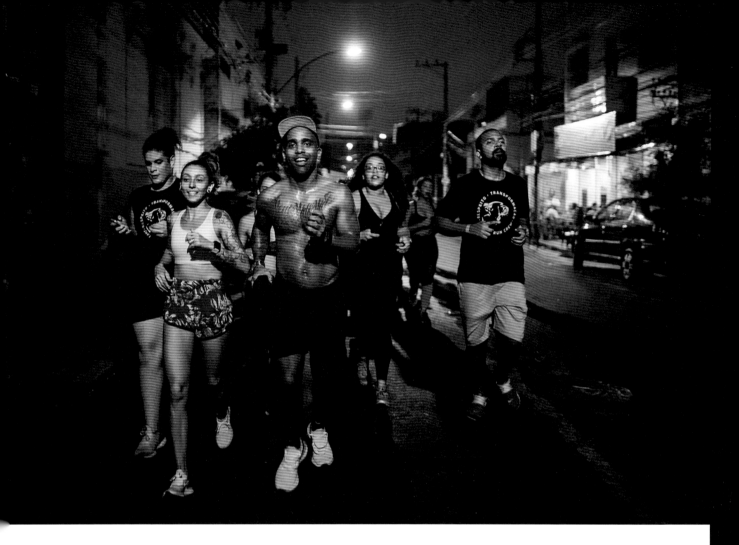

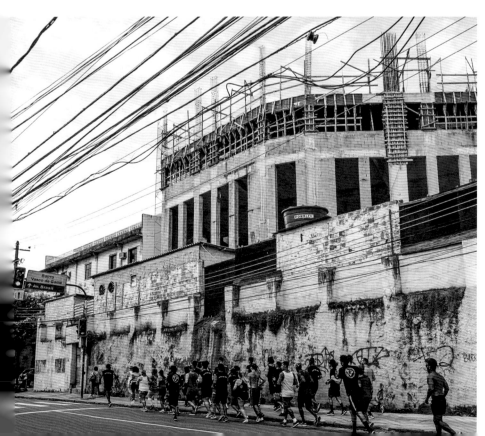

The Ghetto Run Crew originally targeted women as Ghetto Run Girls. The idea was to help young women achieve a sense of place and empowerment in society, through coming together to take over the streets and make others aware of their presence.

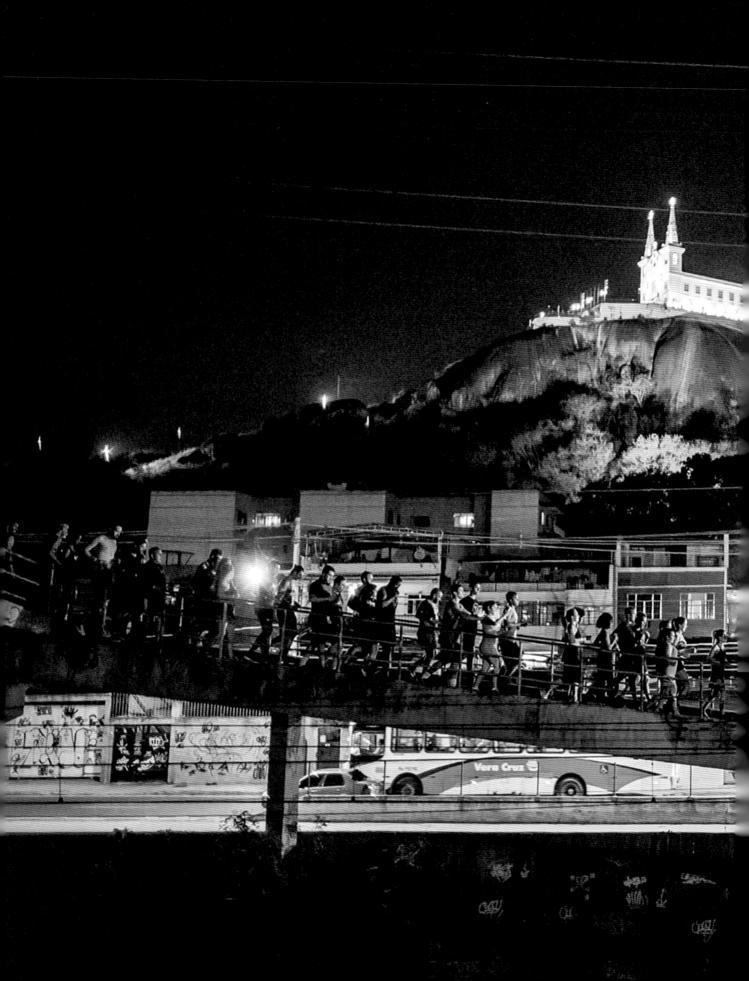

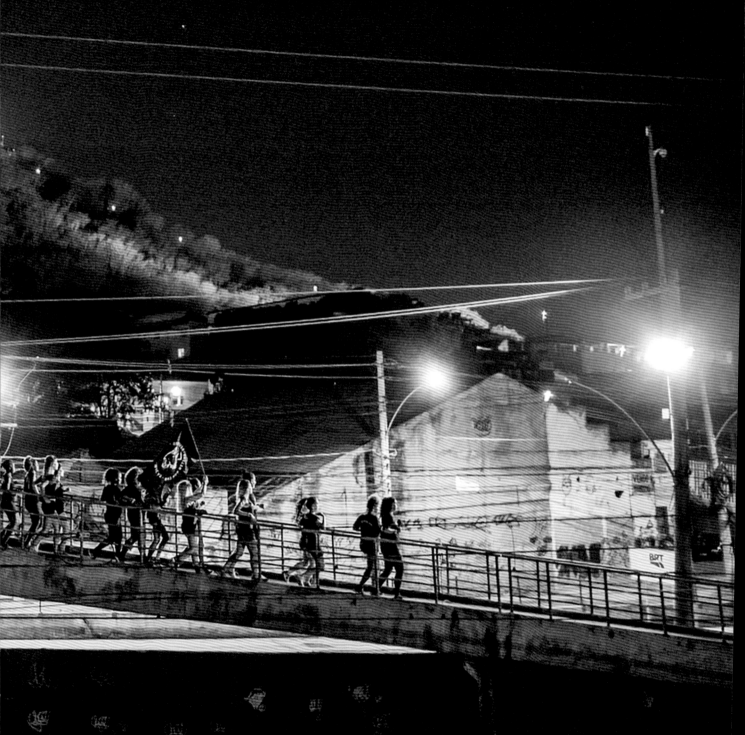

JUNGFRAU-MARATHON

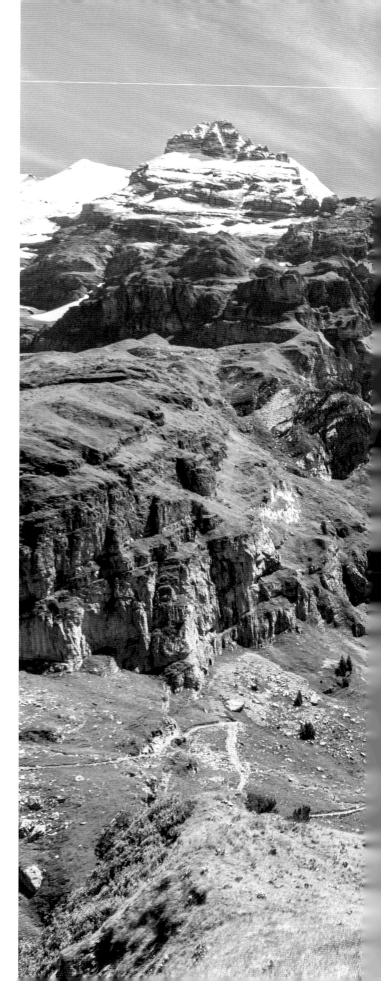

There's no marathon in Europe like it. The Swiss Alps bring you the Jungfrau-Marathon: Alpenhorns, snowcapped mountains, and the knowledge that, after 10 kilometers (6.2 miles), it's nearly all uphill. Join more than 4,000 runners—mad men and women trudging into the clouds.

Advertising itself as "the most beautiful marathon in the world," this is also one of the most popular, despite its many challenges. Places sell out very quickly as a result.

Starting in the mountain-resort town of Interlaken, high in the Bernese Oberland region of western Switzerland, the race climbs nearly 2 kilometers (1.2 miles) in altitude to the finish line at the mountain pass of Kleine Scheidegg, with very little in the way of descent in between. The relentless climb is made rewarding— or at least bearable—by the extraordinary beauty of the region, the enthusiasm of local supporters, and the promise of one of the most dramatic views in running. Those who make it to the final kilometers of the course run the last, grueling stretch under the gaze of three iconic Swiss peaks: the Jungfrau, the Eiger, and the Mönch. ▶

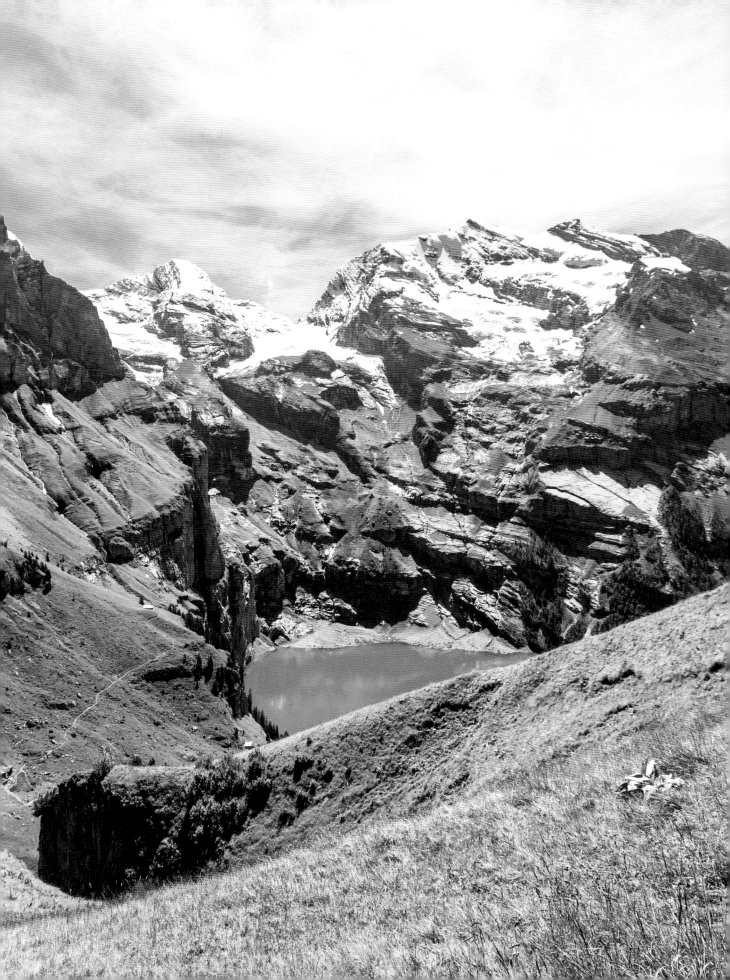

The relentless climb is made rewarding—or at least bearable—by the extraordinary beauty of the region, the enthusiasm of local supporters, and the promise of one of the most dramatic views in running.

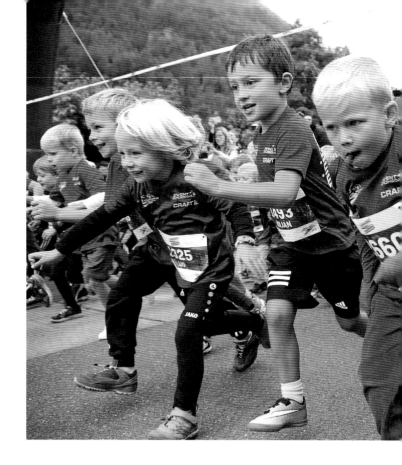

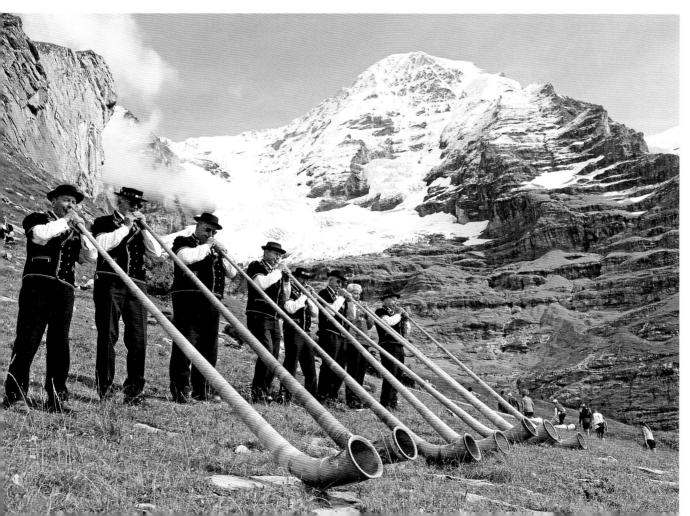

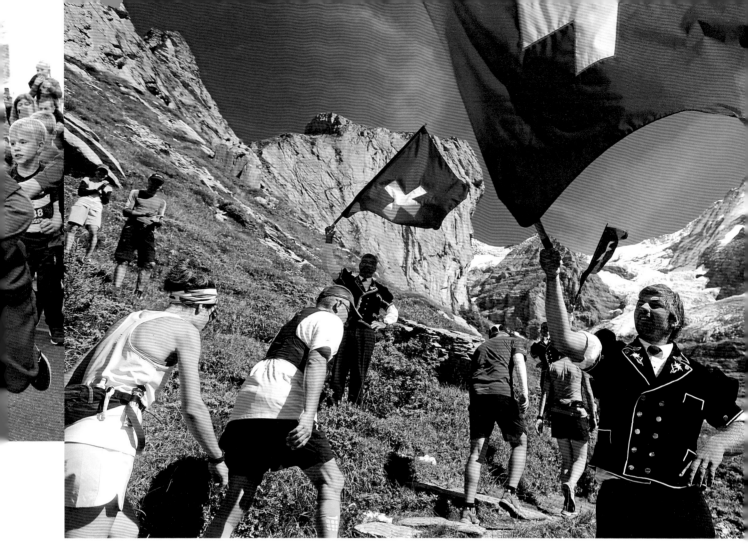

Above: this Swiss event is a truly festive affair, complete with costumed flag bearers. Opposite, top: there is even the Jungfrau-Minirun, with distances of between 200 meters and 1 mile for children up to the age of 16. Opposite, bottom: Alpine horn blowers contribute to the atmosphere.

▶ While this marvellous vista may be the highlight, there is also much to enjoy along this course—the region is a popular tourist destination with an outdoors emphasis, and you can see why. The relatively flat first 10 kilometers (6.2 miles) include a brief stretch along the shores of the turquoise Lake Brienz. On to spectacular Lauterbrunnen, through traditional villages and along wooded trails—Lauterbrunnen village itself is surrounded on all sides by dramatic rock faces, with towering waterfalls tumbling from the rocks. The real climbing begins here, with participants passing through the picturesque village of Wengen on the way to the high point of Eigergletscher at 2,320 meters (7,611 feet). The final 2 kilometers (1.2 miles) only are downhill; runners finish under the famed north face of the Eiger.

Part road race, part trail run, mostly punishing hike, this event is a challenge for everybody. At the elite level, finishing times hover around the 3- to 3½-hour mark, with the course record set by New Zealander Jonathan Wyatt in 2003. However, even amateurs are subject to strict cut-off times, with a 5 hour 35 minute cut-off enforced just before the 38-kilometer (23.6-mile) mark. This, along with the tough terrain, means that the race is not necessarily a good starting point for first-timers; it thoroughly deserves its cult following, nevertheless, and remains a classic. ∎

Length: 4.2 or 42.2 km (2.6 or 26.2 mi)

Location: Interlaken, Switzerland

Date: September

Type: trail/mountainous

Temperature Ø: 10–20 °C (50–68 °F)

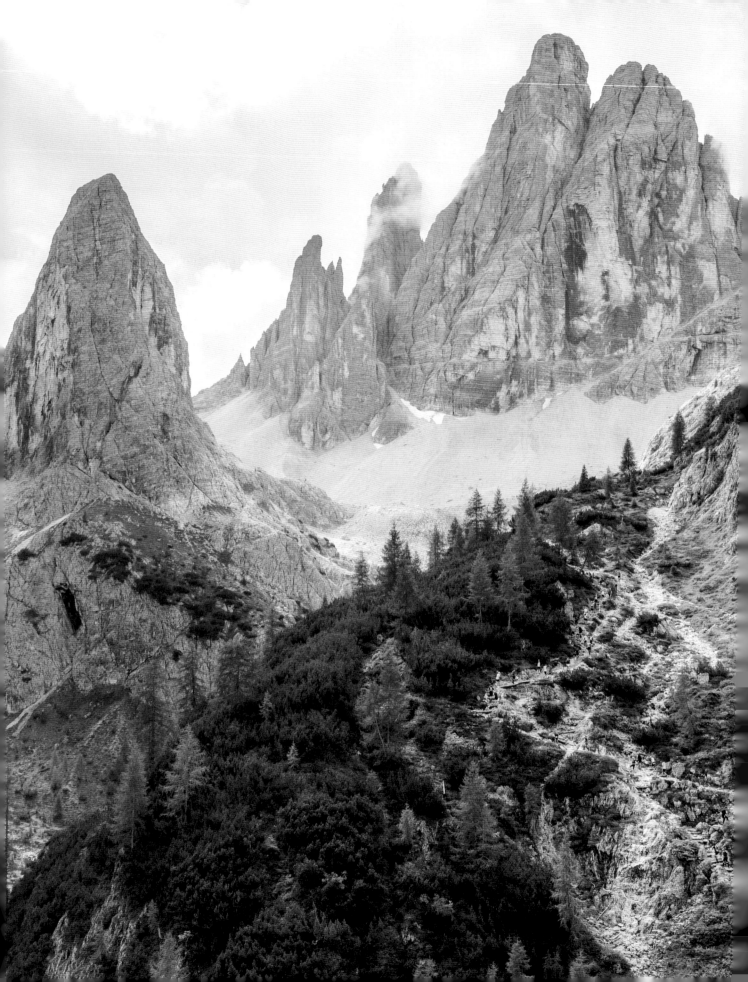

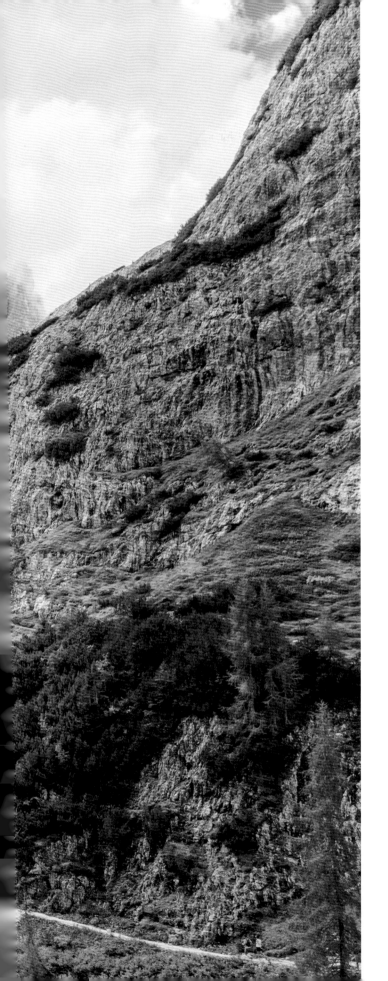

SÜDTIROL DREI ZINNEN ALPINE RUN

Up, up, and away. From the tiny Italian village of Sexten, through the high pines of the foothills of the Dolomites, to the famous Three Peaks Nature Park on the Italian-Austrian border. It's only 17 kilometers (10.6 miles), but it feels like hundreds. The views make every painful step worth it.

Run over a distance of up to 17 kilometers (10.6 miles), and with an altitude differential of 1,333 meters (4,373 feet), the Südtirol Drei Zinnen Alpine Run demands an extremely high level of fitness. No matter how experienced you are in this kind of running, you'll be puffing within a kilometer. Often, mountain running involves at least some downhill, but you're out of luck with this one—it's up, up, up, and more up.

The village of Sexten (or Sesto), where the race starts, is nestled in the Dolomites, in the South Tyrol region of Italy. If you've seen stunning images of the area on Instagram, it's likely this part of the world is already on your bucket list, and rightly so. The rugged and sharp mountains here are part of a Unesco World Heritage site, with the Three Peaks Nature Park a particular highlight. The three summits that give the run its name—and ▶

The start of the race has a fantastic atmosphere (helped by the dumpling party held the evening before), with a particularly committed group of runners brought together at the line.

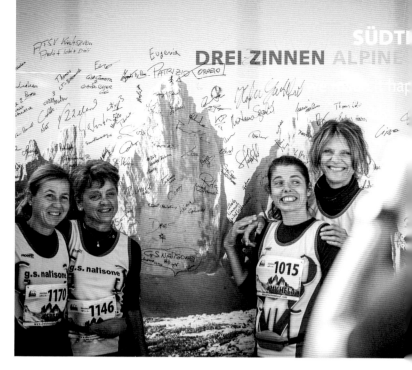

Above: jubilant runners pose for a photograph, having successfully completed the course. Below: participants pace themselves as they start their ascent, with the five Dolomite peaks, known as the Sexten Sundial, behind them.

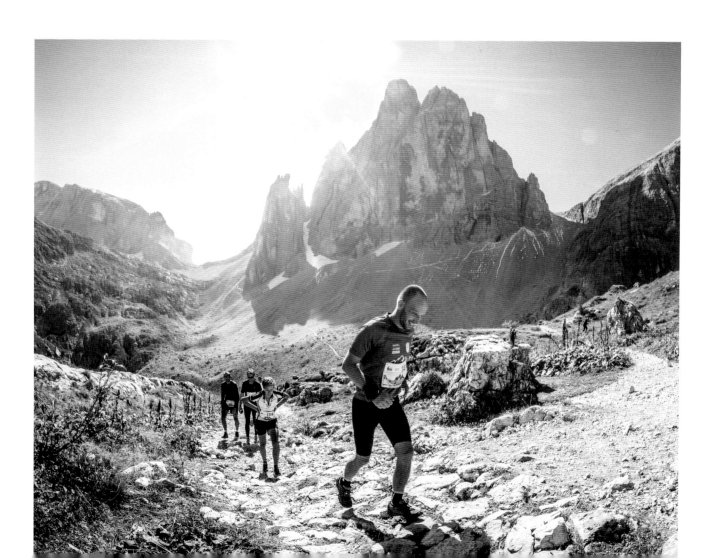

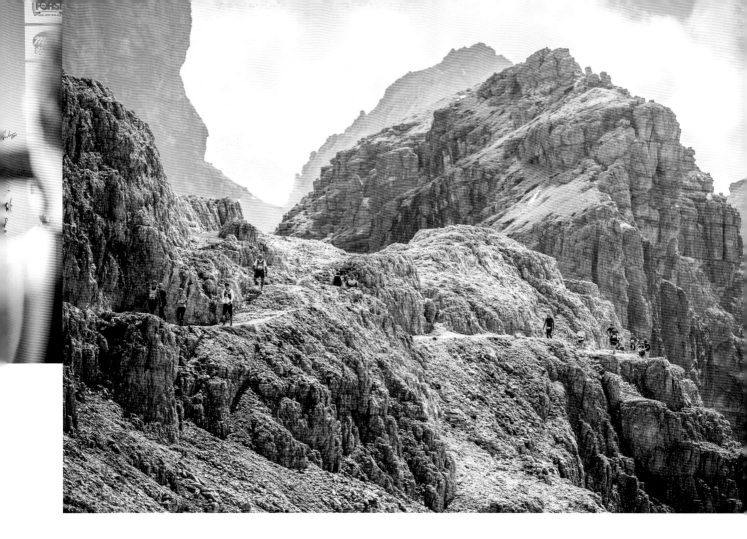

which can been seen from the finish line—are Kleine Zinne (Cima Piccola), Grosse Zinne (Cima Grande), and Westliche Zinne (Cima Occidentale), and they are all almost 3,000 meters (9,800 feet) tall.

The start of the race has a fantastic atmosphere (helped by the dumpling party held the evening before), with a particularly committed group of runners brought together at the line. They loop around the village before heading into the nearby Fischleintal (Val Fiscalina). In green alpine fields, with cows grazing nearby, the mountains rise above and, before you've settled into your stride, you'll be panting for breath, ascending fast. The trail is road initially, but a few kilometers out of the small ski resort and into the mountains, it is littered with large boulders and rocks to navigate.

The 800 athletes taking part in this ascent follow a route that was set out at the race's inception, more than 20 years ago, zigzagging along trails, past a series of mountain retreats, to the high point of the Büllelejoch (Forcella Pian di Cengia) at 2,522 meters (8,273 feet). They continue, passing above the Laghi dei Piani—two beautiful lakes—to the finish line at the Rifugio Antonio Locatelli—S. Innerkofler mountain hut.

Because the finish line is positioned on high, all the runners who finish toward the front of the pack are able to cheer and support those behind them. After finishing, all participants slowly make their way, with sore knees, back down to the village. This journey is twice as long as the ascent—but there's a very welcome pasta party when they get back.

This classically Italian race is cheap to enter and mesmerisingly beautiful, with entrants in for a real treat on blue-sky days. The altitude and steep ascent are a killer—so don't let the short distance fool you into skimping on training. But remember, it's the best way to see the Dolomites up close. ∎

Length: 17 km (10.6 mi) (2019)

Location: Sexten, Italy

Date: September

Type: road/city

Temperature Ø: 12–25 °C (54–77 °F)

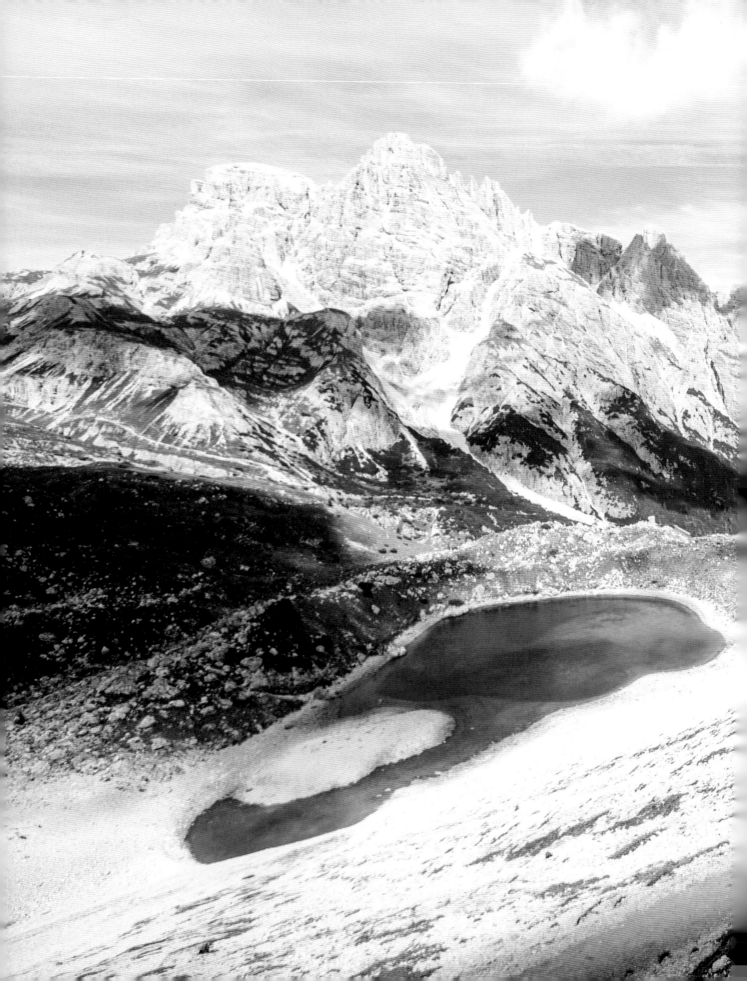

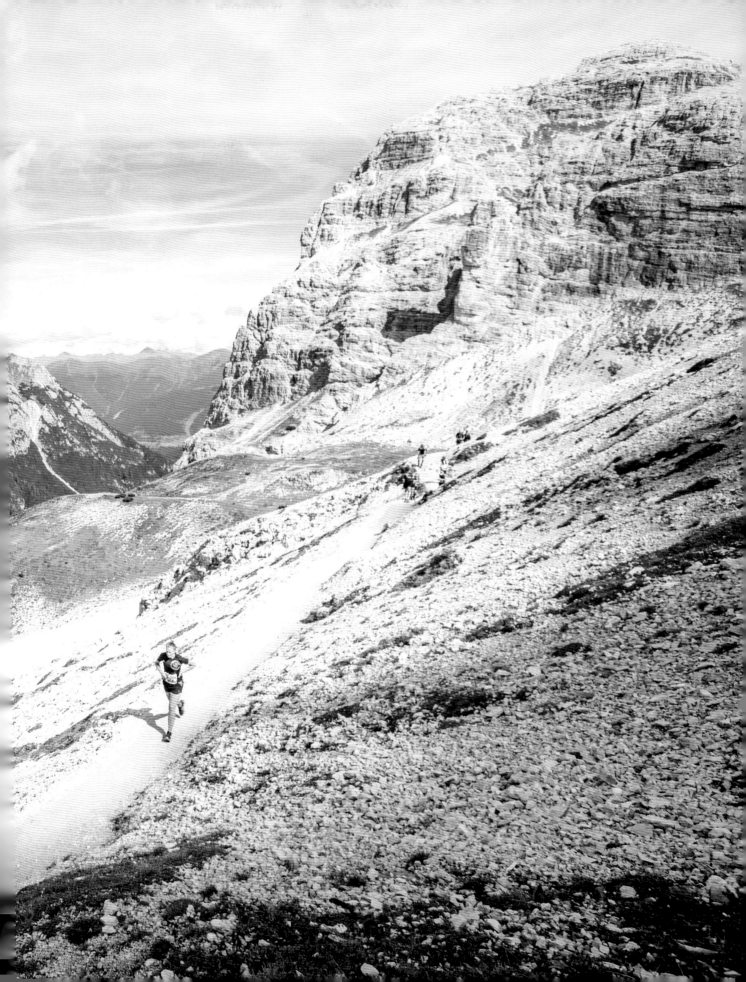

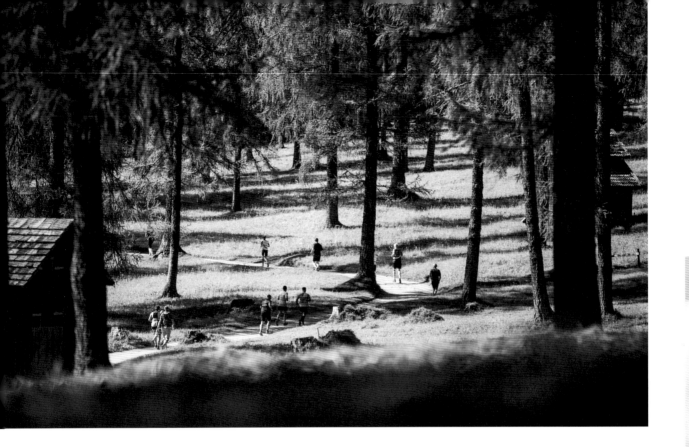

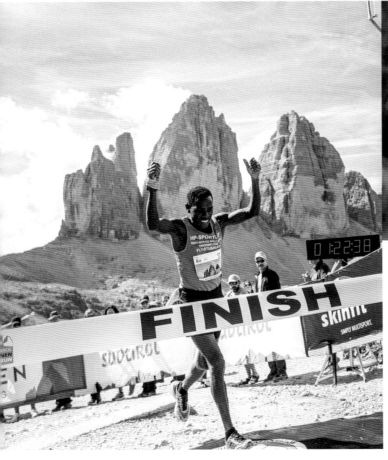

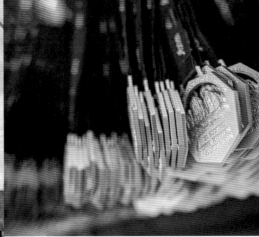

A medal awaits all who cross the finish line at the Rifugio Antonio Locatelli—S. Innerkofler mountain hut—that and the stunning views across the rugged mountains that give the run its name.

The altitude and steep ascent are a killer—so don't let the short distance fool you into skimping on training. But remember, it's the best way to see the Dolomites up close.

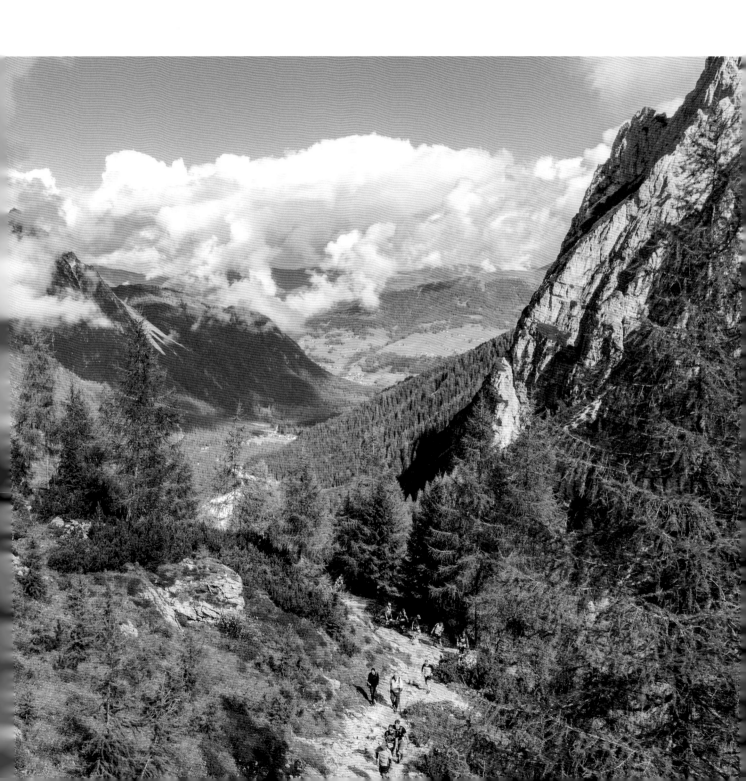

Rising Above: High-Altitude Runs to Take Your Breath Away

Running in the heights needn't mean pure endurance without respite. These locations offer intensely beautiful scenery, adventure, and, in the mountainous regions of Bhutan and Nepal, a sense of calm that's far removed from the strains of daily life (and urban running culture).

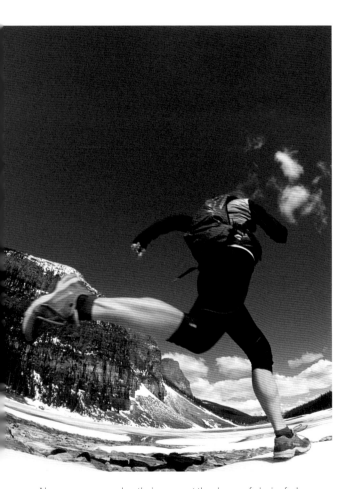

Above: a runner makes their way past the shores of glacier-fed Moraine Lake in Banff National Park. Opposite: one of the trails in the park rises onto a hill that offers unobstructed views of Moraine Lake and the Valley of the Ten Peaks.

Banff National Park

The Canadian Rockies region—specifically this area, Canada's oldest national park— offers miles of mountainous landscape studded with sapphire-blue glacial lakes, picture-perfect towns and villages, and scenic lookouts. Summer brings mirror lakes and lush forest, while winter presents a stunning sub-zero winter wonderland, with sports like ice hockey a particular attraction.

Give the full loop near Sulphur Mountain a go. You will cover 20 kilometers (12.4 miles), with nearly 900 meters (3,000 feet) of climb. If you'd like to run a little further, try heading from Sunshine Village to Shadow Lake; this should give you a full marathon distance with about 2,000 meters (6,500 feet) of climbing. It is a tough one, though.

Another option is to take the 10-kilometer (6.2-mile) route from the hamlet of Lake Louise to Mount Fairview. The peak offers 1,000 meters (3,281 feet) of climbing and your reward for reaching the summit, by way of a delicate larch forest, is a view of the Plain of Six Glaciers and Mount Temple. Head up at dawn or dusk with a head torch—you'll be treated to high-altitude treasures.

Blue Mountains

The wonderland of trails here is world-famous. The rugged and hazy blue lands of the Blue Mountains region in New South Wales, Australia, are known for their intensely dramatic scenery. Eucalyptus forests, steep cliffs and waterfalls, and remote valley villages all lie in this region, the gateway to which is the charming town of Katoomba.Easily reached by train from Sydney, Katoomba has small hostels and camping spots, making it the perfect base for many great running adventures—and for a trip to the Australian wilderness that won't break the bank. ▶

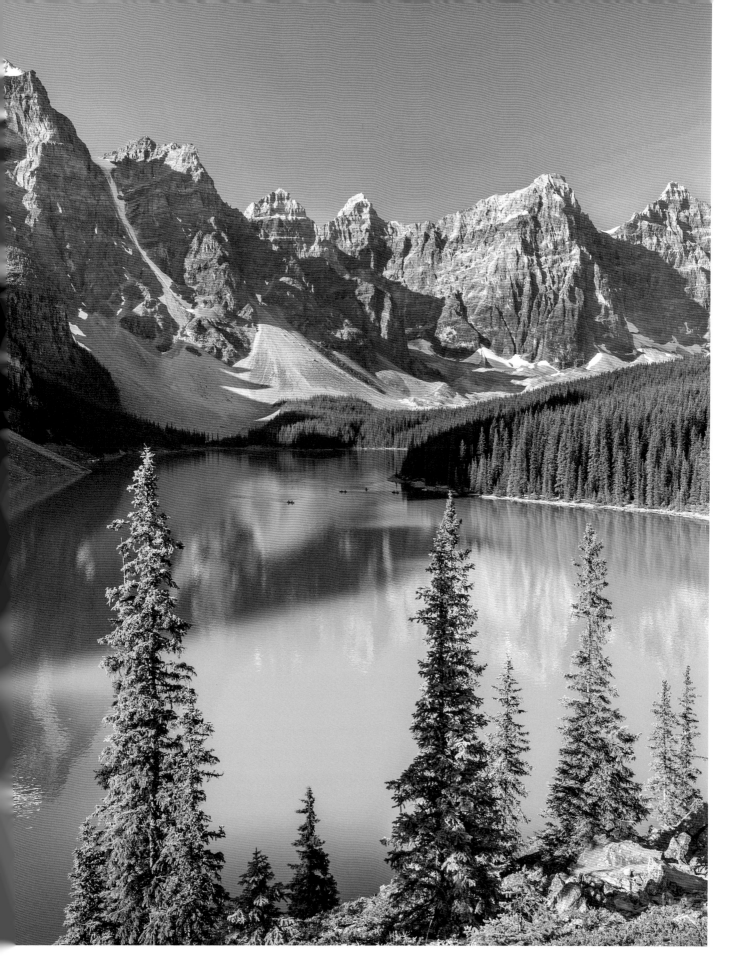

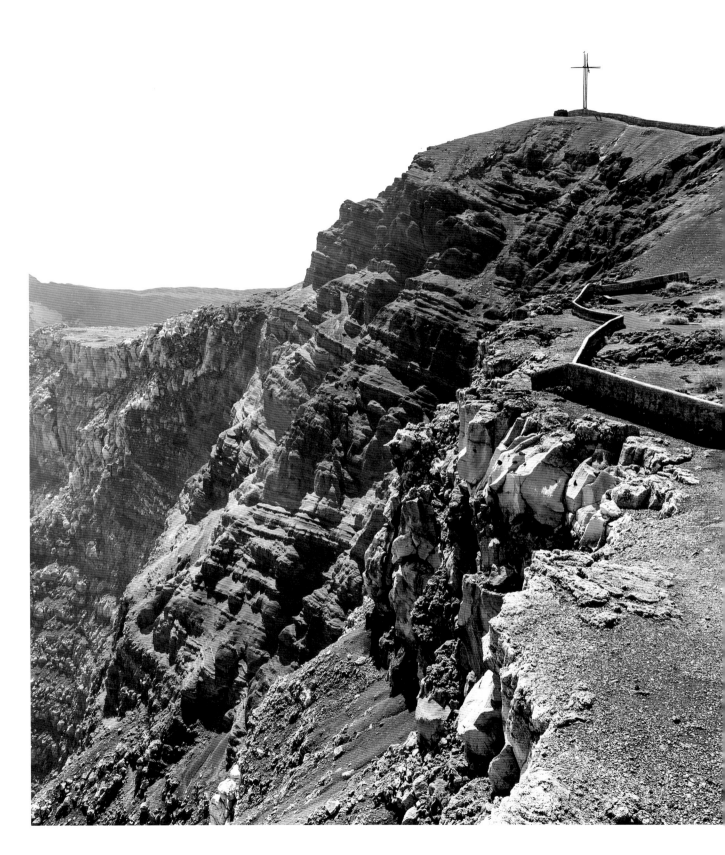

▶ While you're out running, watch out for snakes and rough and treacherous conditions underfoot. Many trails are perfectly formed, others are technical. Start in Katoomba, grab a map, and head down the Furber Steps; from here, trails go in all directions. Get lost but keep an eye on the weather.

Masaya volcano

There are very few places in the world where you can visit an active volcano and sit practically on the rim. The red-hot lava below performs a ballet of light, while a cloud of white smoke fills the active crater.

The impressive volcano is 20 kilometers (12.4 miles) from Nicaragua's capital, Managua, reached after circling many of the city's picturesque lagoons. After a long climb up a paved route, you can sit for a while and watch the display of lava in the volcano's vent, part of a wider system of craters and calderas. It is best at night, when you can capture photographs of the reds and oranges licking at the edge of the rock. Nearby, it is also possible to run along the side of the famous, and famously vast, Lake Nicaragua, or Cocibolca. It's home to freshwater bull sharks and, with a perimeter of about 425 kilometers (264 miles), is the largest inland body of water in Central America, so don't attempt to run around this one in a day.

And if you like steak for a post-run dinner, the city center offers many tasty and affordable options.

Mountains of Bhutan (Thimphu)

The early-morning training runs, the mad rush to find your race bib on a race day, and the mass crowds of big-city races. If you're looking to escape all this and enjoy ultimate peace, head to Bhutan. It is easy enough to write and ask permission to enter this invite-only nation, and the effort is absolutely worth it.

Bhutan has the fifth-highest capital city in the world: Thimphu. The tallest trees in the mountains are often smothered by clouds. Everywhere, even the roads, presents conditions akin to trail running, and there are plenty of hills. Remember to train extra-hard in preparation for the altitudes of up to 2,255 meters (7,400 feet).

From the moment you land on the tiny runway at Thimphu until it's time to go home, the country oozes peace and harmony. Some of the best running tracks, trails, and abandoned routes are just a walk away from the quiet city center. Whatever distance you're running, it's best to bring food you enjoy and a bag to hold much-needed essentials; depending on how far out you go, Bhutan is sparsely populated. Be sure, also, to keep hold of your entry paperwork, so that you're not removed from the run too early.

If you're traveling in winter, wrap up to the tune of at least five layers. It's hot in summer but very cold in winter.

Below: trail running on the unpredictable terrain of the Blue Mountains region of Australia. Opposite: a low wall marks the boundary between safety and the edge of the crater of Masaya volcano, Nicaragua.

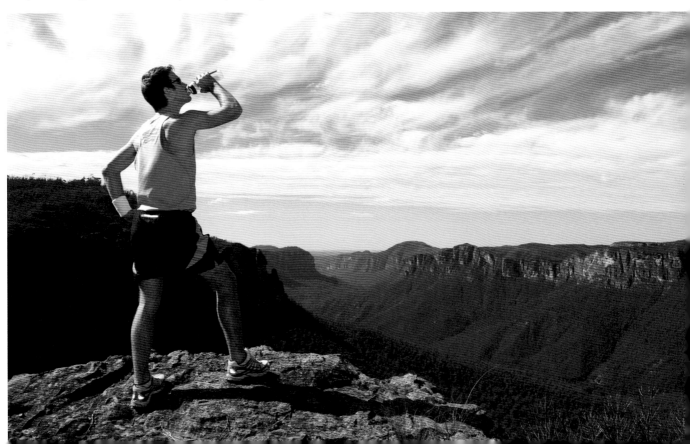

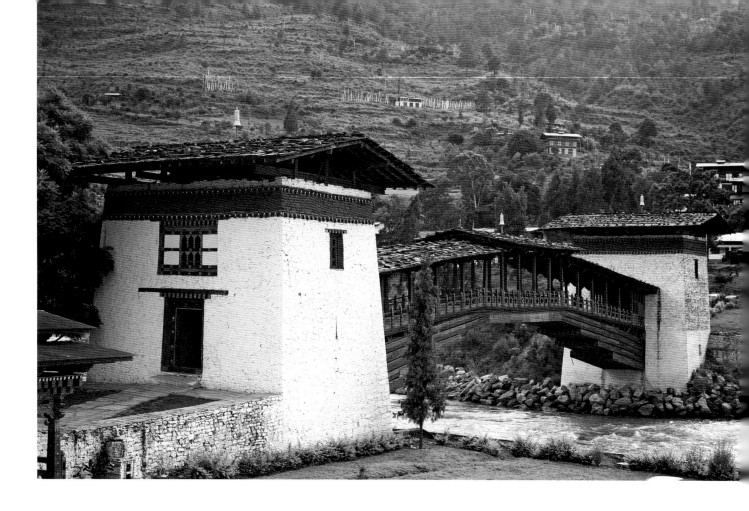

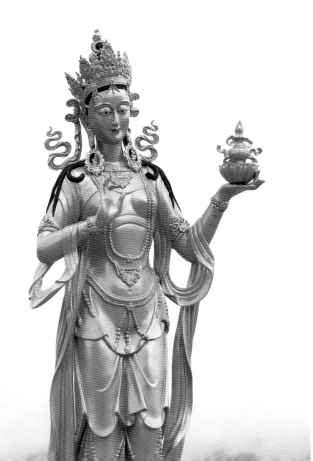

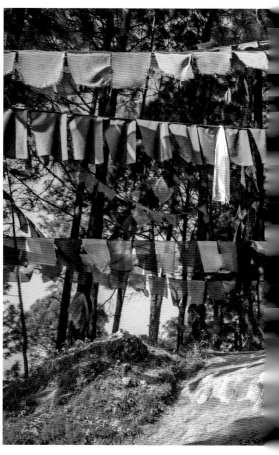

Kathmandu

Nepal isn't just a one-trick pony. Yes, it's home to the incredible Mount Everest, but for those of you who don't have thousands to spend on a trek to Base Camp, fear not—there are plenty of other spectacular and mind-blowing sights.

From hikes in the Himalayas to exploring the bustling streets of Kathmandu, Nepal has plenty to offer. If it's mountain ranges you're after, take the Annapurna Circuit, encircling this snowcapped mountain and its sisters Machapuchare ("fishtail") and Mardi himal, to name just a few. You'll stop at picturesque teahouses along the way and experience beauty you've never seen before as you hike the mountainous terrain.

For local culture, running through the streets of Kathmandu is best. Buildings are festooned with multicolored bunting and prayer wheels line the streets—be sure to run past and roll them right to left for good luck! The local markets fill your senses with bursts of color and aromatic spices.

Nepal is a bundle of bustling culture and spectacular scenery—one for keen photographers as well as runners.

Below: Just outside Kathmandu itself, Shivapuri Nagarjun National Park and the green hills to the south of Lalitpur are popular spots for trail running. Small paths and dirt tracks run between small settlements, taking you past ancient temples and scenes of traditional village life.

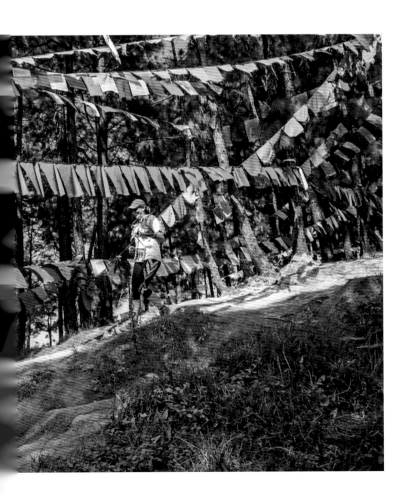

Mountain Runs: The Basics

Banff National Park
Alberta, Canada
Route:
Sulphur Mountain (loop); Sunshine Village–Shadow Lake; Mount Fairview trail
Distance:
10, 20, or 43 km (6.2, 12.4, or 26.7 mi)

Blue Mountains
New South Wales, Australia
Route:
varies; starting point, Katoomba
Distance:
varies

Masaya volcano
Masaya, Nicaragua
Route:
Managua–Masaya volcano–Managua
Distance:
44 km (27.3 mi)

Thimphu
Bhutan
Route:
Thimphu city and the mountains of Bhutan
Distance:
varies

Kathmandu
Nepal
Route:
Annapurna Circuit; Kathmandu city
Distance:
varies

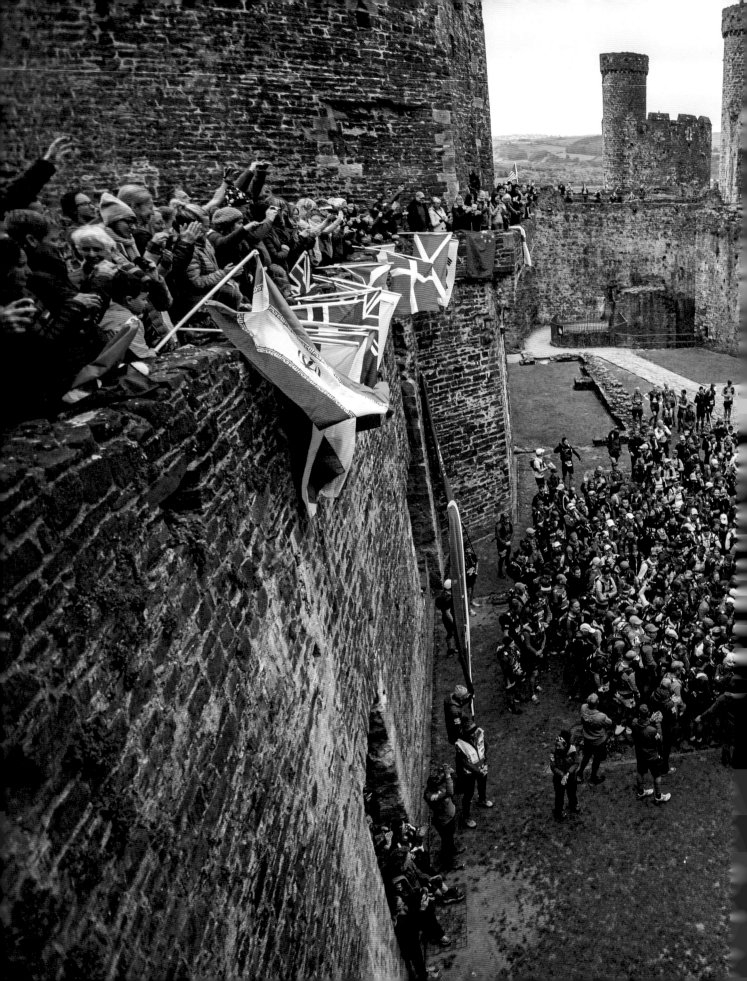

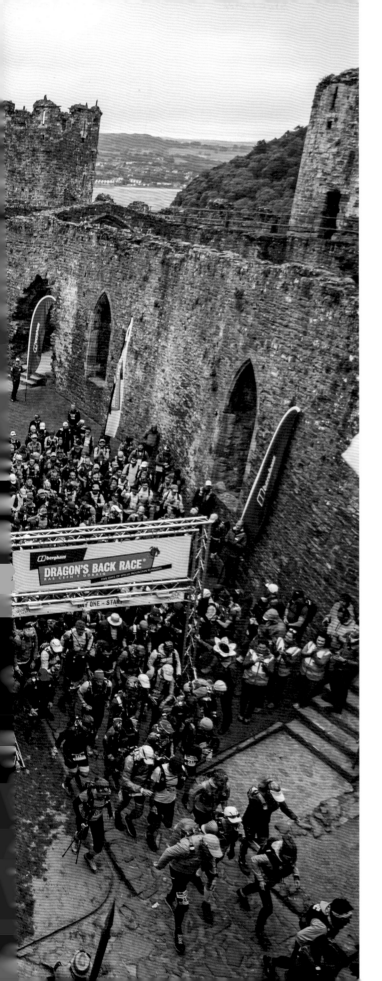

DRAGON'S BACK RACE

Prepare to ride the dragon's back for as long as it will allow you. Join an eclectic mix of beginners and hardened mountain runners picking their way up and down the spine of Wales. And may the weather be in your favor and your campground free of mud.

This legendary race—first held in September 1992, and picked up again 20 years later—inspires mountain runners with fear and awe in equal measure. Known for its "bulletproof" organization, as well as its excruciatingly high level of difficulty, it is becoming an annual event from 2021 (having been held biannually from 2017).

The distance of 380 kilometers (236 miles) is split into six days of running, with daily distances varying between roughly 50 and 70 kilometers (roughly 31 and 44 miles). The whole course incorporates 17,400 meters exactly (57,087 feet) of total ascent, across totally unmarked, wild, and remote terrain. Participants are required to use a map and/or their GPS device to follow the route over the high ridges of the Welsh mountains. It's no wonder that this is known as one of the toughest mountain races globally—the dragon rears its head often. ▶

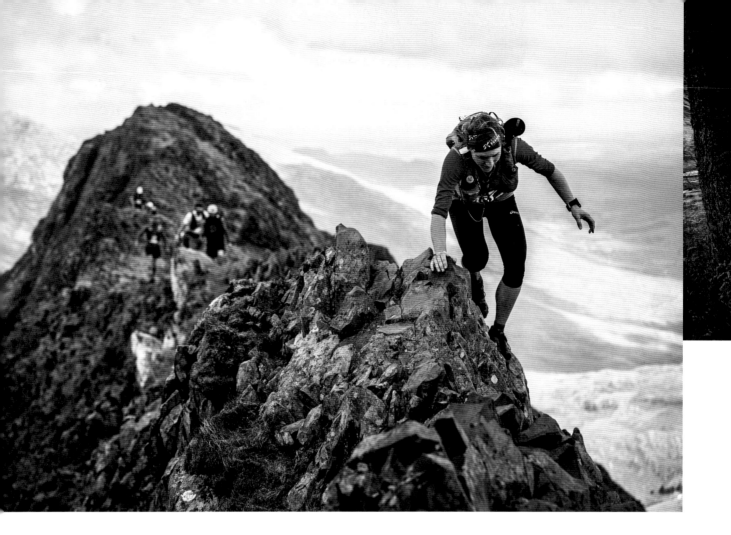

▶ Every racer should be ready for the very technical terrain of northern Snowdonia on day one, and the Rhinogydd region on day two. Even if you are an experienced trail or road runner, the race organizers nevertheless suggest some weekend trips to the mountains to prepare and pre-warn yourself. The average daily distance is not the hard part; throw in a grueling average height gain of 3,100 meters (10,171 feet) and repeat it for six days, and that's when things become challenging. Similarly, what goes up must come down, via perilous descents. If you're afraid of heights or uneasy on your feet, this may not be for you.

Every evening brings a new pop-up overnight campsite, where each runner is provided with a hearty afternoon snack, dinner, and breakfast. This is, of course, a great chance to catch up with fellow participants, get access to the race medics, and, crucially, get a good night's sleep. The race is known for its fantastic resources, including transport for all overnight baggage between campsites, making the running as enjoyable as possible. A wide variety of people run the Dragon's Back Race, so you'll have the chance to share running stories with people of all ages, backgrounds, and levels of experience, plus lots of different nationalities. In all, expect to find a very friendly and supportive atmosphere. Running, as all runners know, is in fact a team sport. Lots of participants end up running large sections of the route together, making friends for life in the process.

This is a rare, difficult gem, but the dragon gives as much as it takes. Unforgettable views are offered for brutal ascents, the pop-up camps in exchange for the harsh weather, and the community of togetherness in exchange for the rocky, ankle-bending ground. With the right preparation, anyone can complete the event if they are willing to suffer for long enough. ∎

Length: 315 km (196 mi)

Location: Wales

Date: September

Type: trail/multi-stage/mountainous

Temperature Ø: 10–17 °C (50–63 °F)

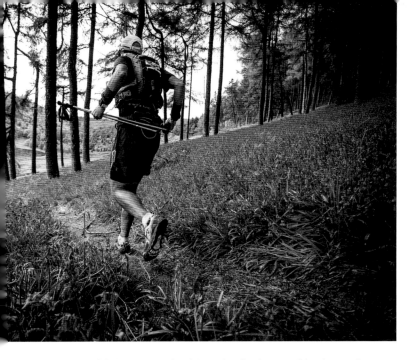

The average daily distance is not the hard part; throw in a grueling average height gain of 3,100 meters (10,171 feet) and repeat it for six days, and that's when things become challenging.

Much of Wales is unpopulated, its ancient landscape wild and rugged. From Crib Goch in the Snowdonia National Park (opposite) to Abergwesyn Common (bottom), roughly halfway through the route, participants can expect everything from precipitous crags to open moorland.

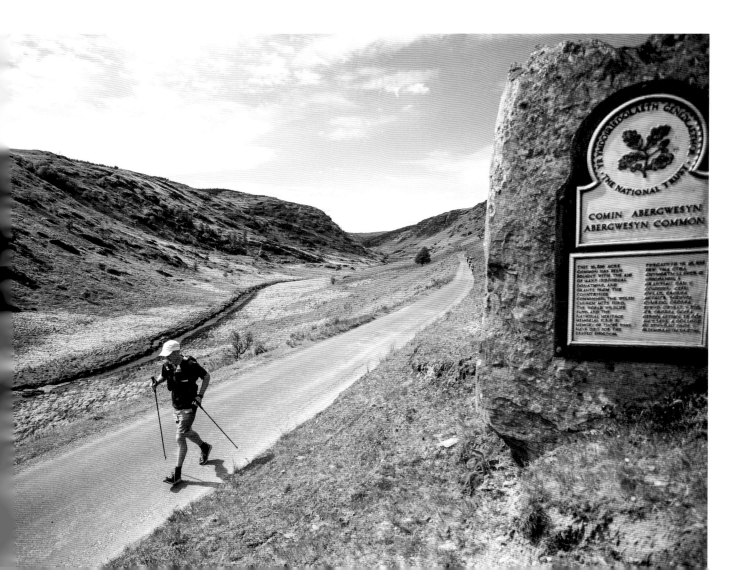

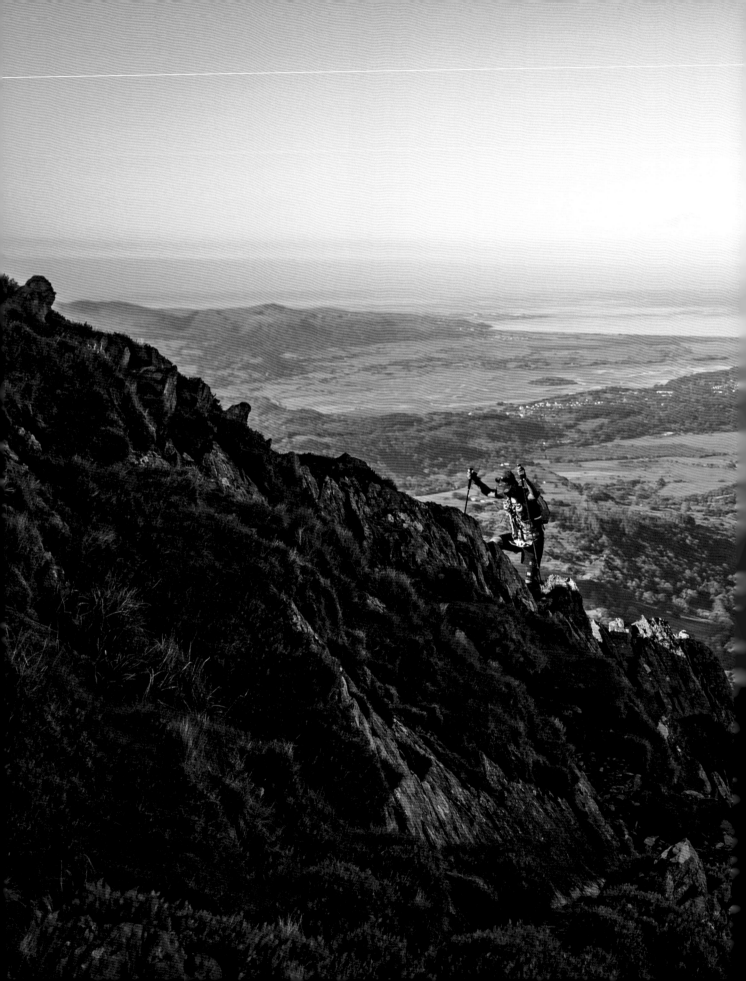

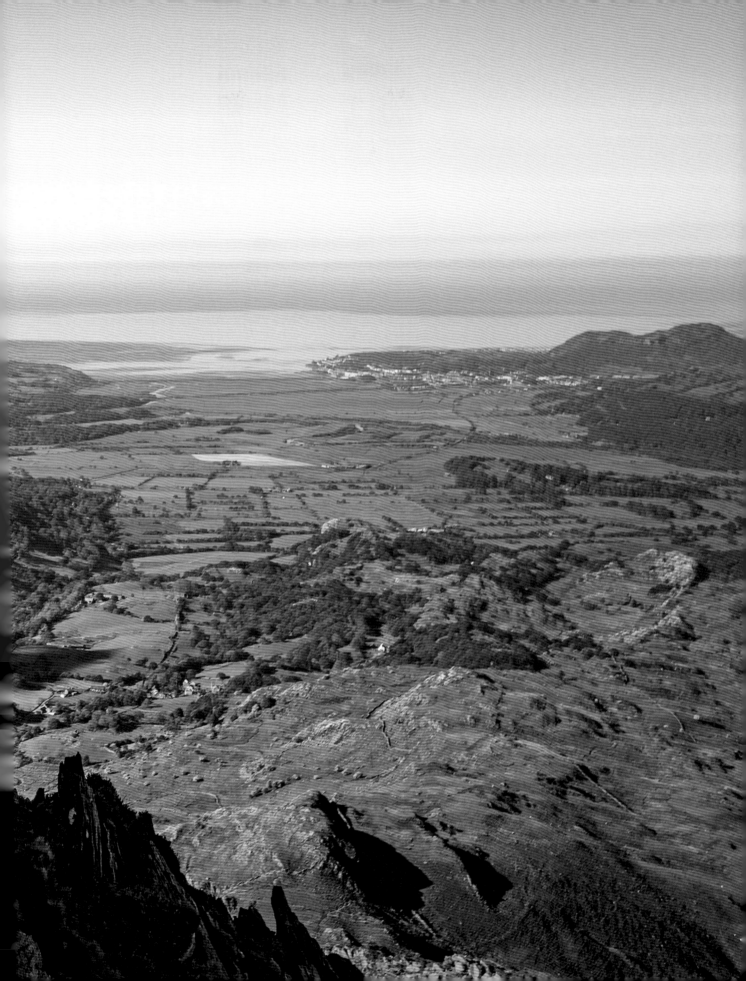

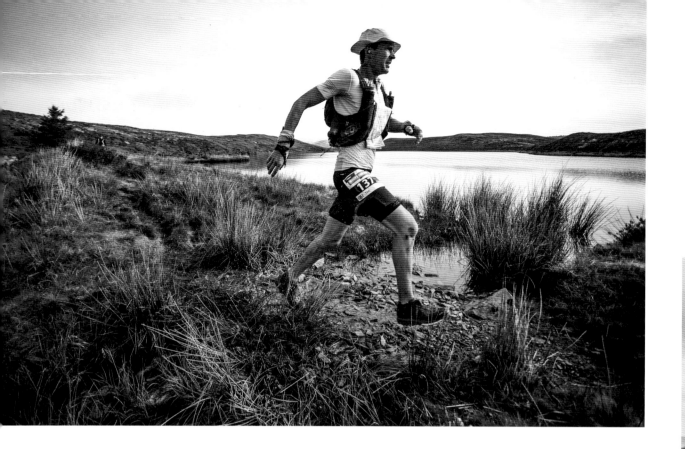

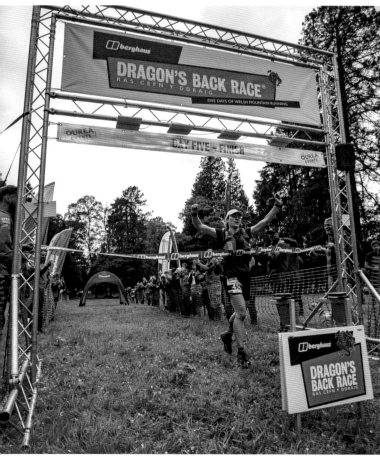

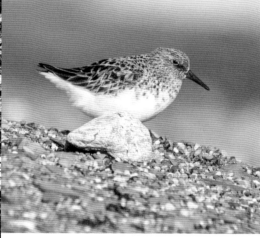

Left: The race runs the entire length of Wales, from Conwy Castle in the north to the finish line near Cardiff in the south. Opposite: by far the most treacherous stretches are in the north, in north Snowdonia.

Every evening brings a new pop-up overnight campsite, where each runner is provided with a hearty afternoon snack, dinner, and breakfast. This is, of course, a great chance to catch up with fellow participants.

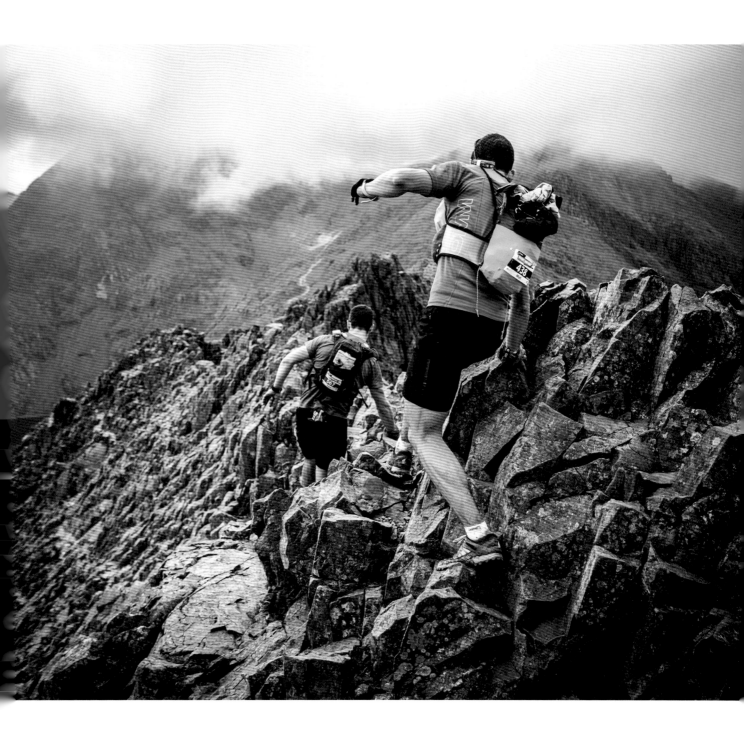

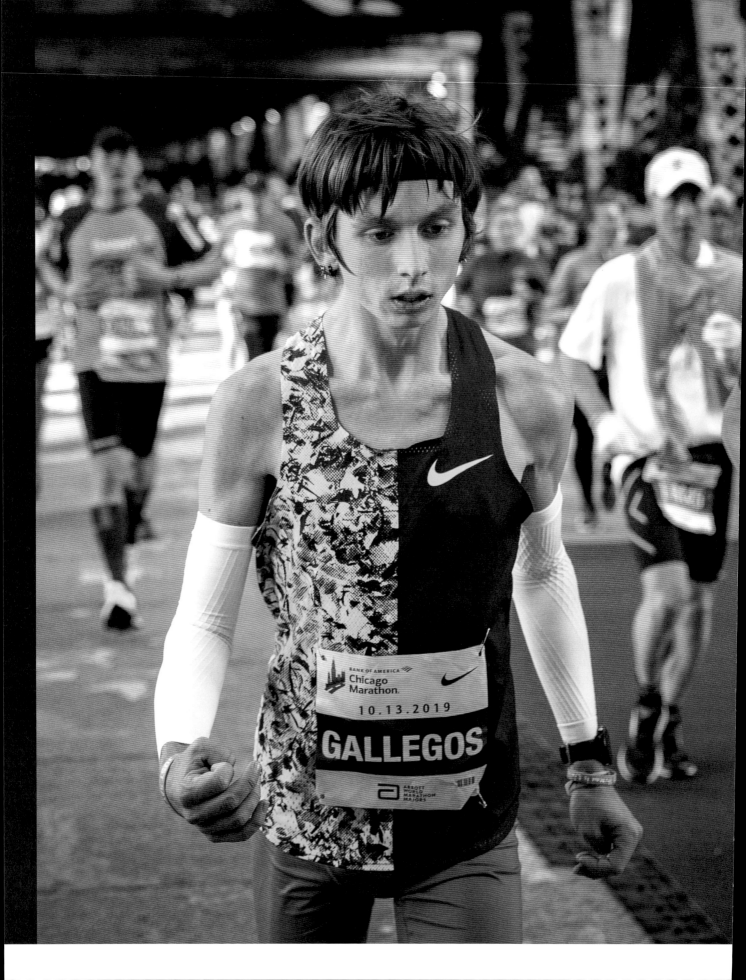

Redefining How the Body Should Move with Justin Gallegos

This runner in his early twenties could have made any number of excuses not to pursue sports. Instead, he became the first professional athlete with cerebral palsy to sign with Nike.

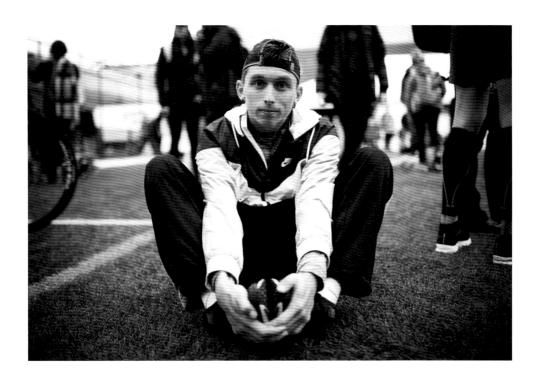

Justin Gallegos needed a walker in order to take his first steps in the world. Born with cerebral palsy, he struggled to bend his knees and lift his legs. When, after finishing preschool, he decided to walk free solo, his limbs had trouble adjusting to their newfound freedom. He fell often. Over the years, his muscles grew stronger and his spills became more infrequent. He participated in karate and equestrian programs designed for children with disabilities. By the time he entered high school, in 2012, Gallegos felt he no longer needed special accommodation. Football was on the cards, though his doctor advised against it, which is reasonable medical advice for anyone, let alone someone with a disability. Encouraged by his father to join the cross-country team, Gallegos initially felt ambivalent toward running. He still remembers his first run. "I fell a lot," he says. "Like, a lot." But he wasn't discouraged: his whole life had been a lesson in getting up and trying again. His goal for the first season was to run 5 kilometers (3.1 miles) in under half an hour. He achieved that in his first race. The more he ran, the more his muscles agreed with his brain. His balance improved. Walking was no longer a burden. "Running really helped improve my quality of life," he says. In November 2015, he ran his final high-school 5-kilometer (3.1-mile) run, this time competing for the varsity team. He crossed the finish line with a time of 26 minutes 23.71 seconds. It was his last race in his hometown of Santa Clarita, California.

The following summer, Gallegos moved upcoast to study advertising at the University of Oregon in Eugene. He joined the school's running club and landed a brand ambassador role at Nike, where he helped develop a shoe for runners with disabilities. He considers the partnership an opportunity to educate people about cerebral palsy. "Many mistake it for a mental illness," Gallegos says. "People told me not to worry about college, even though I had the grades to go."

It can be difficult to describe how it feels to live with cerebral palsy. One online commenter says, "It essentially feels like instead of muscles you have boa constrictors randomly squeezing your ▶

> *"I believe in 'no limits.' Nothing is impossible. I want to be remembered as someone who made a difference, who showed people that what they once thought was impossible is possible."*

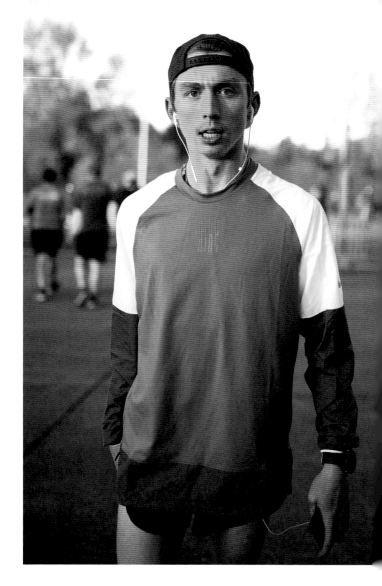

▶ bones into dust … a demon fused to your very DNA." The thing about snakes and demons is that you can vanquish them. In April 2018, Gallegos ran his first half-marathon, finishing in just over two hours. Six months later, Nike offered him a professional contract, making Gallegos the first athlete with cerebral palsy to sign with the company. In October 2019 he finished his most grueling race yet, the Chicago Marathon, buoyed by the example of his hero, Kenyan distance runner Eliud Kipchoge, who had run the world's first sub-two-hour marathon a day earlier. The walls of Gallegos's room are adorned with posters of his idols: Muhammad Ali, Metallica, and local former Olympian Steve Prefontaine, whose celebrity made running a spectator sport in the 1970s. "I love Oregon," Gallegos says. "It's my home. It holds a special place in my heart. I want to stay involved with Nike as long as I can."

Gallegos maintains a close relationship with his family in California. He credits his parents with instilling in him the drive to take more from life than his prognosis offered. "My dad never gave up on me," Gallegos says. "He always pushed me to do bigger and better things. He runs with me. He always knows how to see the positives of a situation. He is a fighter and he fights for me." Gallegos tells me about the sacrifices his mom made when he was still tripping over his feet and dealing with friction at school. It is the only time during our conversation that his cadence changes, emotion stifling his voice. "Anyway," he says, "I wouldn't be here without them."

Gallegos currently runs about 322 kilometers (200 miles) a month. "I believe in 'no limits,'" he says. "Before I thought my max was 48 kilometers [30 miles] a week, and now it's 80 [50]. Next year, who knows where I'll be? It could be 113 kilometers [70 miles] a week. Nothing is impossible. I want to be remembered as someone who made a difference, who showed people that what they once thought was impossible is possible." Gallegos is particularly keen to dispel the victim mentality often projected onto people with disabilities, signing off many of his Instagram posts with the hashtag #IAmNotAVictim. "Victimhood isn't waking up one day and saying, oh, I'm a victim. It's other people feeling entitled to tell you what you need to be a victim of, how to live your life," he says. "I'm not a victim. No one has hurt me. Growing up, people treated me like I was glass. 'Be careful around Justin,' they said. In a way, I was a victim of that. But I refused to let that define me."

Gallegos is becoming an increasingly visible figure in the running community, a "mini celebrity," as he puts it. He embraces the privilege of being a role model. "My platform is much more than being a face for Nike," he says. "It's also spreading awareness of cerebral palsy." His biggest impact is empowering others to recognize that, while no one chooses to live with a disability, it is a choice whether to suffer from it. "Pain is inevitable, suffering is optional," the writer Haruki Murakami famously wrote in his ode to running. "I can be a motivational speaker and try to send a powerful message, but I can't help people," Gallegos says. "If someone is in a rut in their own life, it's up to them to make a change. It's possible for anyone with the right mindset." When he graduates after the 2020 school year, Gallegos wants to race and spread his message abroad (he has not traveled outside the U. S.). Within a few years, he plans to publish a book about how distance running transformed his life. "I hope I can inspire people to follow their dreams and not let anything hold them back," Gallegos says. "When hard work meets dedication, you will be rewarded." ■

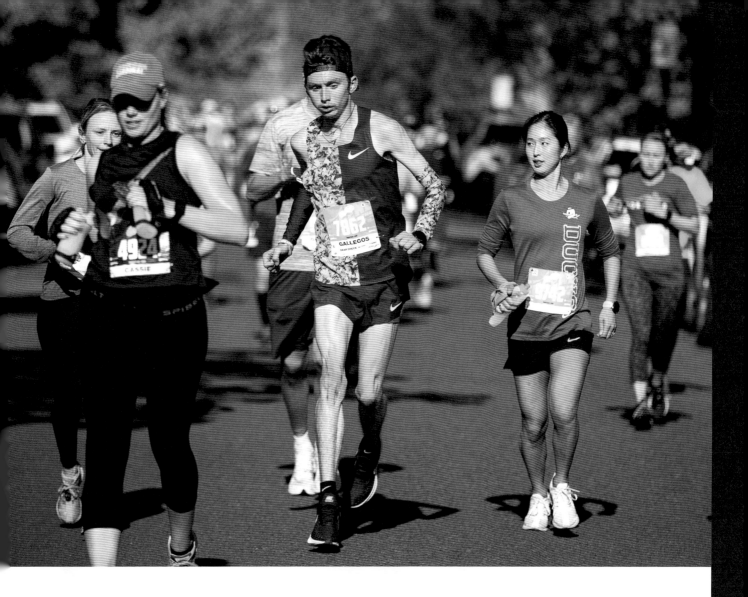

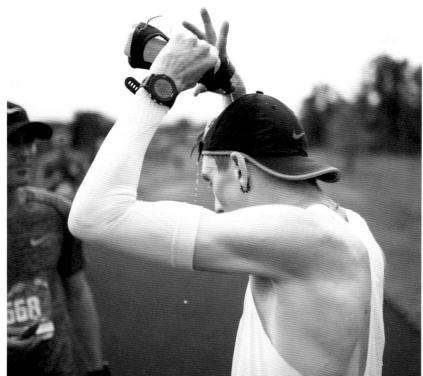

Above: Gallegos competing in the Eugene, Oregon, half-marathon, in April 2019. He crossed the finish line in less than two hours, coming 53rd out of 90 in his age group. His father, Brent, also ran in the event, finishing at the same time.

MIDNIGHT SUN MARATHON

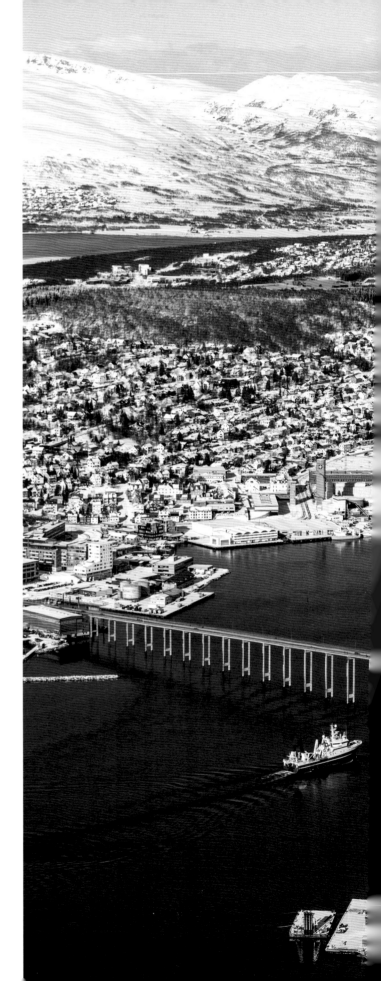

Start your race at night, in daylight, in a historic city where, in June, the sun never falls below the horizon. Runners from all over the world journey to the Arctic Circle to experience this unique run.

There are very few places in the world where you can run a marathon in the middle of the night, yet under the gaze of the sun. The polar day, or midnight sun, is a phenomenon whereby the sun is visible for 24 hours, never setting below the horizon. In Tromsø, Norway, 350 kilometers (217 miles) north of the Arctic Circle, this state of affairs carries on for about nine weeks in mid-summer. Therefore, while the weather may have varied over the 30-year history of the city's marathon, the sun has never been known not to shine. This race isn't mountainous, or technical, but it is special.

The home of this brilliant and quirky race is a major cultural hub of the Arctic Circle; the largest city in northern Norway, Tromsø has a particular reputation for music, theater, and film events. The historic center of the city, on the island of Tromsøya, is also distinguished by its architectural heritage: it has a large number of ▶

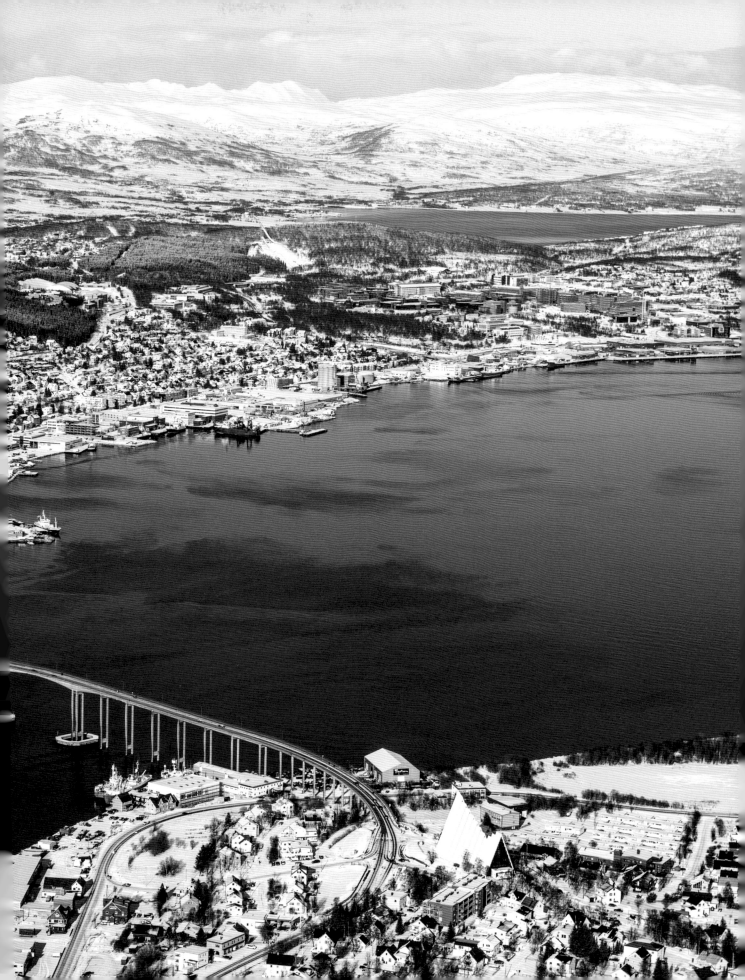

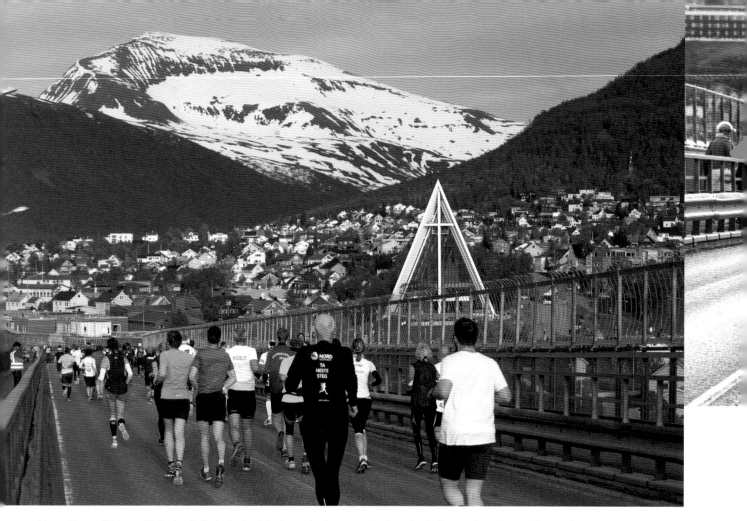

Above: Tromsø Bridge, with the Arctic Cathedral in sight. Opposite, bottom: aside from the challenge of running at nighttime, the course is relatively flat, most of it on roads that hug the coastline.

▶ traditional wooden houses, some of them dating back to the eighteenth century. By contrast, the striking Arctic Cathedral, with its peaked roof and enormous stained-glass windows, is a modern work, only completed in 1965. Marathoners run past this building twice and, unsurprisingly, it's impossible to miss.

The city itself is worth a visit even without the benefit of a runner's high. Racers often arrive a few days early to experience the place in its full glory: a trip in a cable car up the stunning Mount Storsteinen, perhaps, or a tour of the museums, or maybe some pre-marathon hiking. Runners also have the opportunity to attend a banquet-style gathering in the city the "night" before the race—a chance to scoff down some last-minute lasagne and mingle with fellow competitors.

Starting at 8.30 p.m., the race itself takes runners from the hustle and bustle of the city center, over the Tromsø Bridge and towards the cathedral, before looping back, heading round the island to the city airport and then back again. Tromsøya is surrounded by calm waters and rugged, snowcapped mountains, providing beautiful scenery. Happily, the route itself avoids those mountains and is largely run on roads, but it's not all plain sailing. Runners' bodies are ready to sleep, but instead they are attempting a marathon. That in itself means participants will likely not achieve a personal best.

The race is relatively simple, with a positive, fun atmosphere. Locals get involved in the event and its celebrations, helping to alleviate the disorientation of the mix of day and night for out-of-towners. ∎

Length: 4.2, 10, 21.1, or 42.2 km (2.6, 6.2, 13.1, or 26.2 mi)

Location: Tromsø, Norway

Date: June

Type: road/city

Temperature Ø: 7–13 °C (45–55 °F)

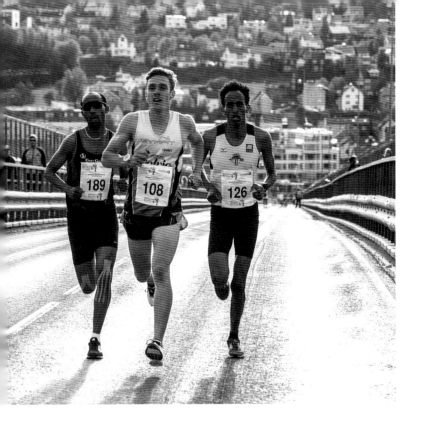

There are very few places in the world where you can run a marathon in the middle of the night, yet under the gaze of the sun. The polar day, or midnight sun, is a phenomenon whereby the sun is visible for 24 hours, never setting below the horizon.

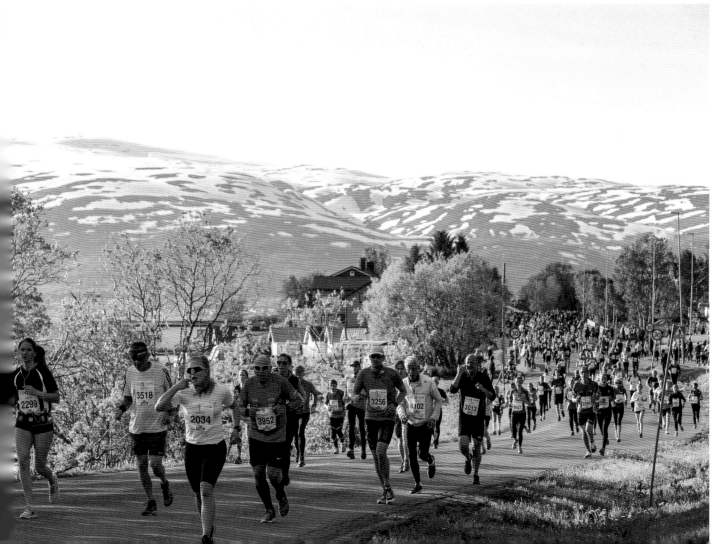

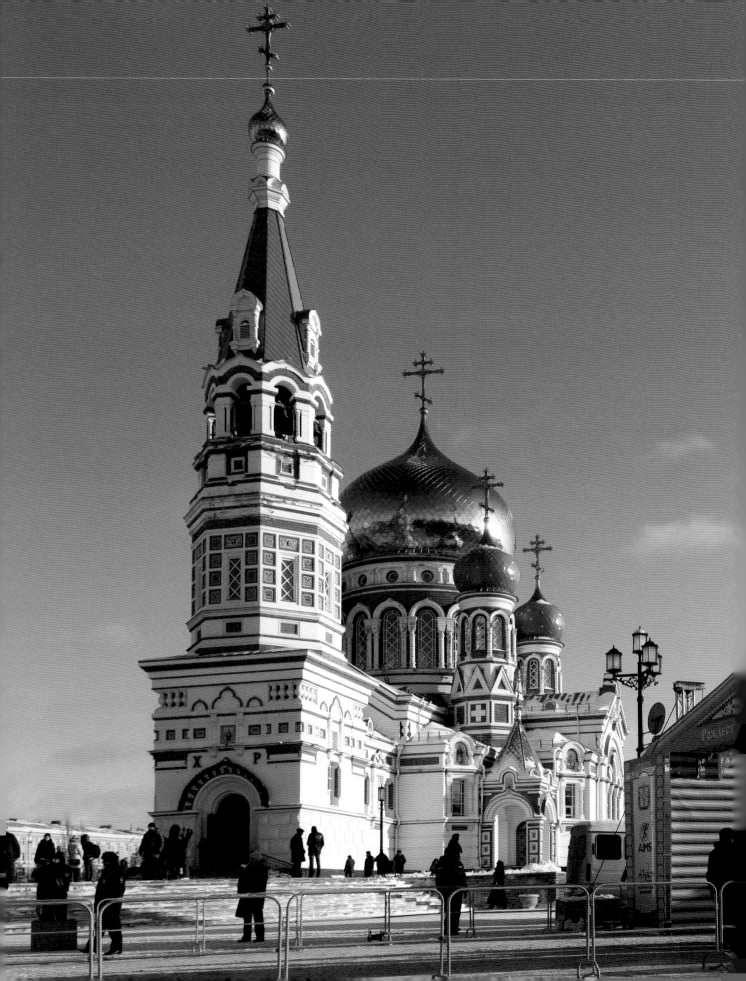

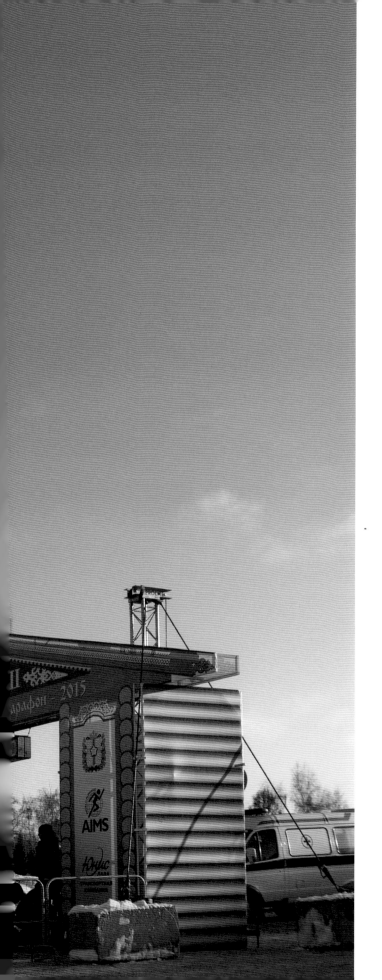

SIBERIAN ICE HALF MARATHON

Snow, ice, big Russian hats, and Siberian architecture. If you're feeling brave enough, take on this route around the wonderland of the city of Omsk in the depths of Russian winter. Since temperatures can reach as low as -45° Celsius (-49° Fahrenheit), a triple-layer approach is recommended. No matter how hard you run, you'll still be cold.

Snow crunching underfoot, ice forming around your face, and hands numb, even with your heart racing. Needless to say, the majority of participants won't need sunscreen for this one—it's likely they'll have no skin on show whatsoever. This is distance running in Siberian winter. What could possibly go wrong?

As it's one of the coldest races in the world, runners can expect to face temperatures as low as -45° Celsius (-49° Fahrenheit). In fact, the extreme weather is one reason Russia has no other comparable major long-distance races in winter. In Omsk, sweat is often seen freezing around the necks and eyelashes of participants, with impressively long icicles forming on beards. Some even say that runners' eyes begin to freeze up. This is one event where it's probably easier to run that it is to watch from the sidelines. Many supporters and locals line the finish area to show support, but ▶

As it's one of the coldest races in the world, runners can expect to face temperatures as low as -45° Celsius (-49° Fahrenheit). In fact, the extreme weather is one reason Russia has no other comparable major long-distance races in winter.

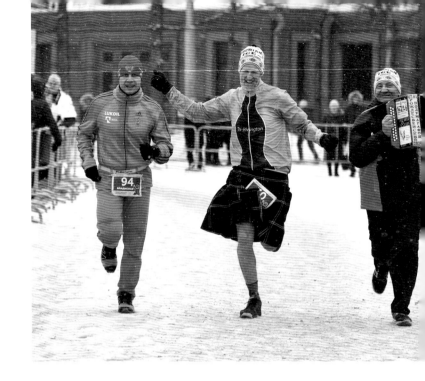

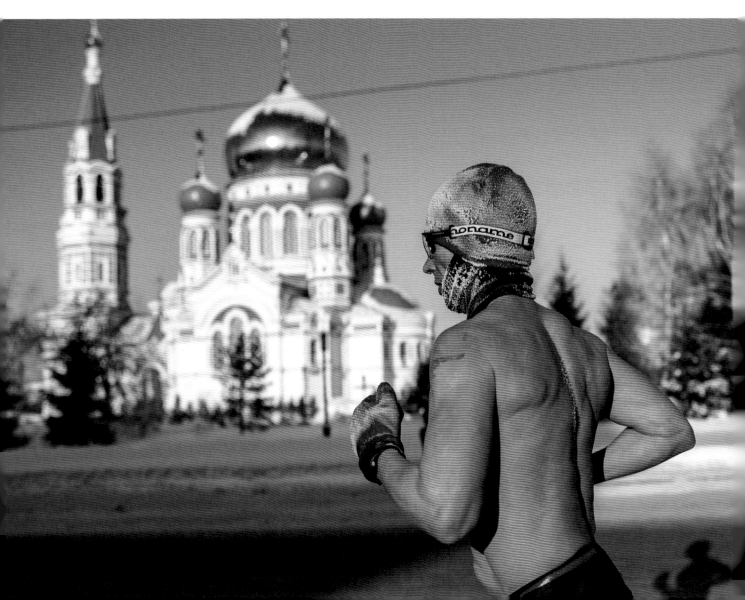

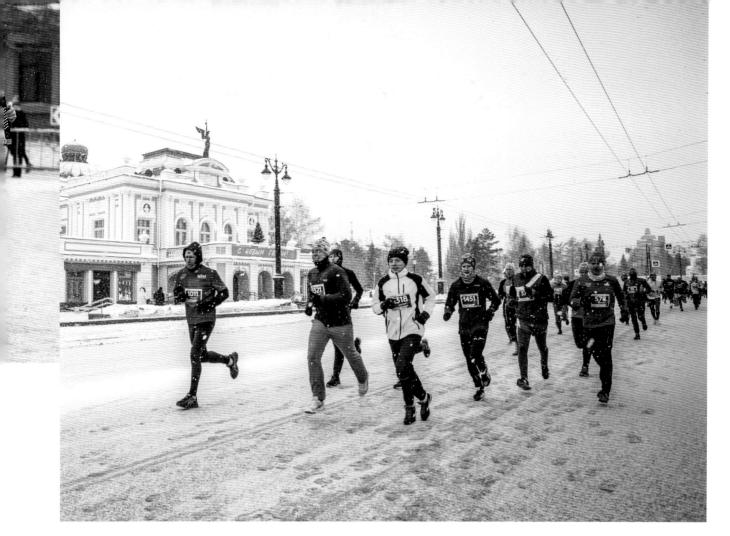

Opposite: although the majority of runners take the precaution of dressing warmly for this event, there are some who choose to wear fancy dress or run bare-chested. There is a prize for the most outrageous costume.

▶ due to the temperature, they quite understandably don't tend to hang around for very long.

Omsk, in southwestern Siberia, is Russia's ninth-largest city, sitting on the banks of the Irtysh River (it's the location of the oldest bridge across the Irtysh). The race passes through its historic center, where wooden houses sit alongside art nouveau architecture, and along the river, though participants probably won't be able to enjoy much of the view, with hoods up, buffs over their faces, and sometimes even goggles donned in preparation for snow starting to fall. At this time of year, the whole city is smothered in snow and ice, with locals keeping out the chill with serious cold-weather garb.

After the race, however, there is a chance to get warm and then try some of the traditionally Siberian winter delights on offer: sledding with huskies, sports shooting, ice swimming—if you're not cold enough already—or relaxing in a Russian *banya* (sauna). Everyone who finishes the race gets a diploma and a medal they can get engraved, as well as a Christmas souvenir (the town will be celebrating Russian Orthodox Christmas), and there are monetary prizes for the top-ranking athletes.

On top of all of this, those who finish become part of the 30-year history of this race, which attracts more than 1,000 hardened athletes from all over the world to compete each year, all keen to face down the cold and take on Mother Nature. ∎

Length: 3, 10.5, or 21.1 km (1.9, 6.5, or 13.1 mi)

Location: Omsk, Russia

Date: January

Type: road/snow

Temperature Ø: -15 – -6 °C (5–21 °F)

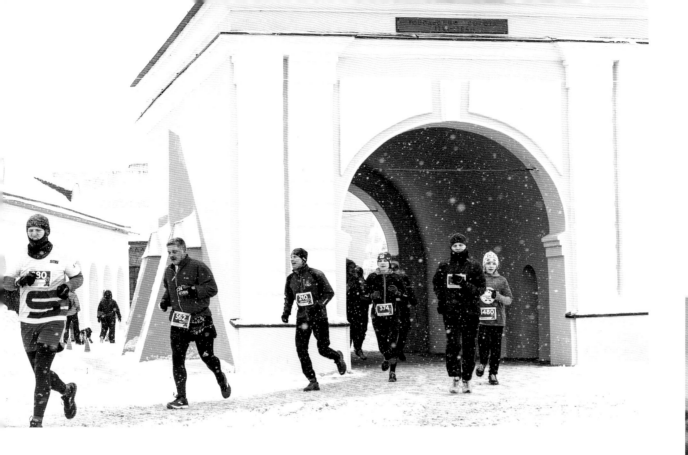

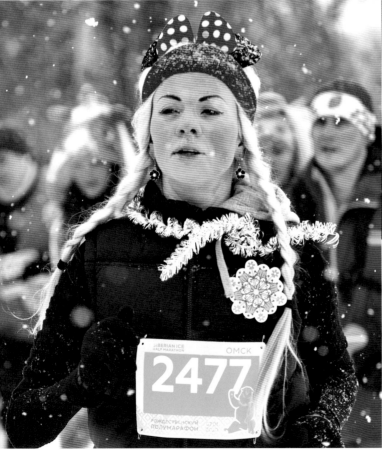

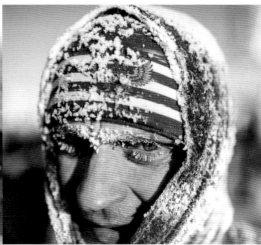

Ice crystals gather on the runners' faces as they complete the 3.5-kilometer (2.17-mile) loops along the embankment of the Irtysh River and through Omsk city center. Hot beverages await the participants as they cross the finish line.

Those who finish become part of the 30-year history of this race, which attracts more than 1,000 hardened athletes from all over the world to compete each year, all keen to face down the cold and take on Mother Nature.

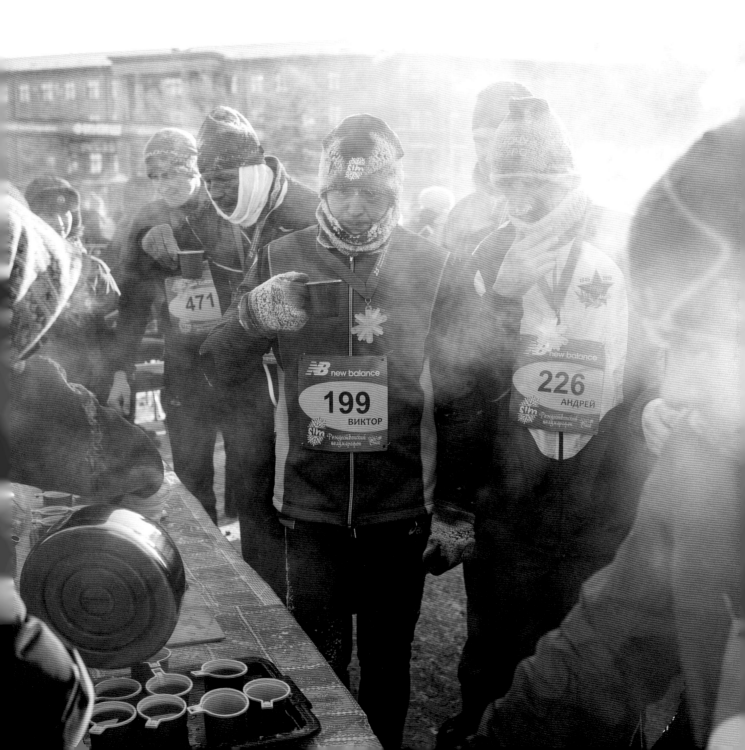

Round the Bend: Weird and Wonderful Runs with a Difference

There's no shortage of variety in today's running world. Alongside the classic races there are plenty of challenges with "extras," from wine tasting to fancy dress to obstacle courses. Creativity and sheer enthusiasm fuel events that include hill climbs and culinary city tours.

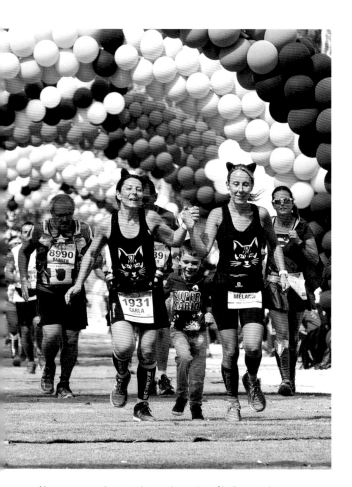

Above: competitors run beneath a series of balloon arches at the Marathon des Châteaux du Médoc, France. Opposite: the Red Bull 400 makes for an amusing sight as competitors scramble up the steep slope, some of them on all fours.

Marathon des Châteaux du Médoc

Want something a bit different? Look no further than the Marathon du Médoc. Classed as the world's longest, booziest race, this quirky trail offers miles of vineyards, incredible scenery, and food. Combine your celebratory post-race drink with the race itself, sampling the delights of more than 20 wines—as well as specialities such as oysters, cheese, steak, and ice cream—along the way.

With pasta parties the evening before and wine instead of the typical granola bar in the finish-line goody bag, this race is pitched as a running event combining "wine, sports, fun, and health." In fact, organizers seem to actively encourage all the things normally discouraged in running.

Don't worry about your traditional kit, fancy dress is practically compulsory in this race and it sends the atmosphere through the roof. Imagine 10,000 runners dressed in costumes ranging from a jar of chocolate spread to a giant romper.

Be prepared for the most unusual marathon you've ever run, and if you're concerned about running with alcohol and food in your stomach, there seems to be just one trick recommended: Imodium.

Red Bull 400

If you're thinking, "400 meters, that's easy, right?", think again. The Red Bull 400 series is one of the most intense competitions out there. The course? A 400-meter (1,312-foot) ski jump, run from base to peak. With individual events spread over three continents, this race is renowned globally for the mental and physical challenge it presents. You'll take on the ski jump in waves, and only those with the top times in each heat proceed to the next rounds. There can be only one winner.

You'll run on an incline increasing up to 37 degrees (75 percent), to the equivalent of 40 stories in height, your heart rate increasing ▶

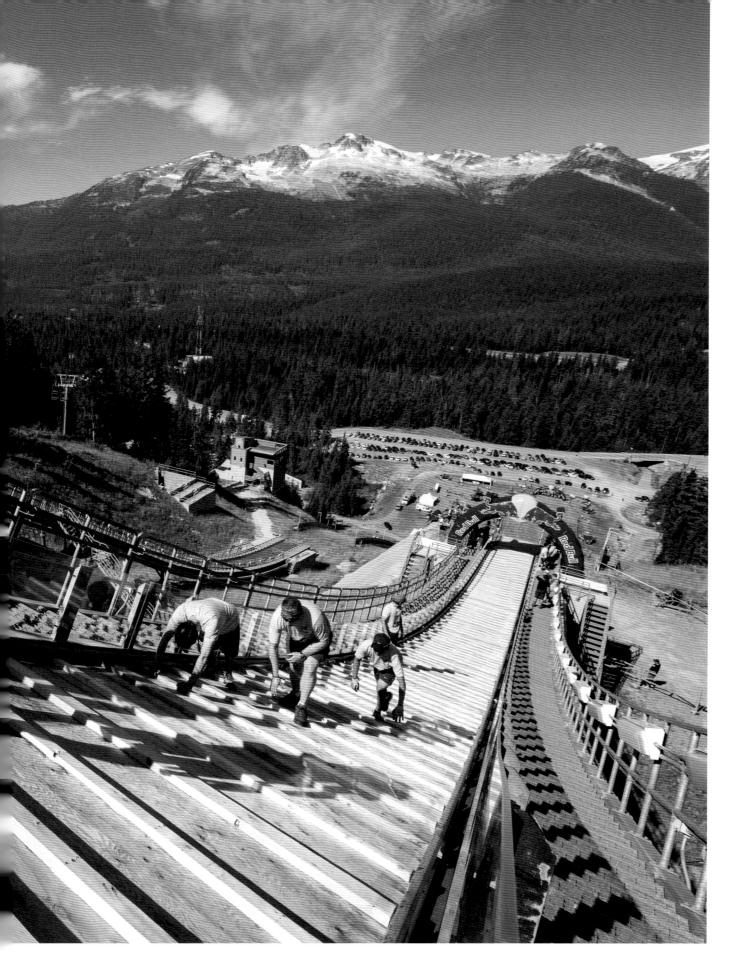

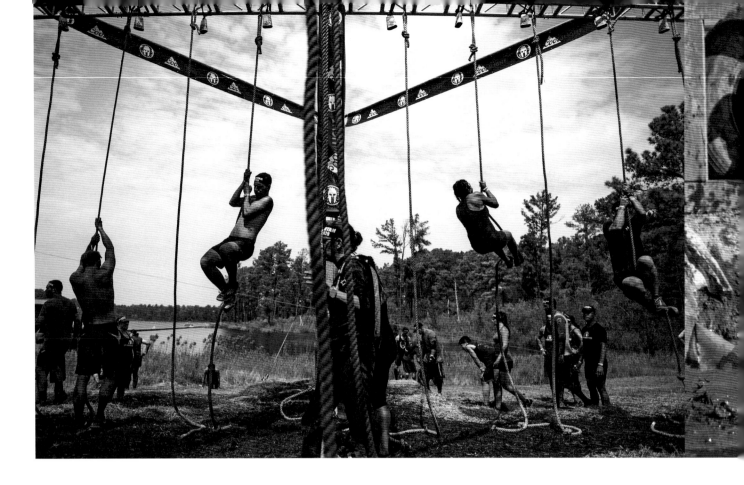
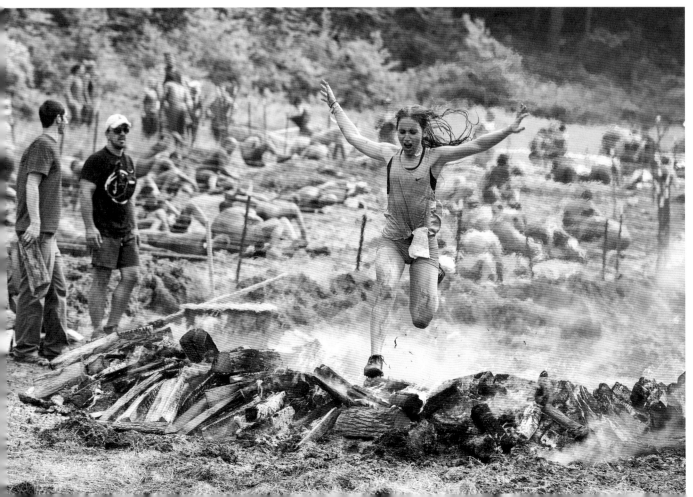

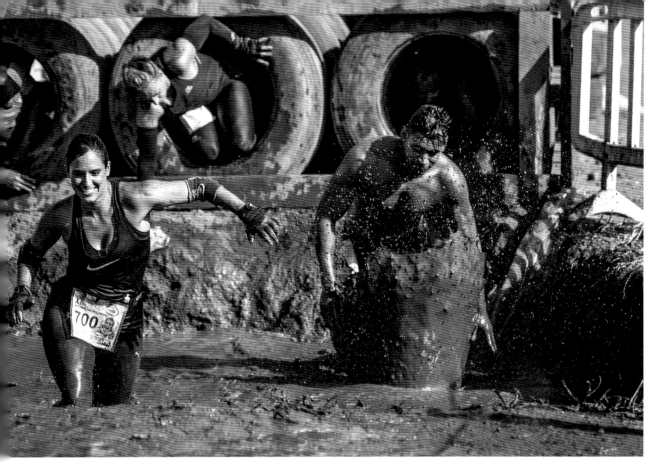

Above and opposite: crawling through huge tires, sloshing knee-deep through mud, rope climbing, and leaping over a fire as the flames lick your legs are just some of the madcap events included in Spartan Race events held across the globe.

▶ from 70 to 200 bpm. The lactic-acid burn in your legs will be overwhelming and you'll start "fire breathing" as your body rushes to increase its breathing rate. By the end of this race you'll probably be crawling on all fours, but what a rush!

Utilizing Olympic-park ski jumps, this race is one in a million, so if you've got big lungs and good endurance, definitely give it a go.

Spartan Race

Do you think you've got what it takes to become a Spartan? With races held globally, this event has come to be known as one of the toughest obstacle courses in the world. Get ready to challenge yourself and push beyond your limits. This one means business.

Due to popular demand, the race has increased its course options around the world to accommodate runners of all levels. From a 5-kilometer (3.1-mile) run with 20 obstacles (the Spartan Sprint), to a 50-kilometer (31-mile) ultra marathon with 60 obstacles, you've got your work cut out.

This is the ultimate challenge when it comes to courage, determination, and strength. With obstacles split into two categories,

including climb and carry or lift, you'll face a range of full-body challenges such as wall climbs, hurdles, rope climbs, spear throwing, tire flips, and even crawling under barbed wire. But don't worry— as the organizers like to say: "There's no Spartan left behind." The energy generated within this race means everyone is in it together and helps each other through. Prove yourself to be a true Spartan— you'll hate it and love it at the same time.

Rifle Run

A U. K.-based event based on a military exercise called a march and shoot—and organized in support of ABF The Soldiers' Charity, the national charity of the British Army— this certainly provides a twist on the usual format for race days. If you like rifles and running, then this is definitely for you.

The first event of its kind, the Rifle Run combines three shooting challenges with a cross-country run, and takes place at two locations in the U. K. Choosing between an air rifle or a shotgun at the starting line isn't usual race protocol, but this is an essential item, as you will be shooting at 20 targets throughout the 10-kilometer ▶

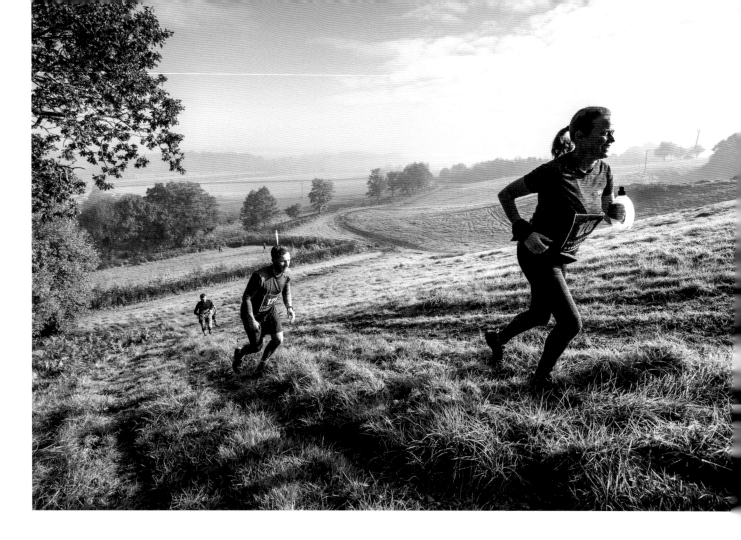
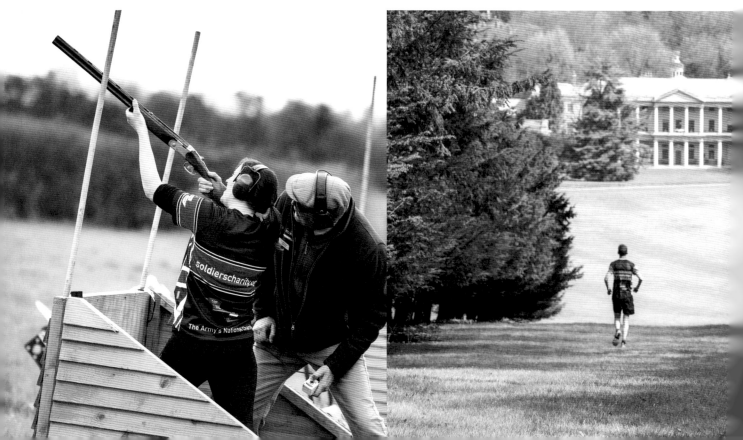

▶ (6.2-mile) run. However, miss a target and you'll face a 250-meter (820-foot) penalty lap, so depending on your skill level, your race could be up to 10 or 15 kilometers (9.3 miles) in length—make sure you're prepared for either. And bring your trail shoes, as things are going to get muddy!

Beer Lovers' Marathon

Calling all beer enthusiasts: we've found the race for you. Sample 16 different Belgian beers as you take part in Liège's fun-filled marathon. Think Oktoberfest combined with a road race.

Against the backdrop of this historic and picturesque city, you'll also have the chance to sample the gourmet offerings that Belgium is known for, such as waffles, chocolate and fries, and you'll be spurred on by live music or a DJ set. But don't dally too long at the stops—the time limit for the race is 6 hours 30 minutes.

Each year this race has a different theme—previous ones have included Wild West and heroes—so be sure to check what the coming year has in store for you. As the miles continue, the drinks flow, and an unforgettable atmosphere builds, you'll find yourself dancing your way to the finish line.

Below: the route of Rifle Run South takes you through West Wycombe estate, including past the elegant Palladian gem of West Wycombe House. Opposite, top: Rifle Run North treats entrants to views of the beautiful Cheshire countryside.

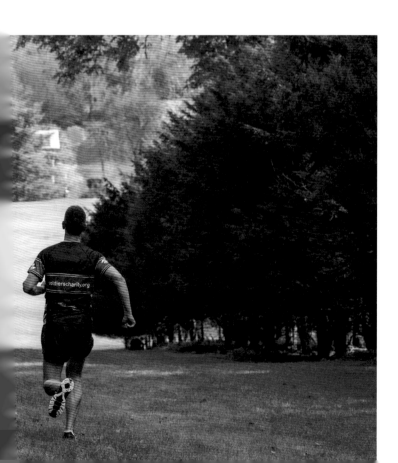

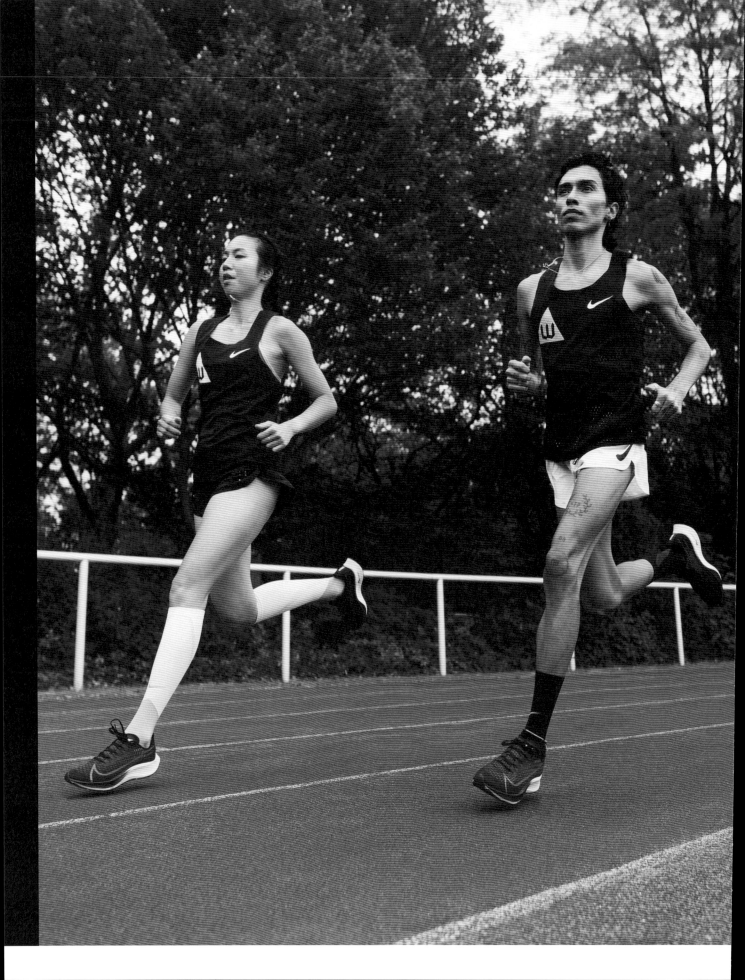

Breaking Down Barriers with the Wayv Run Kollektiv

Meet the duo making space for more diversity in the running world by helping marginalized runners embrace the politics of their bodies.

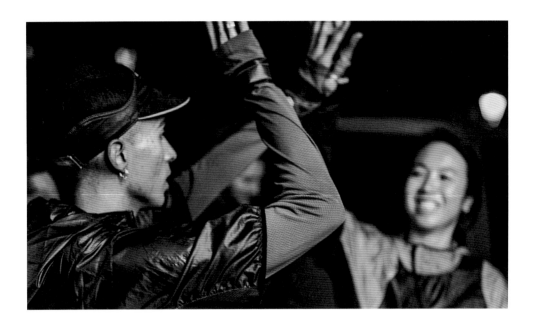

For most people, running is a way to drown out the politics of everyday life. For Thị Minh Huyền Nguyễn and Daniel Medina, running is in itself a political act. Both Nguyễn and Medina grew up marginalized: she in Germany as the daughter of Vietnamese immigrants and he as a queer son of two Colombian parents who moved to the U. S. when he was 11. Medina started running competitively before his teens, Nguyễn a little later, finishing her first marathon in 2016. When the two met at a running club in New York City, they bonded over their activist approach to the sport. "Huyền and I can vouch for how good it is to be able to reclaim ownership of your body and feel powerful," Medina says of running.

After moving to Berlin—Medina in 2017 and Nguyễn a year later—the two founded the running community Wayv Run Kollektiv. Its manifesto is to "support and embrace the politics of putting black/brown, queer, female, trans, Muslim, different, underrepresented, and marginalized bodies into motion." Nguyễn and Medina were always engaged with the issue of representation: she through her studies in media science and he through his writing and visual art. Running allowed them to engage by simply showing up—by putting their bodies in motion just like everybody else—the difference being that, in Germany especially, they are observable outliers in the running community. "We both actively embrace being visible and making sure our space is respected," Medina says. "In running, that is a very political thing."

After Medina ran his first Berlin marathon, he was jarred by the post-race photos, which depicted a sea of white bodies. "[Huyền and I] joke, like, 'Wow, look at all the diversity,'" Medina says. "I think joking is a way of coping with it, but it's scary that people don't notice. Like, no one caught this? No one saw anything wrong with this?" In the running world, black and brown bodies are often featured in top 10s and influencer campaigns. Nguyễn and Medina, competitive runners who collaborate with Nike, have a footprint in this world. "We were privileged enough to have access to the running community at large because we had the bodies we had, and were good at [running] and had the right clothes," Medina says. Sometimes he and Nguyễn feel like "sneaking ninjas," infiltrating a world in which they hope to create space for others. "Going into this, we knew we wanted to share resources. How can we make use of our connections and our platforms to highlight other people and their stories?" Nguyễn says. ▶

> *"On race day, it's just you, but the collective win is so much more powerful than just the individual win. Being a team and having a community makes it so we all experience the same pain."*

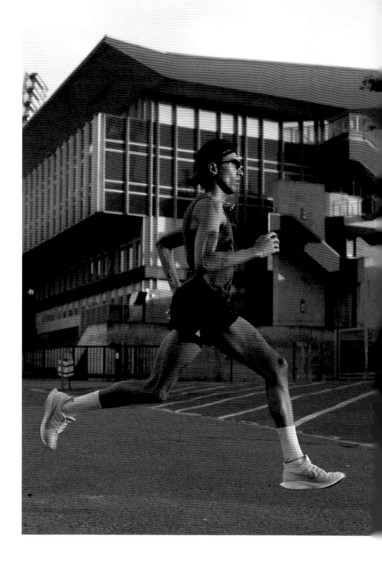

▶ Not everyone who joins Wayv Run Kollektiv is duty bound to lead the struggle. "Because we're dealing with people who are marginalized and underrepresented, it's very difficult to also ask them to be visible," Medina says. "Not everyone has the energy to be visible." This is especially the case while training for a marathon. For many, the most empowering thing they can do is simply run, embrace their body. Running is democratic in ways other aspects of life may not be. It is an equalizer. In *What I Talk About When I Talk About Running*, Haruki Murakami writes, "Your quality of experience is based not on standards such as time or ranking, but on finally awakening to an awareness of the fluidity within action itself." Wayv Run Kollektiv is a gateway to that awareness.

The most common question distance runners are asked is "Why?" Most people do it to prove something to themselves. After all, running is a solo sport. By building a community, Nguyễn and Medina have found a way to make running bigger than any one person. "On race day, it's just you, but the collective win is so much more powerful than just the individual win," Medina says. Running can be a grueling sport. It can demand more than you can give, taking the air out of and from under you. "Being a team and having a community makes it so we all experience the same pain," Nguyễn says. As the saying goes, pain shared is pain divided. The opposite can also be true. A bad race feels heavier when you carry others' expectations. "When there are tough times, the loss is doubly so, because you feel like you've let down all of the brown gay boys," Medina says. "You give people an opportunity to say, 'Oh, you see, they are weak. They can't do it.'"

Nguyễn and Medina often share the less glossy parts of running. Medina talks candidly about his bouts of depression. On Instagram, Nguyễn took followers on her emotional journey to the 2020 Tokyo Marathon—from the euphoria of qualifying for the race to the grief of learning an injury would rule it out (it was ultimately postponed due to the coronavirus pandemic). She regularly reflects on her place in the world—as a woman, as a person of color, as a daughter of immigrants. "My personal is my political," she says. "It is already a political act to survive." In his 1951 book-essay *L'Homme révolté (The Rebel)*, the French philosopher Albert Camus writes, "the only way to deal with an unfree world is to become so absolutely free that your very existence is an act of rebellion." Is there anything more absolutely free than running?

In 2019, Nike Running invited the Wayv Run Kollektiv co-captains to Shanghai for a symposium on global running culture. Nguyễn and Medina designed a shirt for the occasion that includes a quote by the American black feminist lesbian poet Audre Lorde: "Without community, there is no liberation." Under an Instagram post of the event, one commenter, quoting Lorde, wrote, "the master's tools will never dismantle the master's house, right? Y'all should work that angle instead. Nike is my problematic fave as they say." Nguyễn and Medina replied as sneaking ninjas might: "We're not trying to dismantle any houses, but rather build our own. Yes, we work with existing structures at the moment, but with the knowledge and intention of making new ones." By the end of the trip, a local group had been inspired to start a queer running community in Shanghai.

As for what's next, Medina has a vision: "I have this image of a beautiful trans woman of color at the Fifth Avenue Mile in New York just, like, demolishing, wearing our singlet—I would love that so much." ∎

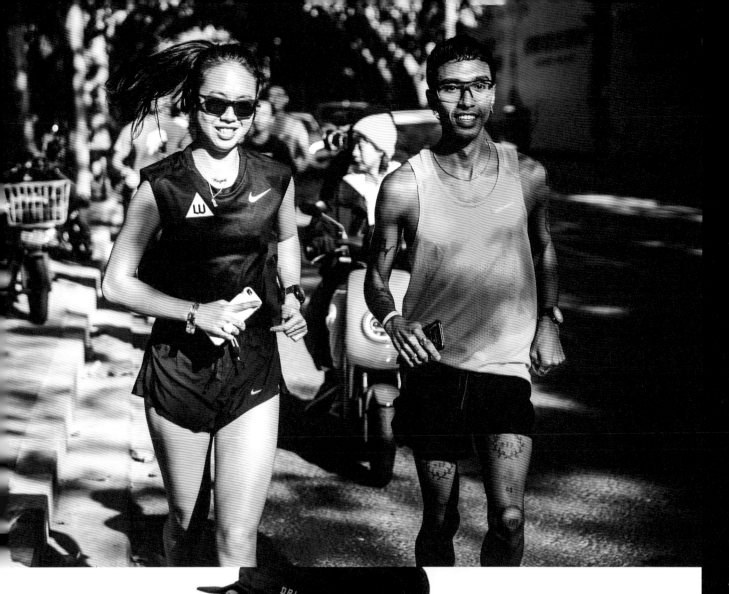

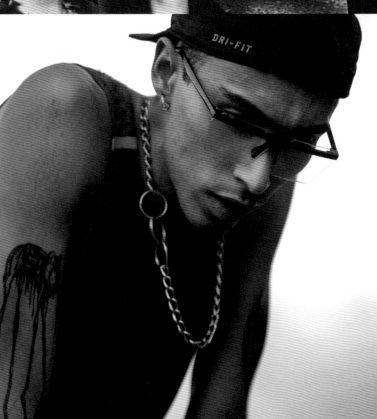

Wayv Run Kollektiv's motto is "Making Wayvs." By encouraging LGBTQI+ and BIPOC people to take to the streets, its founders hope to increase the collective's visibility and thus make it harder for its members to be ignored or overlooked. They want to effect social change through diverse leadership.

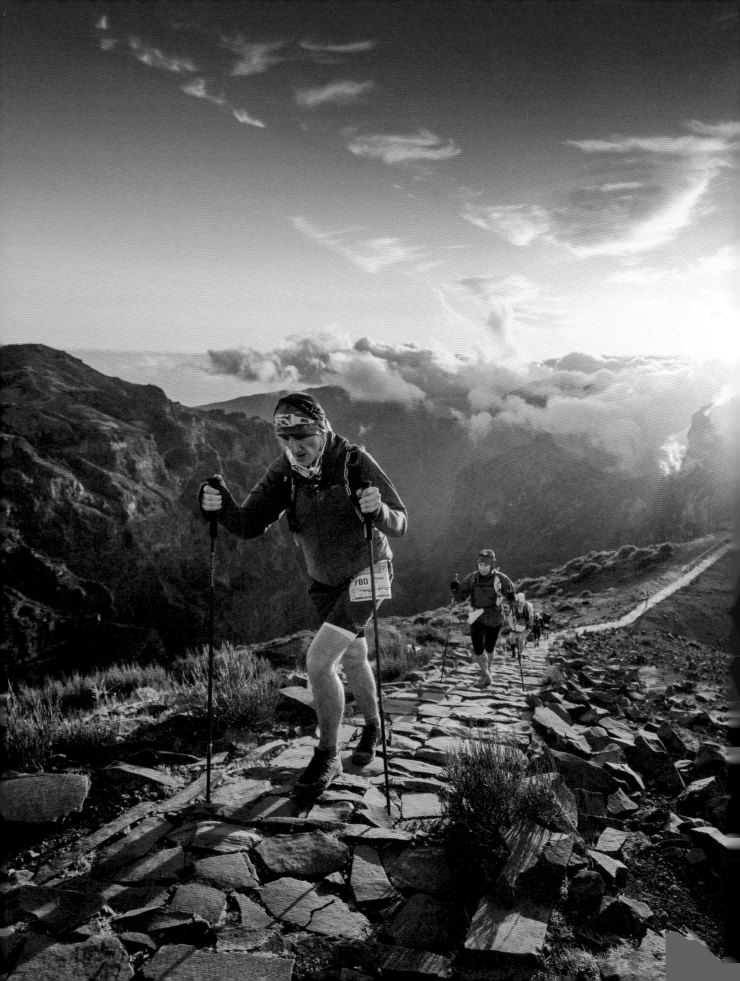

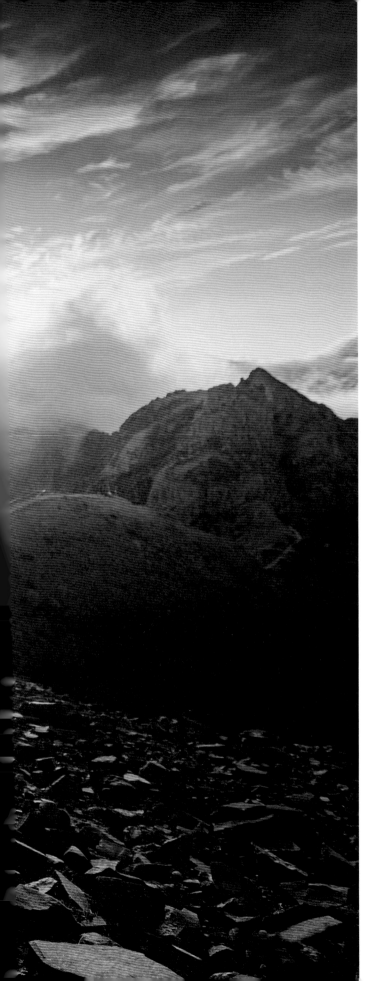

MADEIRA ISLAND ULTRA-TRAIL

It rarely gets much better, or harder, than this—running from sea to sea via the steepest mountainous peaks of the island of Madeira. A young race compared to many and often overlooked, it is well organized, with some of the most beautiful scenery in the world. One to consider.

The island of Madeira is a popular tourist destination, visited by about a million holidaymakers every year. They come to this tiny island in the Atlantic for its mild and sunny climate, mountainous beauty, and rich culture. Madeira is a paradise for wildlife enthusiasts especially, and the trails and *levadas* (man-made water channels) that cut across the rocky island wind past waterfalls, rockpools, and subtropical forests, including the Laurisilva—the ancient laurel wood that stands on the north side of the island and is a protected Unesco World Heritage site.

Arguably, however, the best is saved for participants in this family of trail-running events, which takes runners deep into the island interior and away from coastal tourist hotspots. Emerging from an annual tradition that took hold among the island's trail-running enthusiasts, the first official version of the Madeira Island Ultra-Trail ▶

The trails and levadas (man-made water channels) that cut across the rocky island wind past waterfalls, rockpools, and subtropical forests, including the Laurisilva—a protected Unesco World Heritage site.

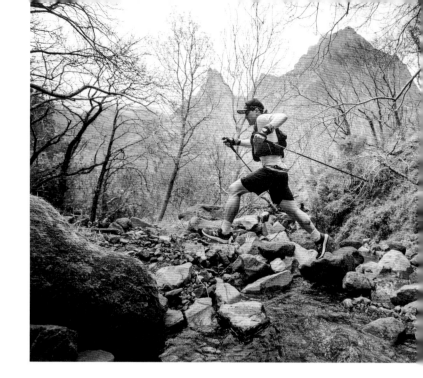

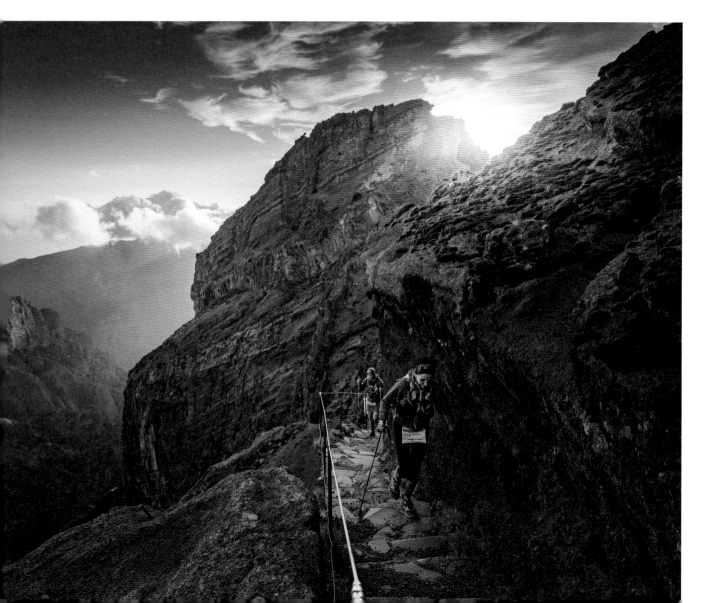

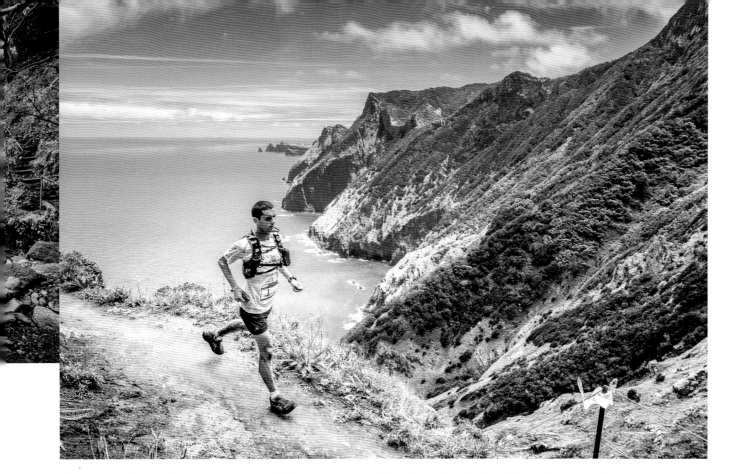

Starting and ending at sea level, the coast-to-coast MIUT course runs almost the entire length of the island, from northwest to east, scaling peaks in the stunning central mountainous massif at the heart of the island.

▶ (MIUT) took place in 2008 with 141 racers, the route stretching from the lighthouse at Ponta doPargo, on the island's westernmost edge, to the city of Machico in the east. The route has been through several permutations, but, since 2013, has stuck with the format that takes participants from Porto Moniz in the northwest to Machico; it is now part of the formidable Ultra-Trail World Tour and tempts about 2,500 runners each year.

There are now a variety of distances on offer, starting from 16 kilometers (10 miles), not all of them overlapping. The three longest routes—60, 85, and 115 kilometers (37.3, 52.8, and 71.5 miles)—require some pedigree, with entrance dependent on having completed another run with a certain number of International Trail-Running Association (ITRA) points.

The full ultra distance, though not as long as some of the trail runs featured in this book, is undoubtedly tough, with 7,000 meters (22,966 feet) of total climb and a high point (at Pico Ruivo) of 1,790 meters (5,873 feet). Starting at midnight, participants immediately face some of the toughest climbing, up to the points of Fanal and Estanquinhos. However, as is typical of this race, there are rewards along the way: cheering spectators on the bridge over the Janela River, and picturesque stands of centuries-old trees lining the trail.

In the central mountainous massif, again, technical and punishing climbs are accompanied by breathtaking views across the valleys and plateaus of the island. Although the ascents aren't over, the final third of the race is arguably less technical and runs past the Funchal Ecological Park, finishing on leafy forest tracks with stunning ocean lookouts along the route.

Running Madeira is truly a fantastic experience. If you manage to complete the full ultra, you will be rewarded with four points towards taking part in the Ultra-Trail du Mont Blanc—just in case you haven't had enough of running up mountains. ■

Length: 16, 42, 60, 85, or 115 km (10, 26.1, 37.3, 52.8, or 71.5 mi)

Location: Madeira

Date: April

Type: trail/mountainous

Temperature Ø: 13–20 °C+ (55–68 °F+)

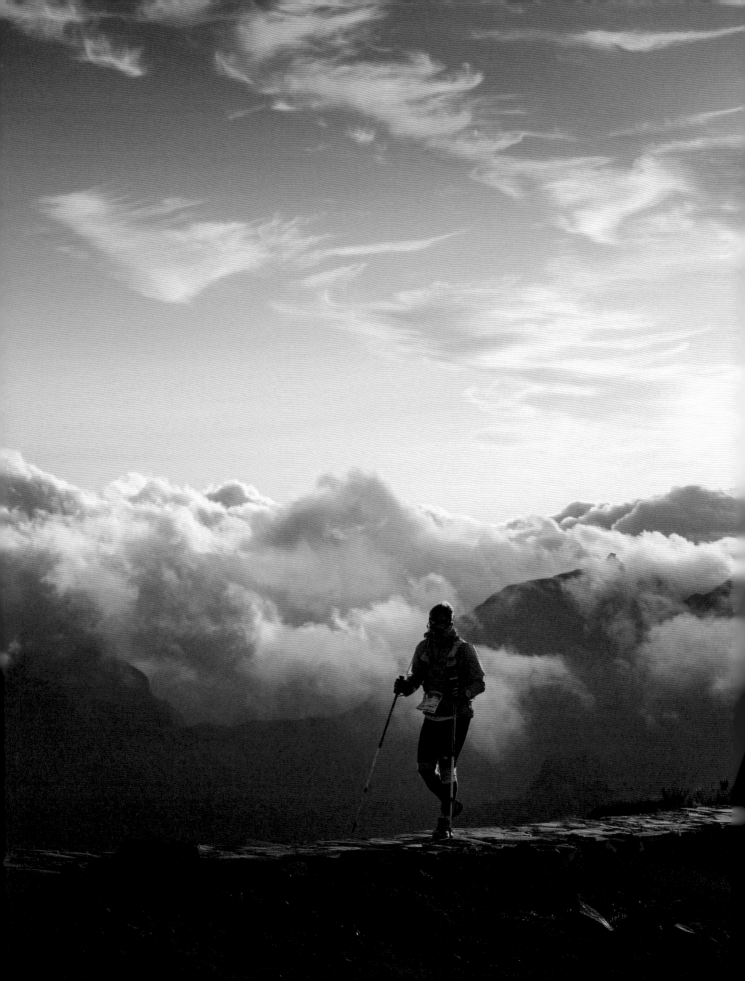

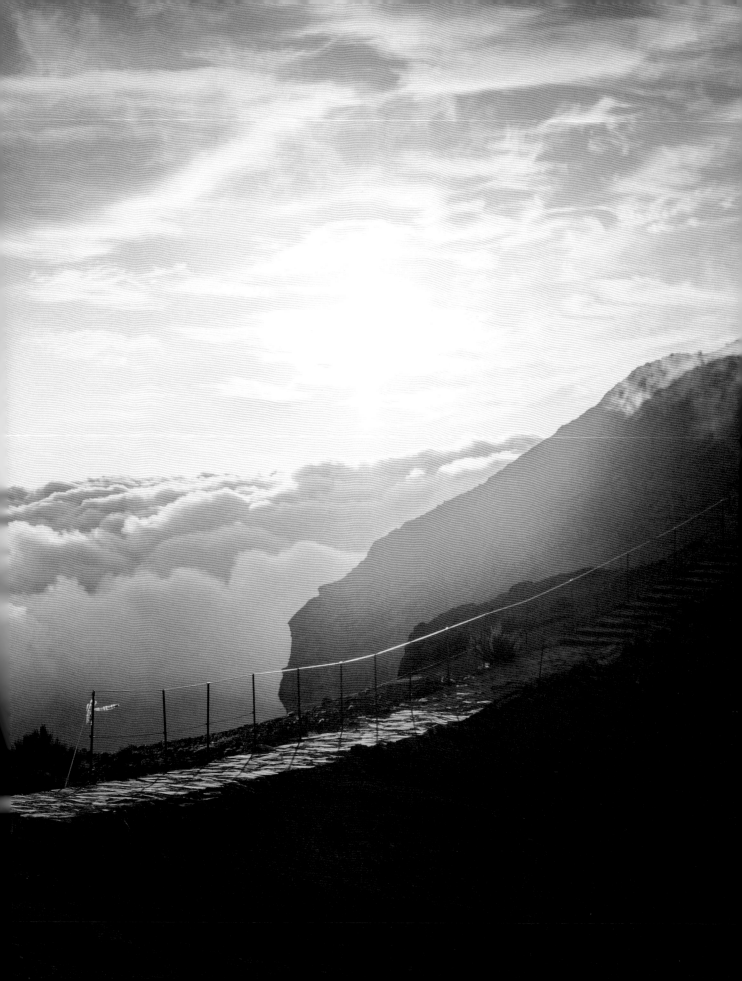

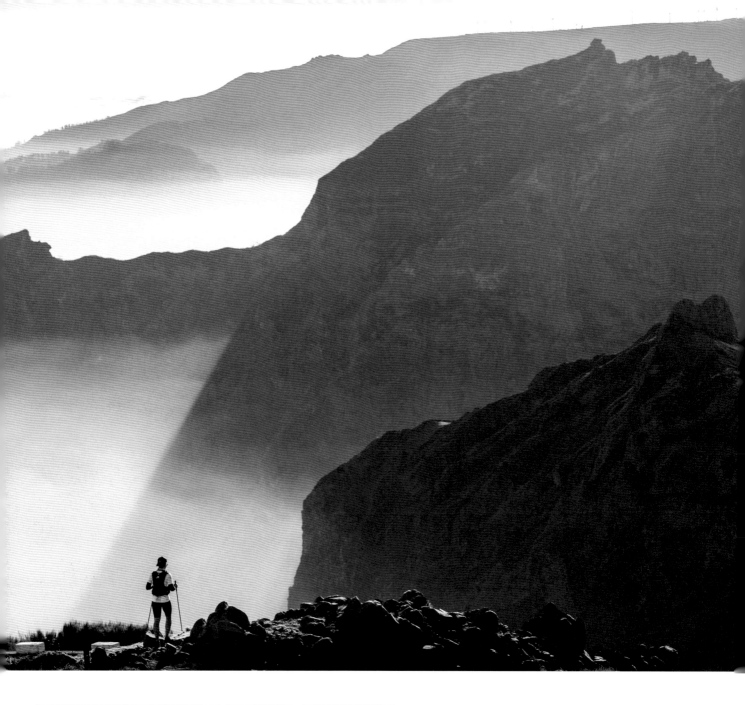

There are rewards along the way: cheering spectators on the bridge over the Janela River, and picturesque stands of centuries-old trees lining the trail. In the central mountainous massif, again, technical and punishing climbs are accompanied by breathtaking views across the valleys and plateaus of the island.

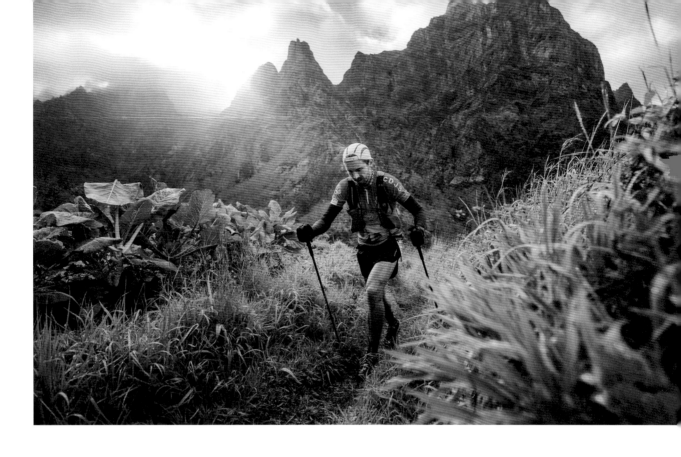

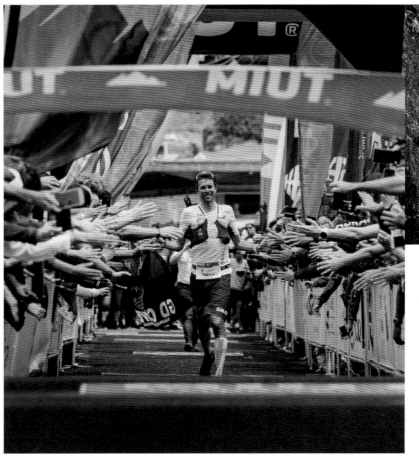

Madeira packs a huge amount of challenging terrain into its tiny size. By the time the trail runners reach the finish line in Machico, they will have scaled steep mountains—some with alarmingly precipitous paths—trekked through enchanting forests, and crossed numerous streams.

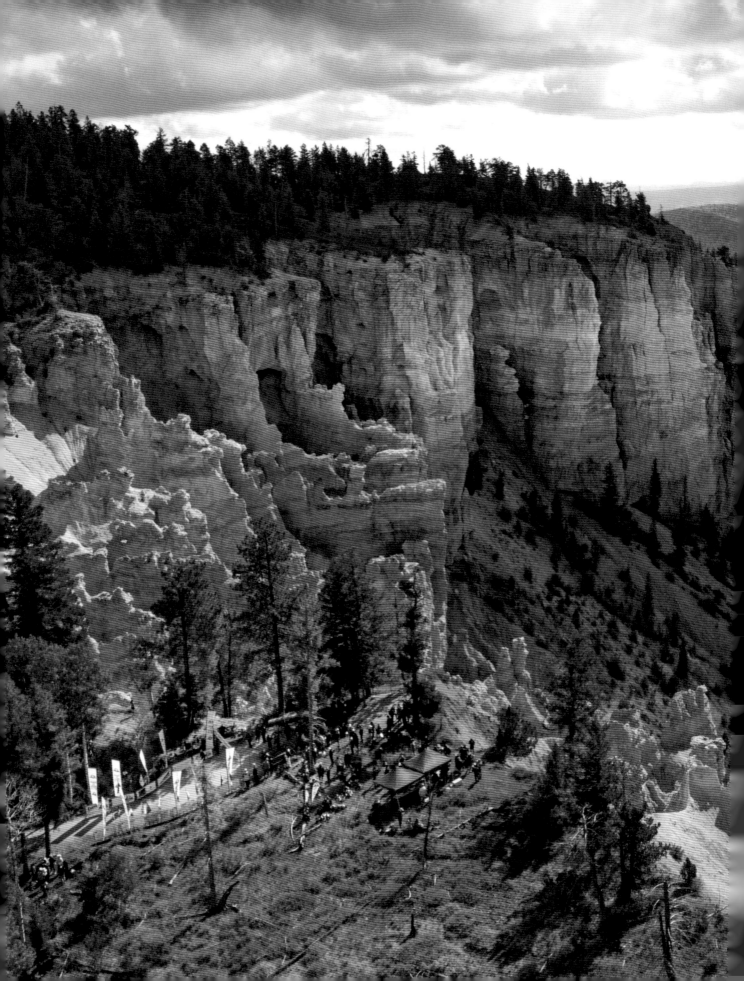

GRAND TO GRAND ULTRA

Run one of the Seven Natural Wonders of the World. The enthusiasm and collegiate feeling of runners flooding through the Grand Canyon combines with the quality of the organization to produce a real treat for both runners and spectators. This is American ultra running at its finest.

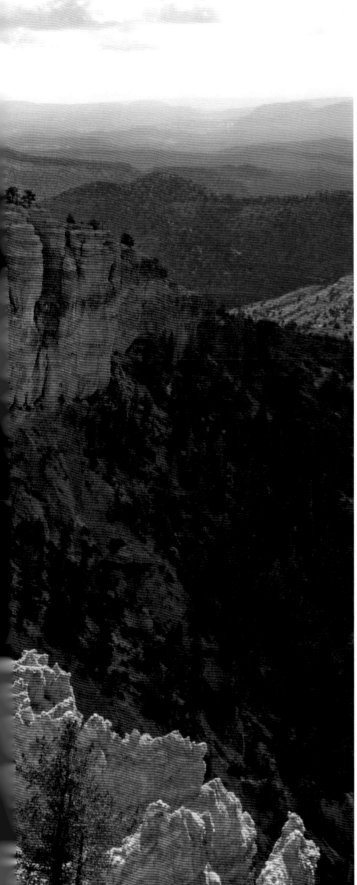

This self-supported, multi-stage ultra through and beyond the Grand Canyon is a truly extreme event. Competitors run 273 kilometers (170 miles), in six stages, over seven days, proceeding from the north rim of the Grand Canyon, in Arizona, to the summit of the Grand Staircase, Utah. Between the two, they pass through an astonishing ancient landscape, running over sand dunes, along forest trails, and up rocky ascents until they reach a final altitude of 2,651 meters (8,698 feet) and look back, taking in a panoramic view of the whole course. The total ascent over the route is a massive 5,499 meters (18,041 feet).

It's worth pausing over this world-class course, as its variety, extremity, and beauty are all on a "grand" scale. Areas of outstanding national importance along the route include the Kaibab National Forest, Zion National Park, and Dixie National Forest. Zion especially, ▶

This ultra through and beyond the Grand Canyon is a truly extreme event. Competitors run 273 kilometers (170 miles), proceeding from the north rim of the Grand Canyon, in Arizona, to the summit of the Grand Staircase, Utah.

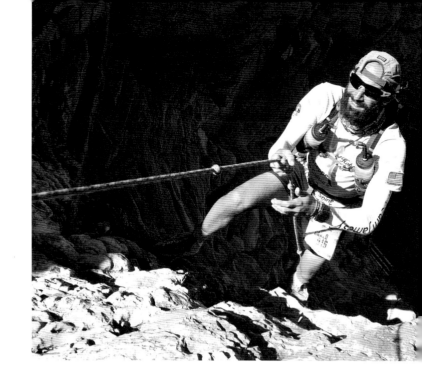

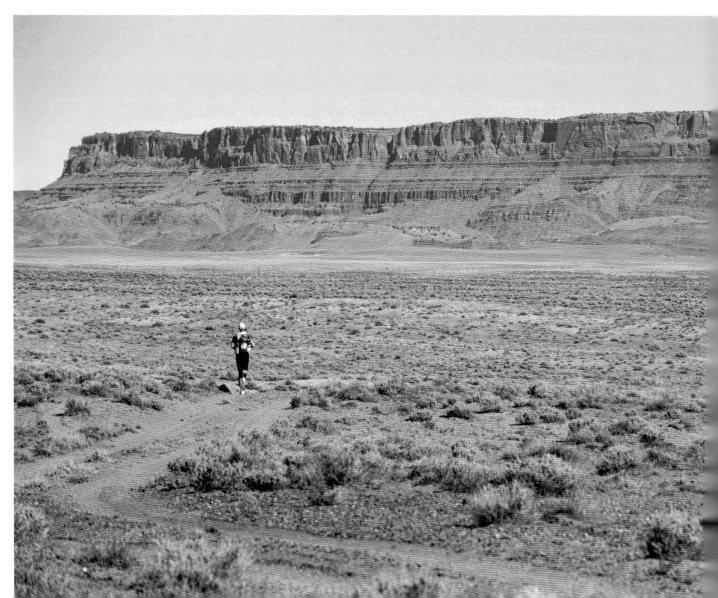

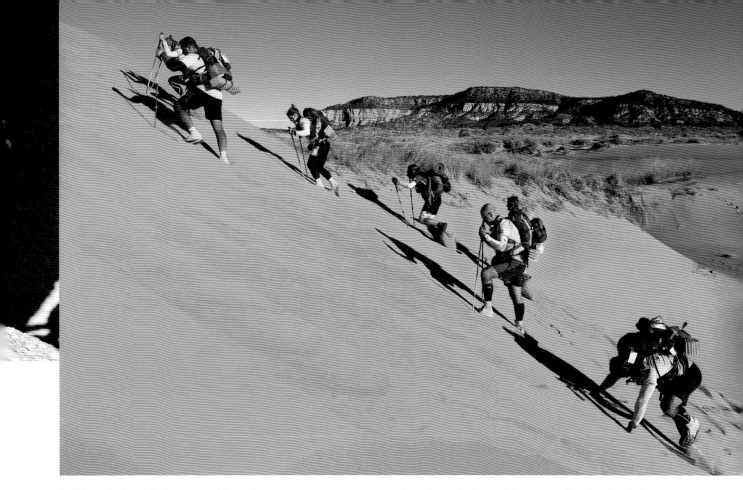

As if the punishing daily distances and fluctuating temperatures are not enough of a challenge for the participants of the Grand to Grand Ultra, they also find themselves scaling cliff faces, hiking across sand dunes, and navigating forests.

▶ constitutes a spectacular part of the course, with its diverse wildlife and geological formations including mountains, mesas, rock arches, buttes, monoliths, and slot canyons. The region is also home to creatures including desert bighorn sheep and the critically endangered California condor, which was declared extinct in the wild in 1987 but has been reintroduced to this area through careful management. Dixie is a forest covering almost 2 million acres and incorporating four officially recognized wilderness areas—a true national treasure.

Lucky for runners that there is so much natural beauty on display, given the hardships of this course. Both overheating and hypothermia are risks—temperatures drop dramatically at night—as are altitude sickness, blisters and dehydration, and stings and bites—rattlesnakes and scorpions are common on the course. Each entrant is required to carry all of their own food and equipment, including mandatory items listed by the organizing body, along the route. The long stage of the race alone is approximately 80–85 kilometers (50–53 miles) in length and partly run in darkness, requiring competitors to wear headlamps and warning lights.

The (ultimately cancelled) 2020 race had only 170 spaces available, with nationality quotas. Despite the challenging nature of this run, there is a waiting list every year, so it's worth getting your application in early if you want to avoid disappointment. What is the appeal? Given the strength and dedication required, not just for the race itself, but for the arduous training and preparation it requires, there is inevitably a strong sense of camaraderie on this trail, which is cemented by the experience of running alone and at the limits of endurance in one of the last great wildernesses. As one former participant put it, "We all started out as strangers and ended the week as one big family." ■

Length: 273 km (170 mi)

Location: Grand Canyon, Arizona, U. S.

Date: September

Type: trail

Temperature Ø: 20–30 °C (68–86 °F)

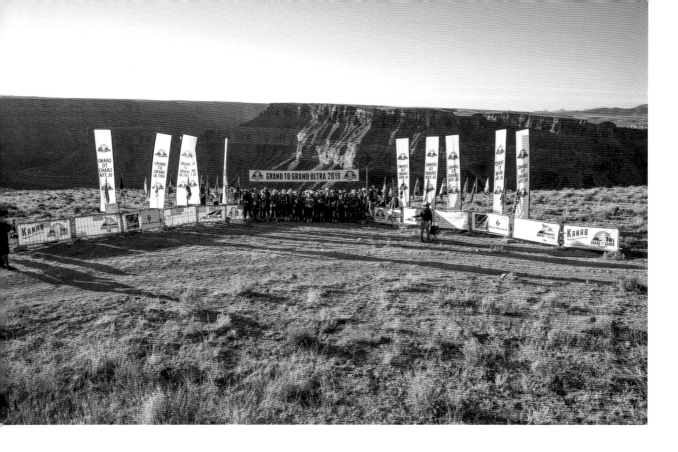

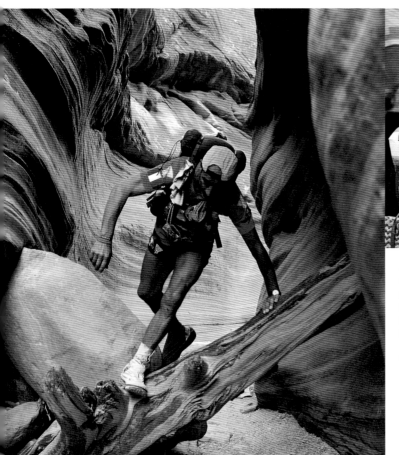

Besides forging great friendships, Grand to Grand Ultra competitors are rewarded with running across one of the most remote regions of the planet amid landforms untouched for millennia. This event is a real opportunity to reconnect with nature.

They pass through an astonishing ancient landscape, running over sand dunes, along forest trails, and up rocky ascents until they reach a final altitude of 2,651 meters (8,698 feet) and look back, taking in a panoramic view of the whole course.

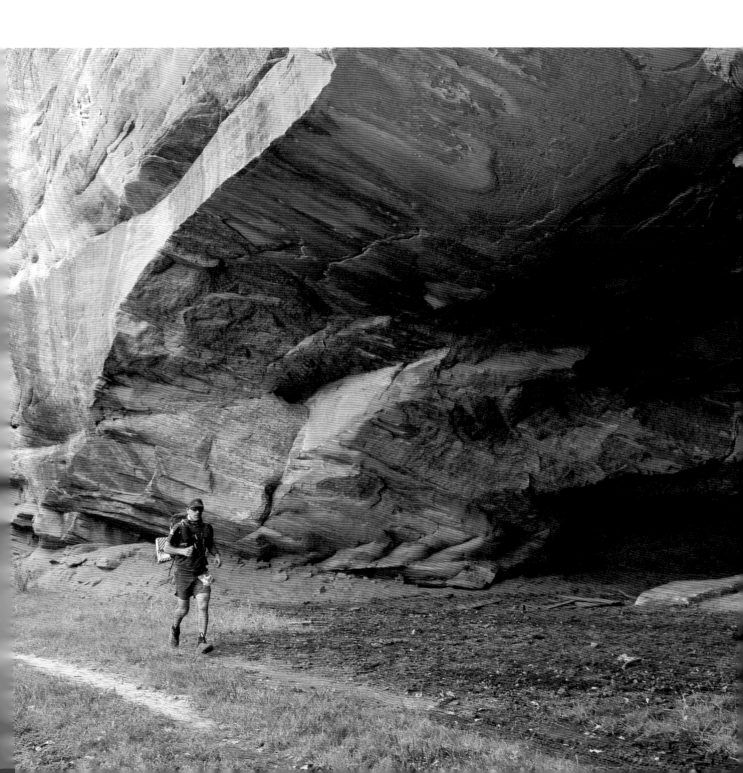

MONGOLIA TRAIL RUN

An ultra run (and walk) for all levels of ability. The emphasis here is on adventure, with feet as the mode of transport. Mongolia has a lot to offer, and this six-day, multi-stage race showcases natural wonders and cultural highlights.

Taking place on the remote steppes of central Mongolia, this trail run—a relatively new event, created in the wake of the success of 2019's Mongolia Stage Race—covers 174 kilometers (108 miles), with participants sleeping in traditional *gers*, or yurts, over six stages and running or walking the distances in between. It's designed for amateur runners of all levels, as well as walkers, with an emphasis on seeing the country and enjoying its cultural heritage.

Starting in the Elsen Tasarkhai ("piece of isolated sand") dunes of the Bayangobi desert, and finishing at what is estimated to be the oldest-surviving Buddhist monastery in Mongolia, Erdene Zuu in the Orkhon Valley Cultural Landscape (a Unesco World Heritage site), the trail is a large "hook," taking in a variety of terrains and a wealth of historic sights. From true desert to wooded valleys, highlands to mountains, past hot springs (where time is set aside on ▶

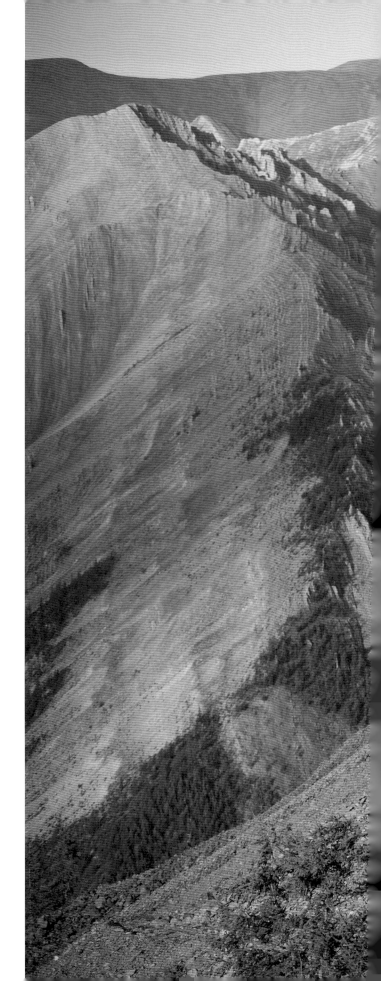

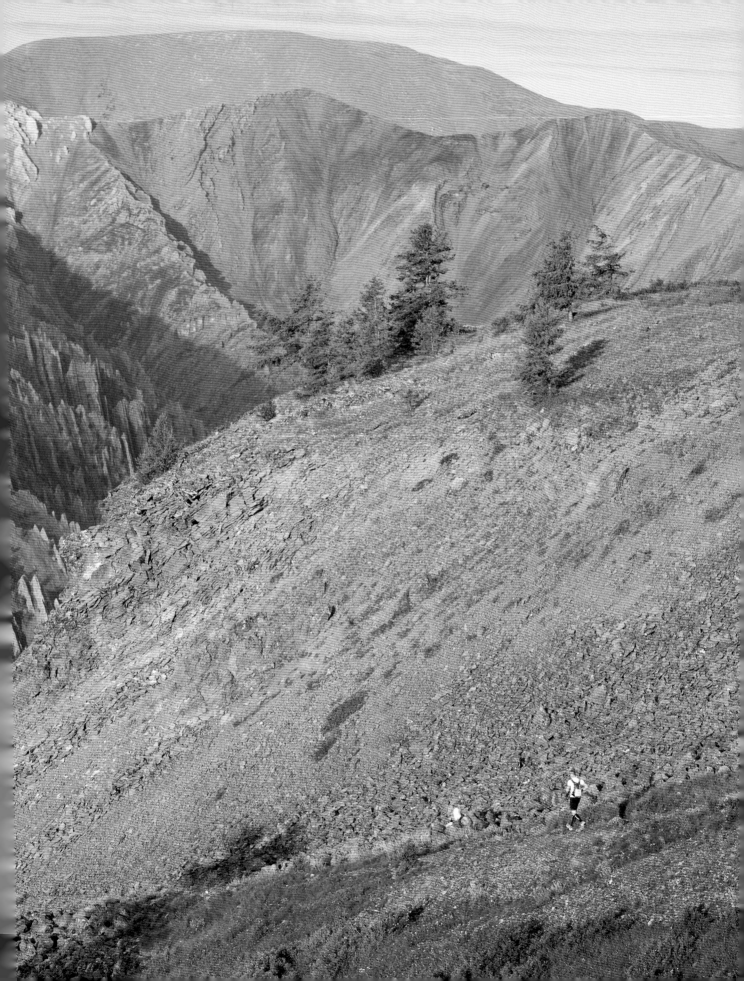

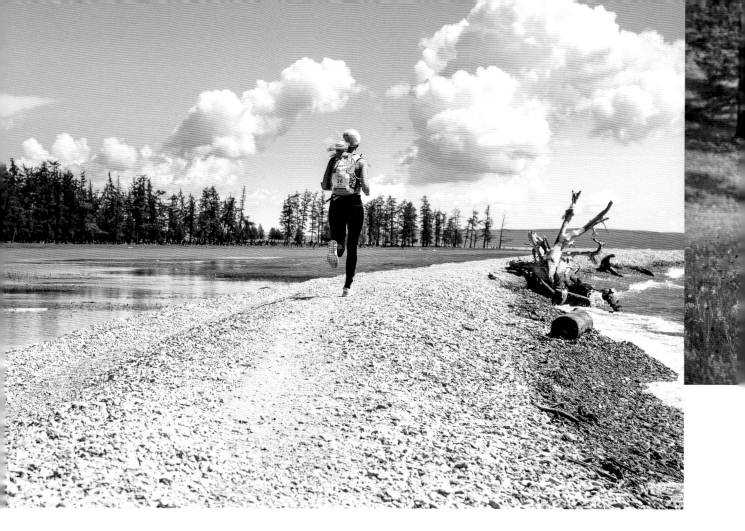

▶ the third day to take a dip), lakes, and small nomadic settlements, the richness of the setting makes this more akin to an all-inclusive adventure trip than a traditional ultra.

Wildlife and natural wonders dominate the first part of the run: Lake Ugii, reached at the end of the first stage, is a significant waterfowl breeding area, with 150 types of birds visiting the site annually. Along the Orkhon and Tamir rivers, in stages two and three, familiar herd animals—deer, goats, horses, and sheep—can be seen, while vultures and eagles soar overhead. The evenings are packed with trips to towns, monuments, and museums: day two, for example, ends with a trip to the towering Galdan Zuu temple, which houses a 7-meter-tall (23-foot) statue of the Buddha.

Day six is the lightest of all the stages, with just under 14 kilometers (8.7 miles) of running, and the emphasis on enjoying the ancient city of Karakorum, the capital city of Genghis Khan's empire in the thirteenth century. Here you can see the ancient Great Hall archaeological site, as well as stone monuments including the turtles (symbols of eternity) that once marked the boundaries of the city.

The schedule is exhaustive and the organization rigorous, but so is the running, for those who want to push their limits. The difficulty of the trail running increases day by day, with the fifth day covering nearly 40 kilometers (25 miles), with 1,443 meters (4,734 feet) of ascent. The organizers downplay this element somewhat in their notes, with details about provisioning and navigation relegated to race regulations, while racers are advised, when they "have no strength left" in mountainous stage five, to look to the Ovoos—sacred stone heaps used as shrines—for some distraction.

For athletes who wish to test themselves while simultaneously devoting time to the cultural and historic experiences offered by a host country, this kind of trip is ideal. ∎

Length: 174 km (108 mi)

Location: Bayangobi desert, Mongolia

Date: August

Type: trail

Temperature Ø: 10–22 °C (50–72 °F)

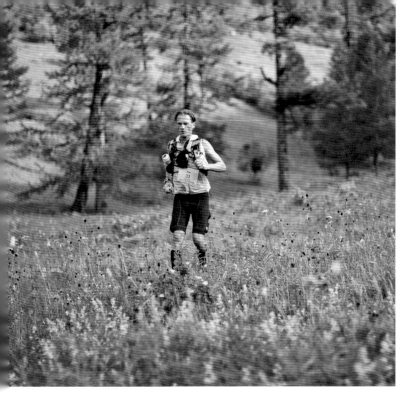

From true desert to wooded valleys, highlands to mountains, past hot springs, lakes, and small nomadic settlements, the richness of the setting makes this more akin to an all-inclusive adventure trip than a traditional ultra.

With a route that takes you from the Elsen Tasarkhai sand dunes of the first stage, through gentle valleys and woodland, and around the shores of two great lakes, the Mongolia Trail Run is known for its unforgettable, mostly verdant backdrops.

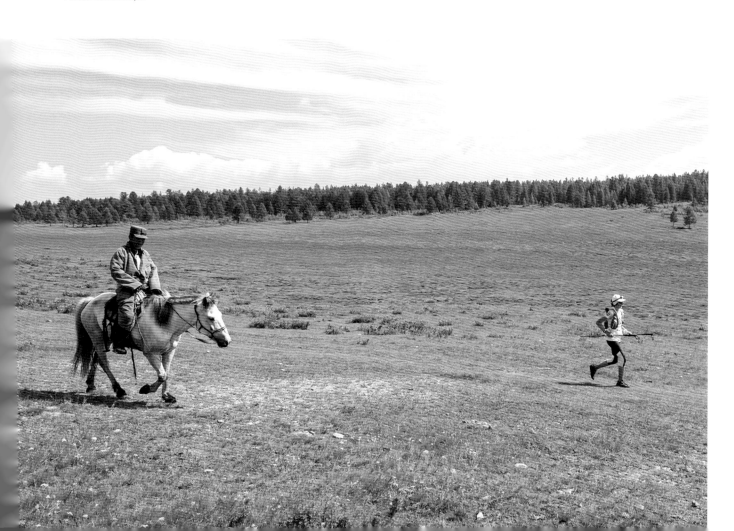

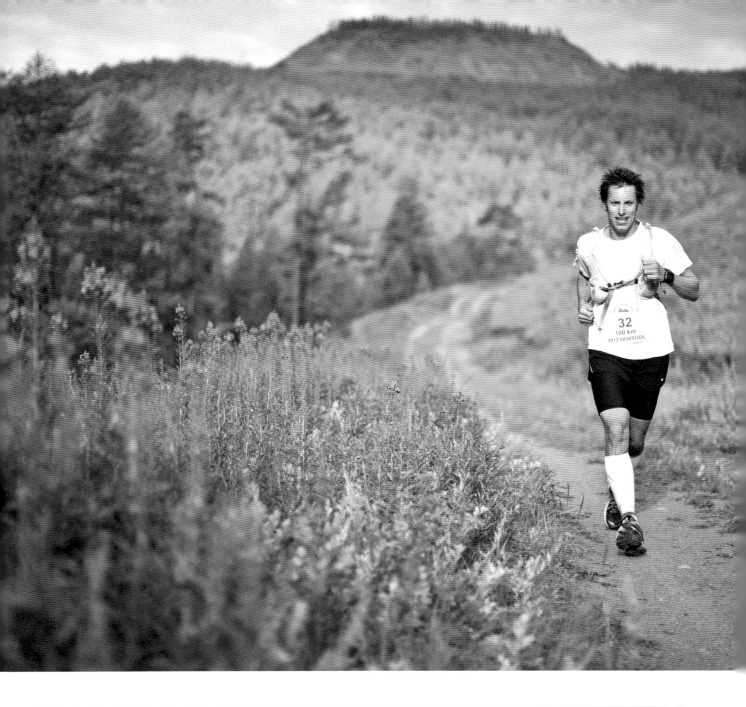

Wildlife and natural wonders dominate the first part of the run: Lake Ugii, reached at the end of the first stage, is a significant waterfowl breeding area, with 150 types of birds visiting the site annually.

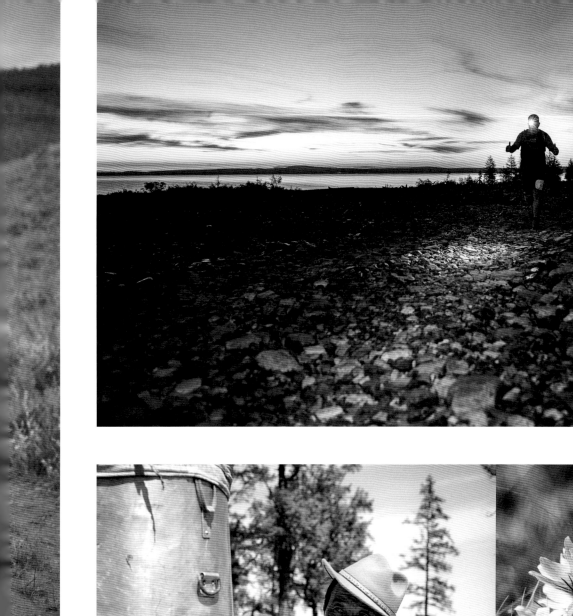

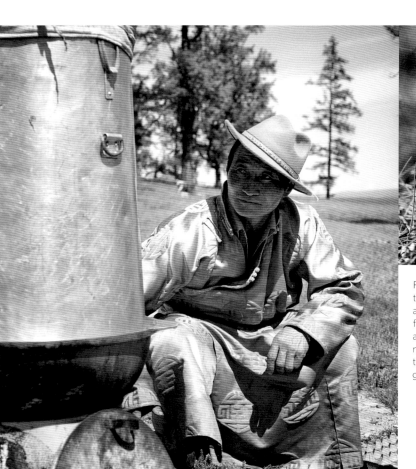

Participants in the race through this vast Mongolian landscape are treated to stunning flora and fauna at every turn. They might also encounter members of nomadic tribes living simply from the land, as they have done for generations.

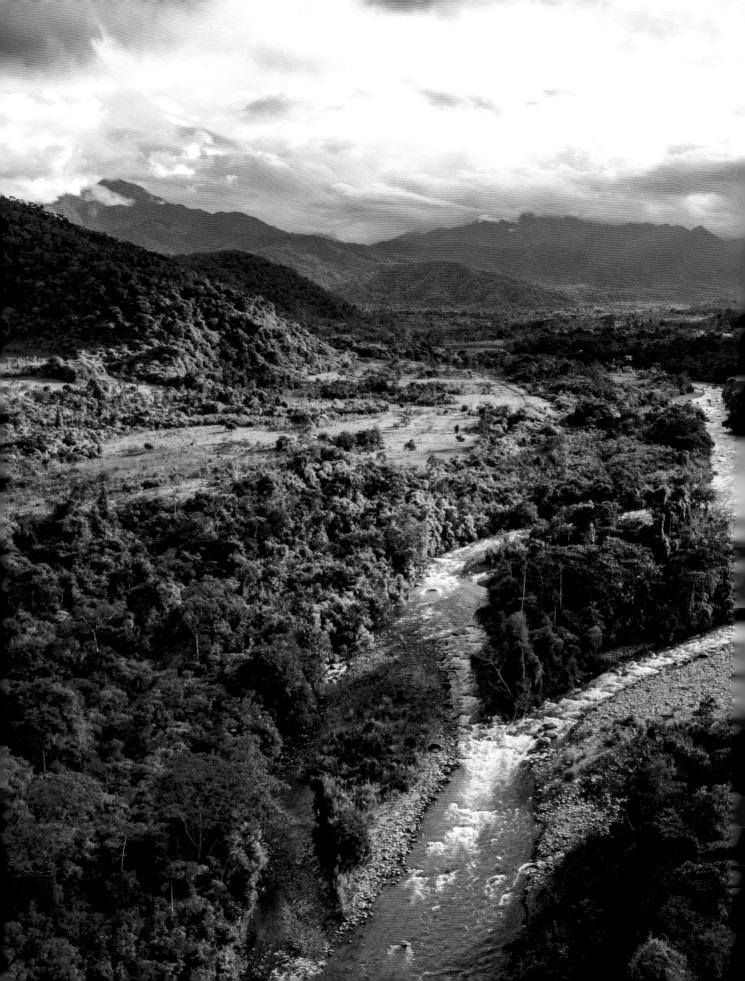

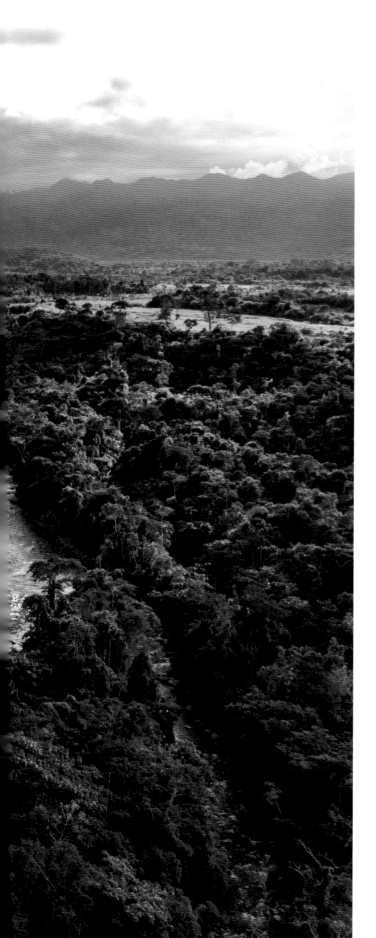

JUNGLE ULTRA

From cloud forest to Amazon jungle, this epic, multi-stage race is for the toughest of the tough—even desert and mountain runs cannot compare. In case the bugs, mud, and rain aren't challenging enough for you, this one is a self-supported run, so pack light.

This is unique terrain. Humidity levels reach nearly 100 percent in the jungle, so sweating won't help you as you run the demanding 230 kilometers (143 miles) along this mostly descending route. "Run" is not quite the word, however—this is more of a scramble, or a crawl in places. There's knee-high mud, raging rivers, uneven and overgrown trails—and that's before you even consider the bugs.

Base camp, organized by Beyond the Ultimate, is high in the Andes, with roiling clouds beneath you in the forest canopy. Runners gather at the start line and stare down the single track that marks the first leg of their descent to the village of Pilcopata in Madre de Dios province, many miles distant. Along the way they'll spend four nights in the research stations and lodges. They will contend with intense heat and sudden and torrential downpours, they'll ford rivers and clamber under waterfalls, climb scree and slide down ▶

Manú National Park is the setting for the adventure—a Unesco World Heritage site and the protected home of a number of diverse ecosystems, from rain forest to grasslands. It's the former that ultra racers contend with.

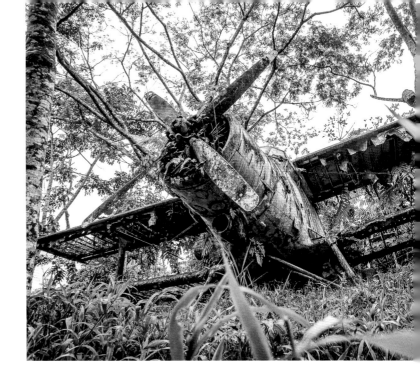

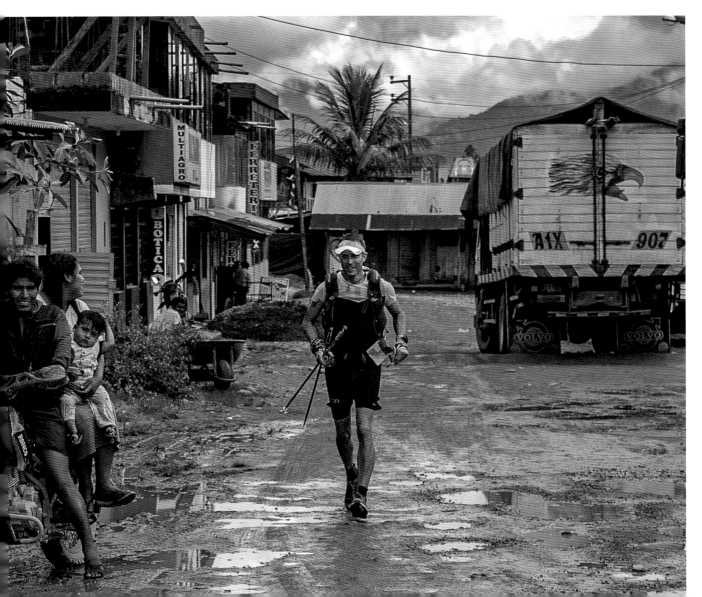

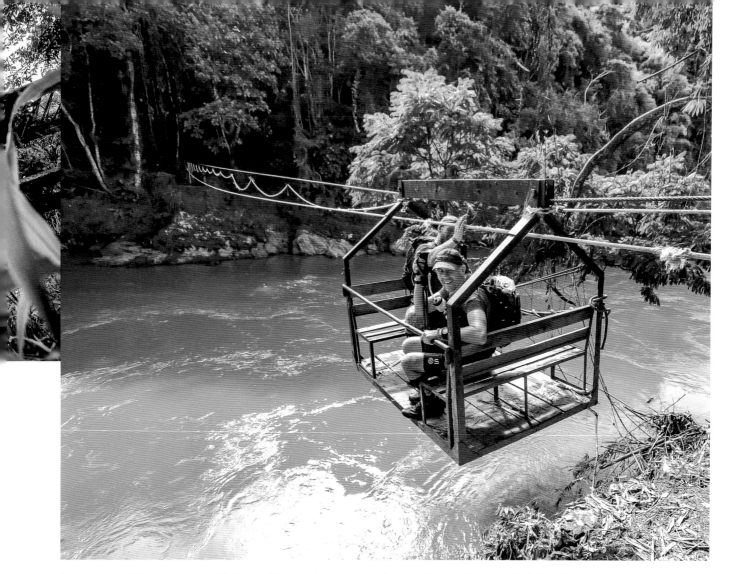

Above: race participants cross up to 70 rivers and streams—in some cases using a zip-line to get from one side to the other.
Opposite, bottom: in the few villages through which the race passes, locals stop to watch the spectacle.

▶ muddy trails, all among rain forest foliage. Given the havoc this kind of landscape wreaks on your pace, it's likely you'll also run a good portion of the trail in the dark.

Manú National Park is the setting for the adventure—a Unesco World Heritage site and the protected home of a number of diverse ecosystems, from rain forest to grasslands. It's the former that ultra racers contend with. In the lower altitudes alone, animals known to live here include marmosets, jaguars, capuchin monkeys, pumas, sloths, and armadillos. And more than 1,000 bird species make their homes in the trees. So if you have time to look up, there is plenty to see.

This race is self-supported: for five days you will be carrying your own hammock, food, clothing, safety equipment, and a minimum of 2.5 liters of water, which can be topped up at checkpoints. This requirement, in combination with the climate, means that this is a race where, more than ever, preparation and adequate training are of paramount importance. As one veteran has put it: "In the jungle, distance is meaningless." Even if you've run a comparable amount, this will be a unique challenge.

Run it, scramble it, and survive it to collect your medal. ∎

Length: 230 km (143 mi)

Location: Manú National Park, Peru

Date: June

Type: jungle

Temperature Ø: 17–30 °C (68–86 °F)

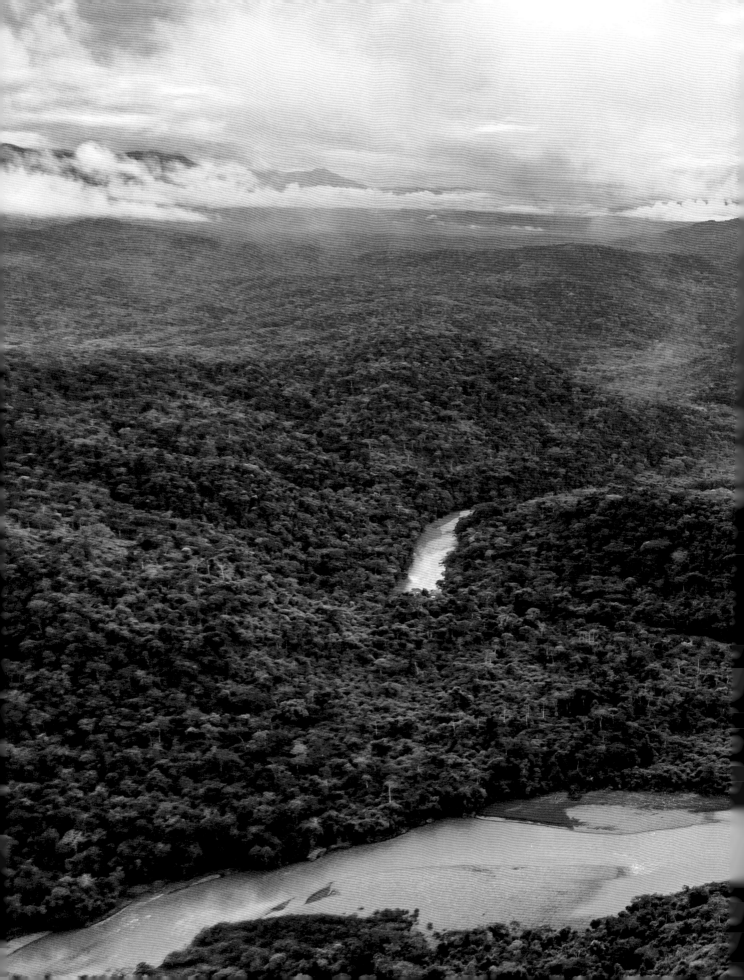

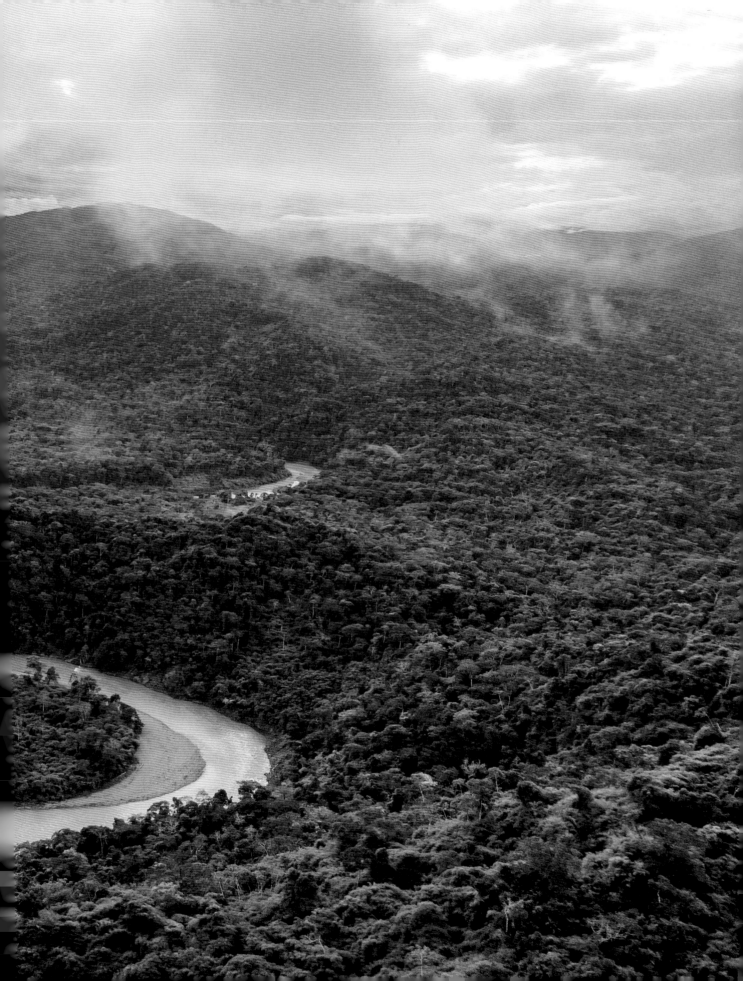

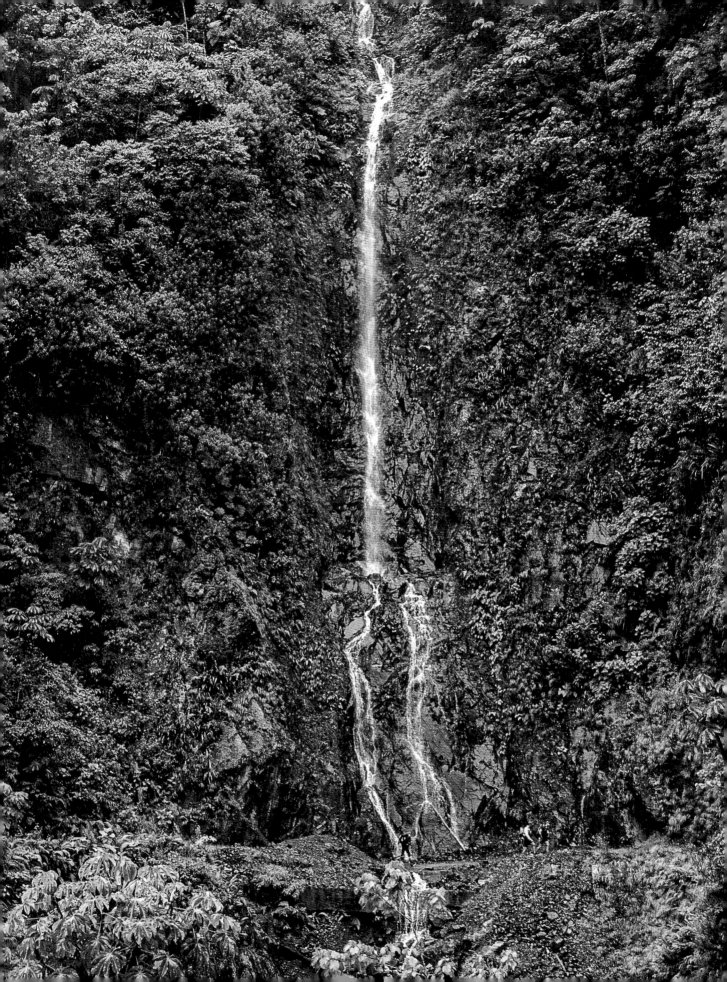

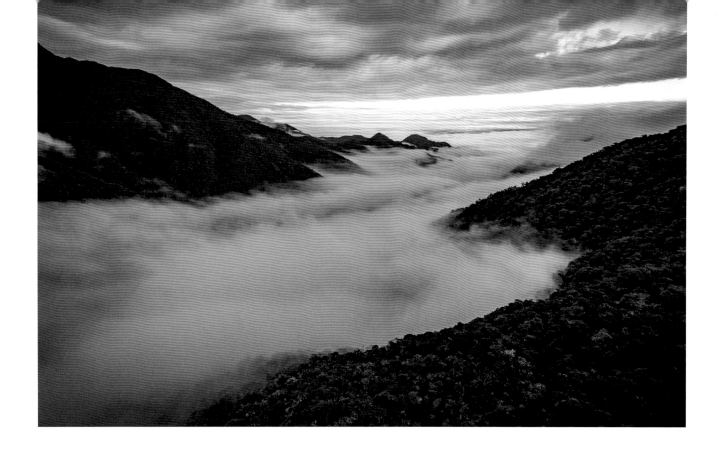

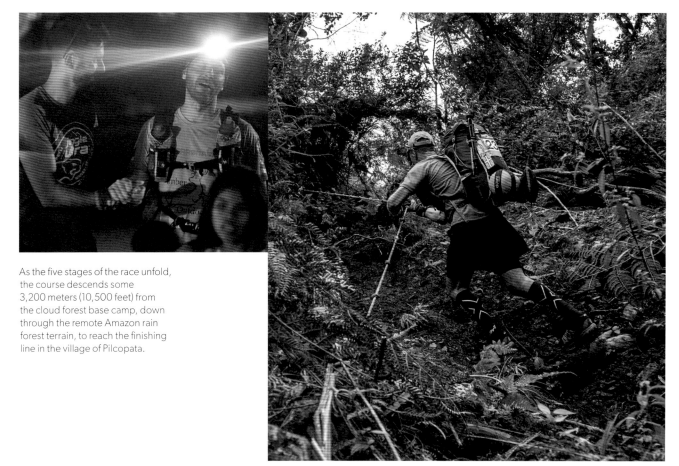

As the five stages of the race unfold, the course descends some 3,200 meters (10,500 feet) from the cloud forest base camp, down through the remote Amazon rain forest terrain, to reach the finishing line in the village of Pilcopata.

GUATEMALA IMPACT

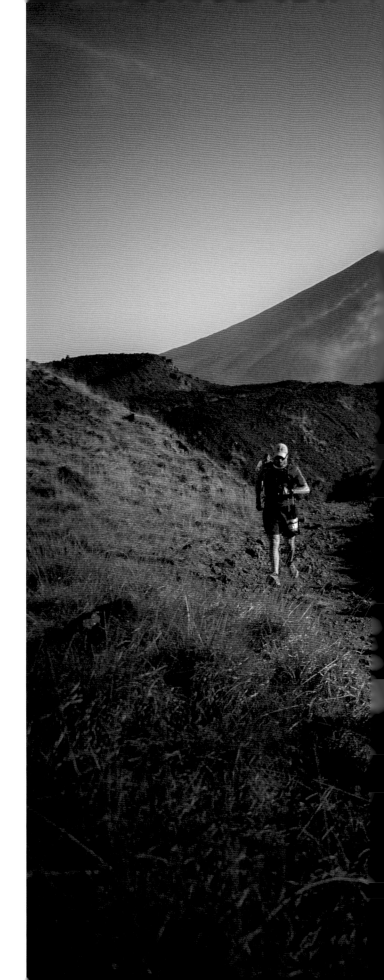

So much more than a race, this week-long event in Guatemala combines a unique run—across the lava fields of a live volcano—with work in the community. It's the brainchild of Impact Marathon, whose mission is to harness the power of running to "uplift communities and empower runners."

A life-changing week of stunning trails, with runners committing to making an impact and empowering a community through work with two local charities. Organized by Impact Marathon—whose speciality is this kind of socially engaged, international race—this event in Guatemala has a focus on work with youth. The two local partners are Caras Alegre, which provides an after-school club in a small community adjacent to a prison, and SERES, a group that works across all sections of the community to develop young leaders.

The first fews days of the Impact event, held in the Antigua region of Guatemala, combine training runs with visits to sites of social action. Projects that welcome the group include the Resilience Farm, which focuses on sustainable land use on the slopes of Fuego volcano, and the SERniña children's initiative in the schools of ▶

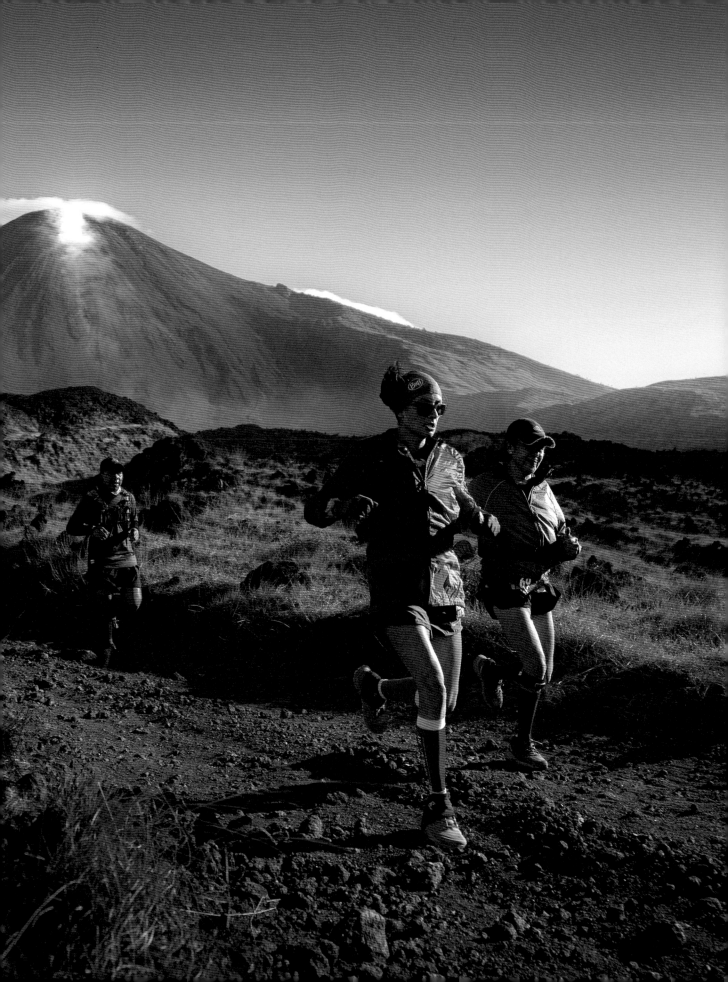

Organized by Impact Marathon—whose speciality is this kind of socially engaged, international race—this event in Guatemala has a focus on work with youth.

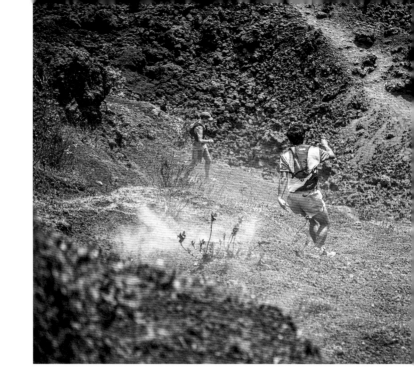

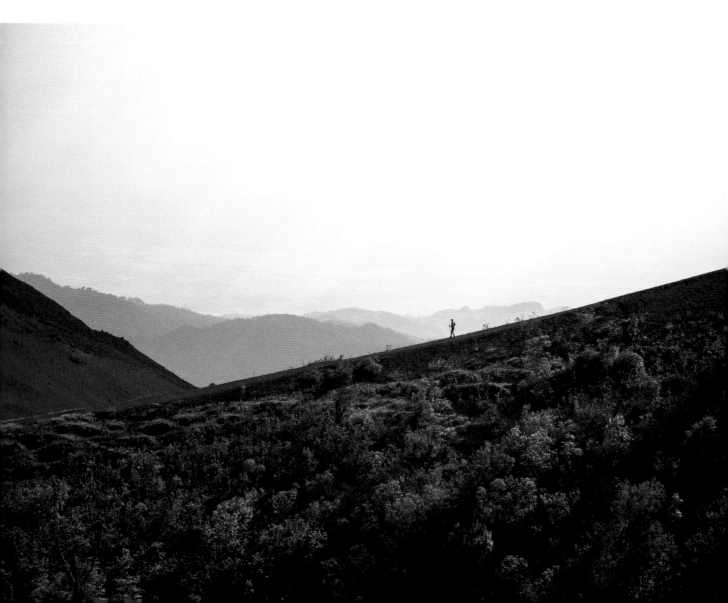

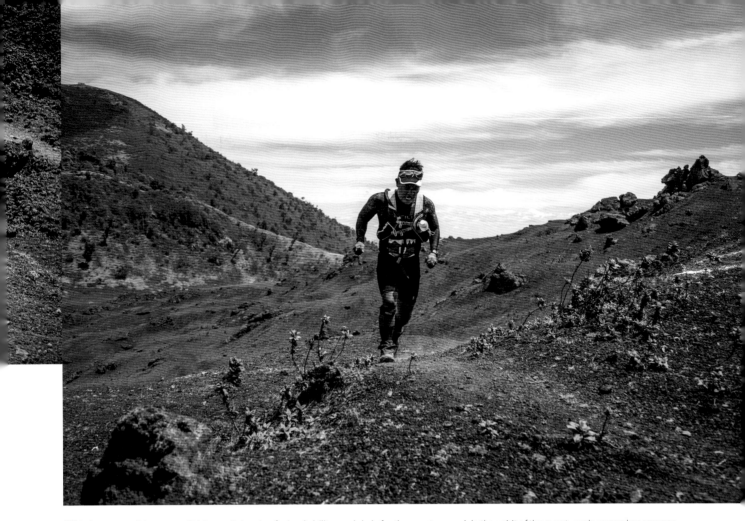

With three race distances available, participants of mixed ability can join in for the greater good. In the spirit of the event, each course has a name: The Beast of Pacaya, 42.2 kilometers (26.2 miles); I 'Lava' This Race, 21.1 kilometers (13.1 miles); and I 'Finca' That's Enough, 10 kilometers (6.2 miles).

▶ El Hato. A rest day in the town of Antigua is followed, on day five, by the climax of the week—race day.

Pacaya volcano, within the Pacaya National Park, has been active since 1961. The Impact course that covers its flanks takes you on winding trails through local fincas, or homesteads, across the lava field, and for those completing the full marathon length, right up to the crater at the summit, at an altitude of nearly 2,400 meters (7,874 feet). Returning to the finish via the southern lava field is compared to "running on the moon." This is the hardest trail in the Impact series.

Four different packages and levels of accommodation are available across the five-day trip from El Hato to the finish, from an outdoor-camping option to the treehouses of the athletes' village, which is one of the most appealing in the Impact series. The view from this high-altitude site is remarkable, taking in three volcanoes, including Pacaya, which often offers up a glowing red lava show after dark: the perfect view to enjoy as you recuperate from your run.

Participants in Impact series events are each asked to raise a minimum of USD 1,300 to support the NGOs and charities of the host country, with the stated aim being to help that nation achieve its UN Global Goals through practical, local action. This emphasis may be different to that of other endurance events, but the running is no less rigorous and the sense of camaraderie no less pervasive. Crossing the finish line with new friends and fellow runners, the organizers tell us, feels more like a "victory lap" than a race, and marks your entrance into a global running movement. ∎

Length: 10, 21.1, or 42.2 km (6.2, 13.1, or 26.2 mi)

Location: Antigua, Guatemala

Date: March

Type: trail/road

Temperature Ø: 13 – 26 °C (55 – 79 °F)

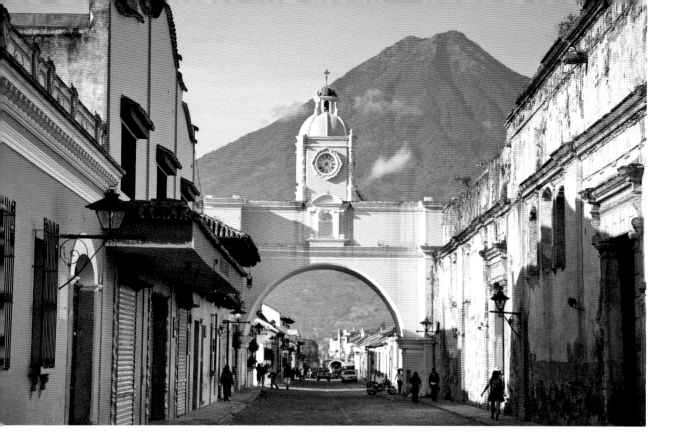

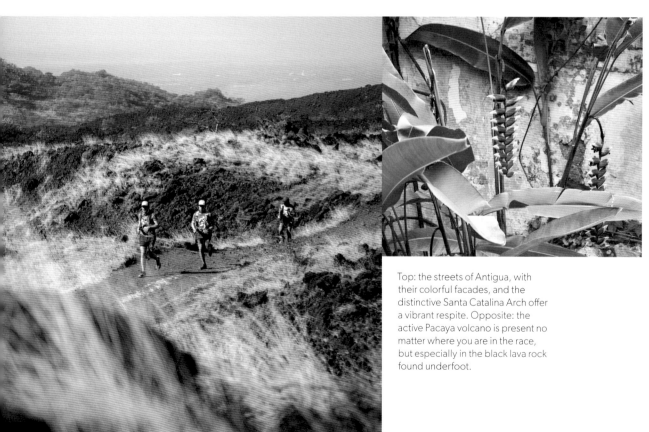

Top: the streets of Antigua, with their colorful facades, and the distinctive Santa Catalina Arch offer a vibrant respite. Opposite: the active Pacaya volcano is present no matter where you are in the race, but especially in the black lava rock found underfoot.

Pacaya volcano has been active since 1961. The Impact course that covers its flanks takes you on winding trails through local fincas, or homesteads, across the lava field, and for those completing the full marathon length, right up to the crater.

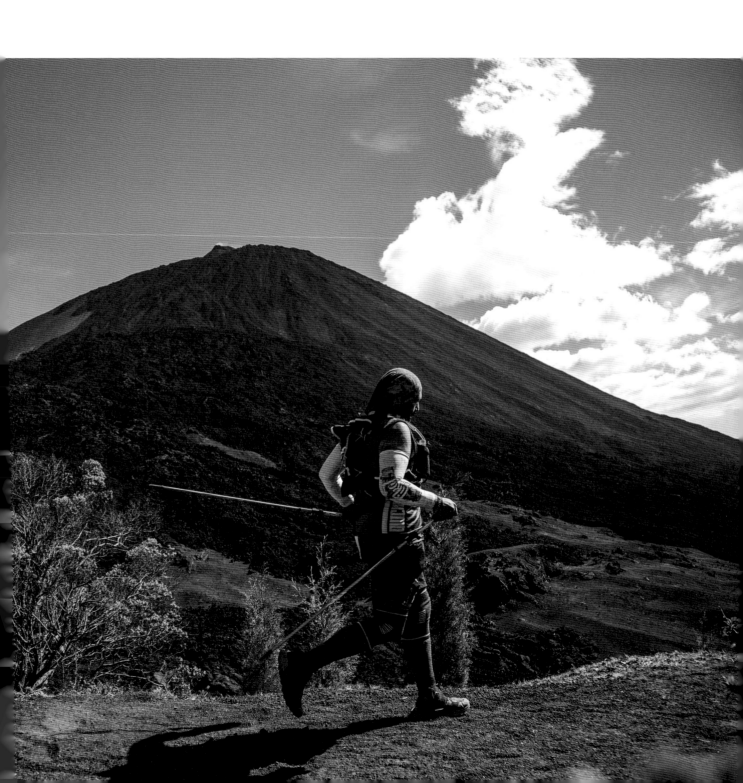

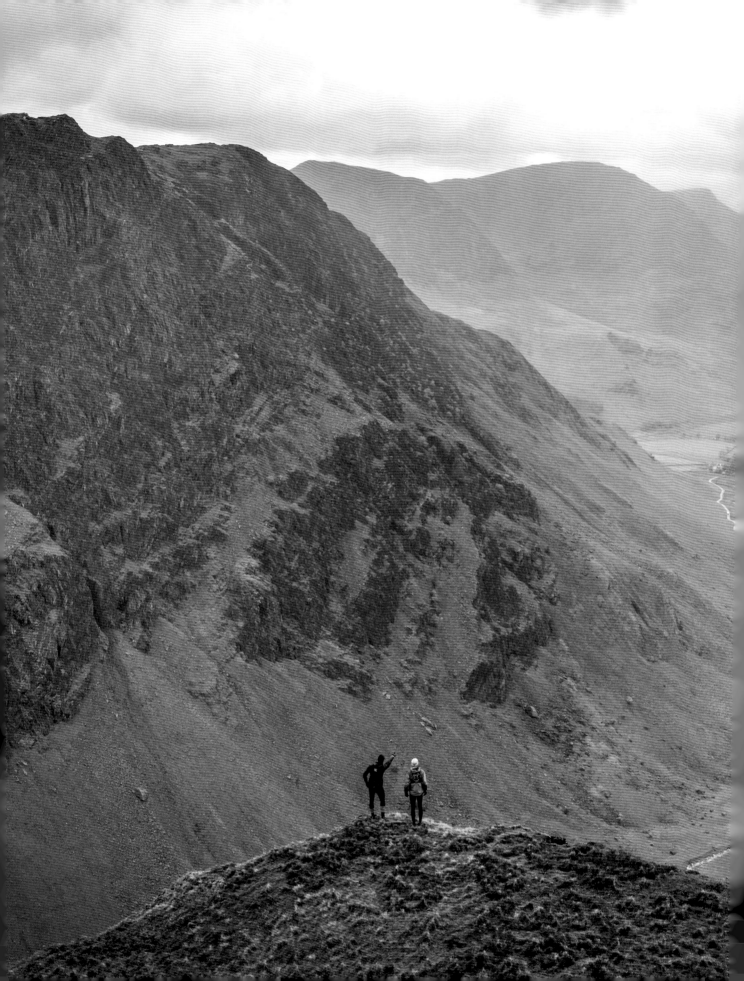

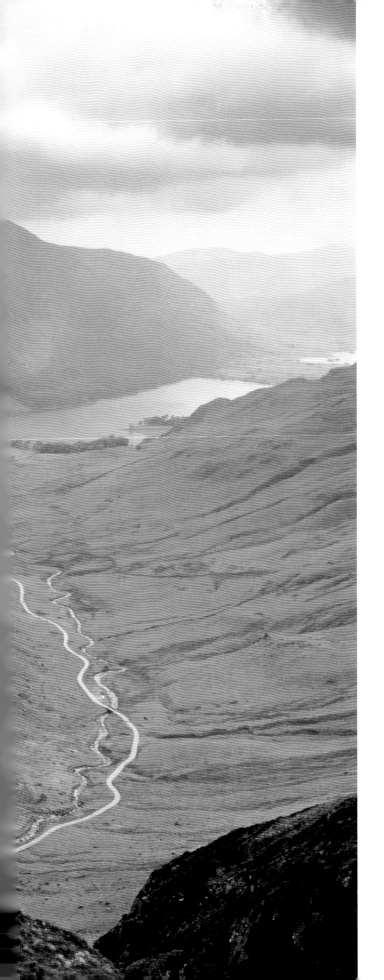

BOB GRAHAM ROUND

English fell running at its finest. Do Bob Graham proud by taking to the mountains of the U. K.'s Lake District to challenge yourself against the clock and the inclines. Your challenge? Run 42 peaks in 24 hours. No way markings, no aid stations, just you and the mountains.

The Bob Graham Round is a classic British 24-hour challenge, covering 42 of the best fells of the picturesque Lake District. It is attempted by about 200 fell runners each year, with about one in three attempts being successful. The harder it is, the greater its allure, it seems. It is a peerless way to enjoy the British countryside.

One of the "big three" mountain runs of the U. K.—the Paddy Buckley Round in Snowdonia, Wales, and the Scottish Ramsay Round being the other two—the Bob Graham is not strictly a "race," nor is there necessarily a fixed course to be followed. It is "open" to contenders at all times of year (though winter attempts are less common), and while the Bob Graham 24 Hour Club—formed to promote safe long-distance fell running in the area as a whole—administer the official run and keep records, there is nothing stopping runners from attempting part or all of the challenge, ▶

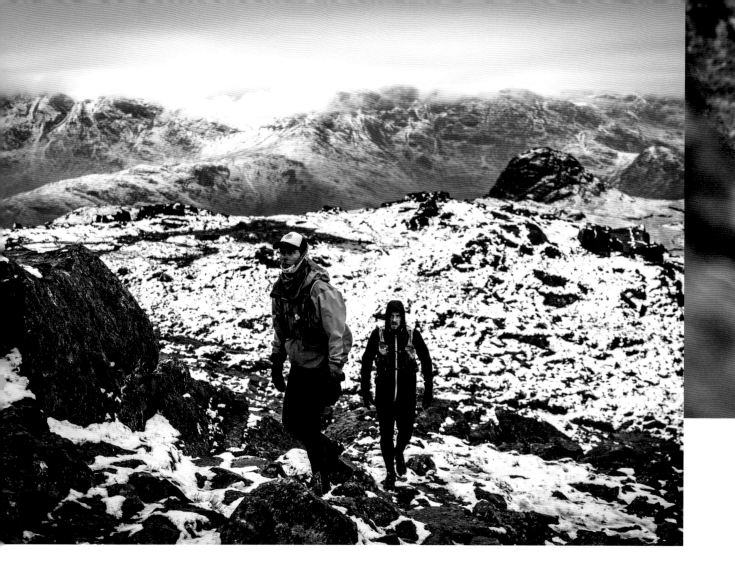

▶ or a variant, on their own, unofficial terms, "for fun." And what better way to experience the stunning landscapes of the Lakes? May the weather, the lakes, and the mountains permit you.

This region has a long and storied tradition of fell running—one that stretches back more than 150 years—with the first recorded long-distance round of the famous peaks completed by a Reverend J. M. Elliott of Cambridge in 1864 (he managed nine of them). Keswick guest-house owner Bob Graham attempted the informal challenge of running up and down as many Lake District hills in 24 hours as possible in June 1932. His record of 42 peaks was only officially beaten in 1960, by Alan Heaton, who completed a slightly modified version of Graham's run in 22 hours 18 minutes, setting the classic course as many run it today, lured by the combination of distance running and summiting high mountains.

Traversing these 42 fells, starting and ending at Moot Hall, Keswick, involves approximately 106 kilometers (66 miles) of fell running, 8,199 meters (26,900 feet) of which are ascent. The fastest time over the course is a record currently held by legendary mountain racer Kilian Jornet: he made it in 12 hours 52 minutes in 2018. The current women's record stands at 14 hours 34 minutes, and was set by Beth Pascal in 2020. A separate challenge, in which runners

attempt to increase the number of peaks covered in 24 hours, also continues, with 78 peaks the current figure to beat.

Most runners who attempt the round have a support crew, offering food, water, and witnesses. The Bob Graham 24 Hour Club requires that participants are accompanied at each summit—data from GPS devices is not accepted—to verify their successful attempt. Otherwise, its list of official rules is simple: Respect the route. Respect those who live and work along the round. Respect the history, traditions, and ethos of the route. And, most importantly, don't mess things up for others. ■

Length: 42 peaks in 24 hours, approximately 106 km (66 mi)

Location: Keswick, U. K.

Date: all year round

Type: trail/self-navigation

Temperature Ø: any British weather (rain likely)

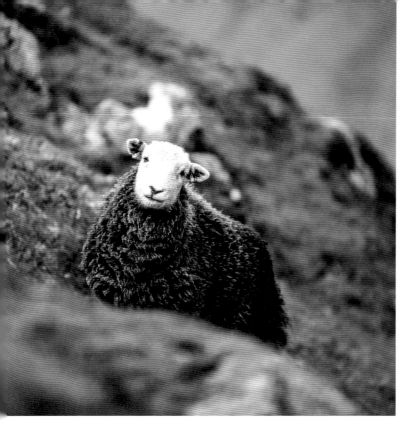

The Bob Graham Round is a classic British 24-hour challenge, covering 42 of the best fells of the picturesque Lake District. It is a peerless way to enjoy the British countryside.

There is no set time of year for running the Bob Graham Round. In recent years, wintertime has grown in popularity, despite the route often being harder to negotiate due to wind, snow, and rain.

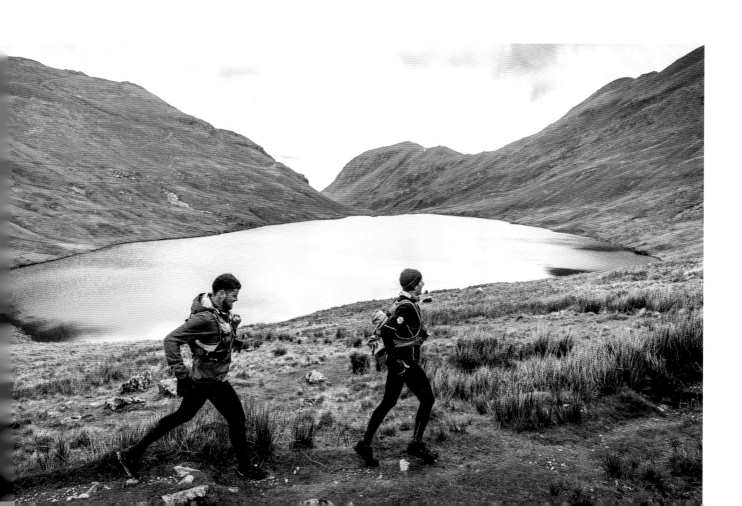

The list of official rules is simple: Respect the route. Respect those who live and work along the round. Respect the history, traditions, and ethos of the route. And, most importantly, don't mess things up for others.

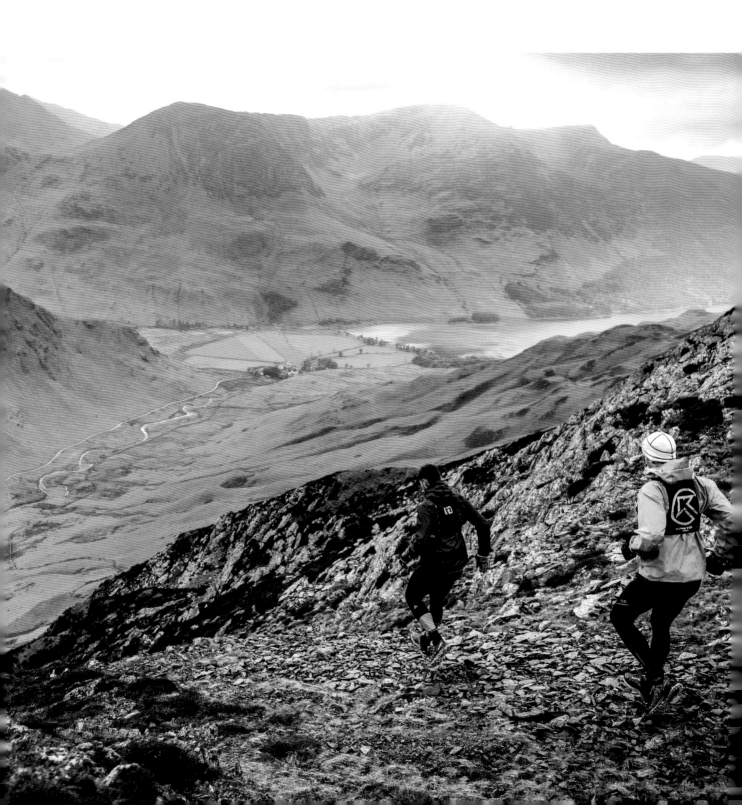

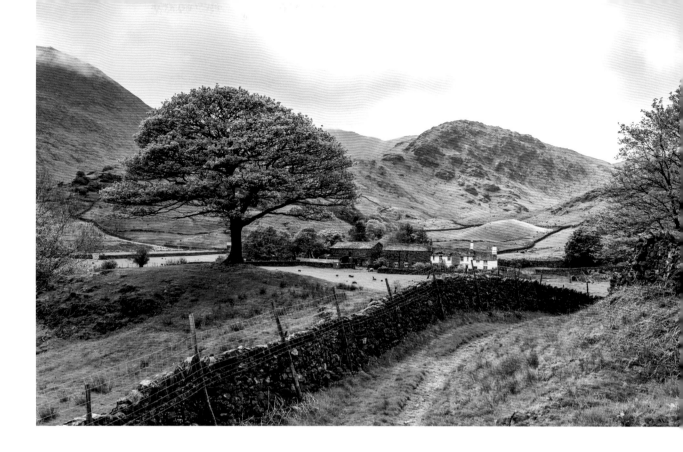

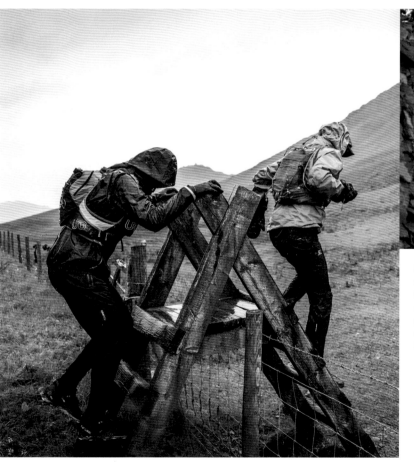

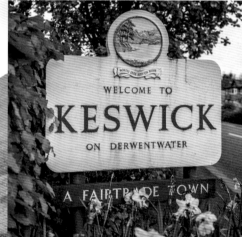

Opposite: There are a number of very steep ascents and descents to the course. To verify the successful mounting of each summit, each participant is accompanied on each stage by a club member who has run the route before.

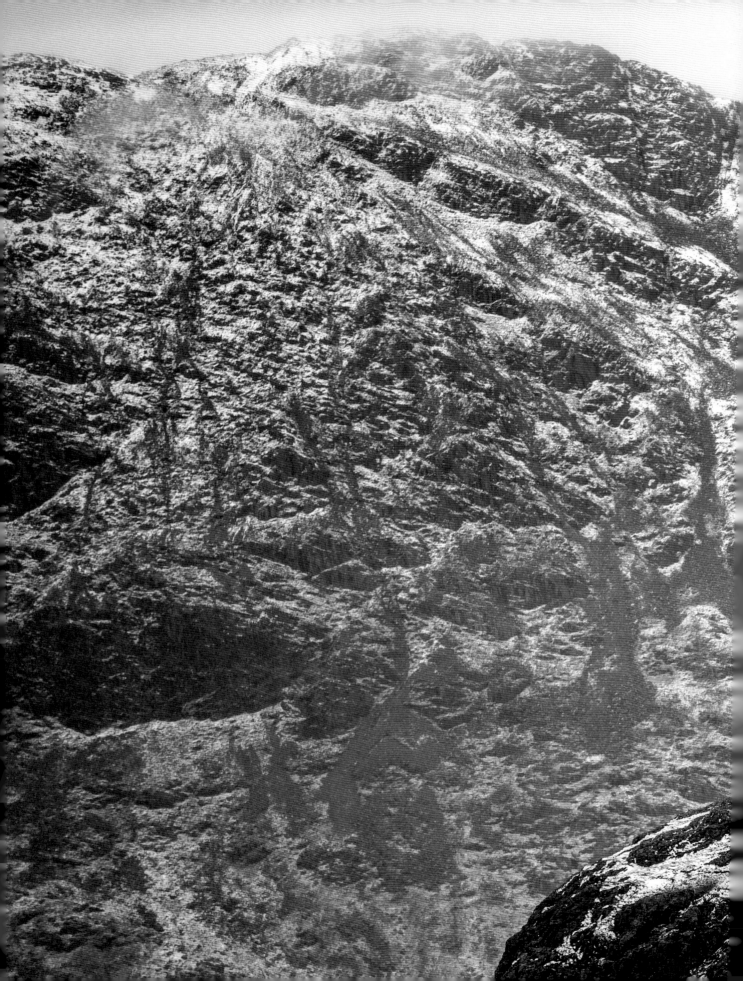

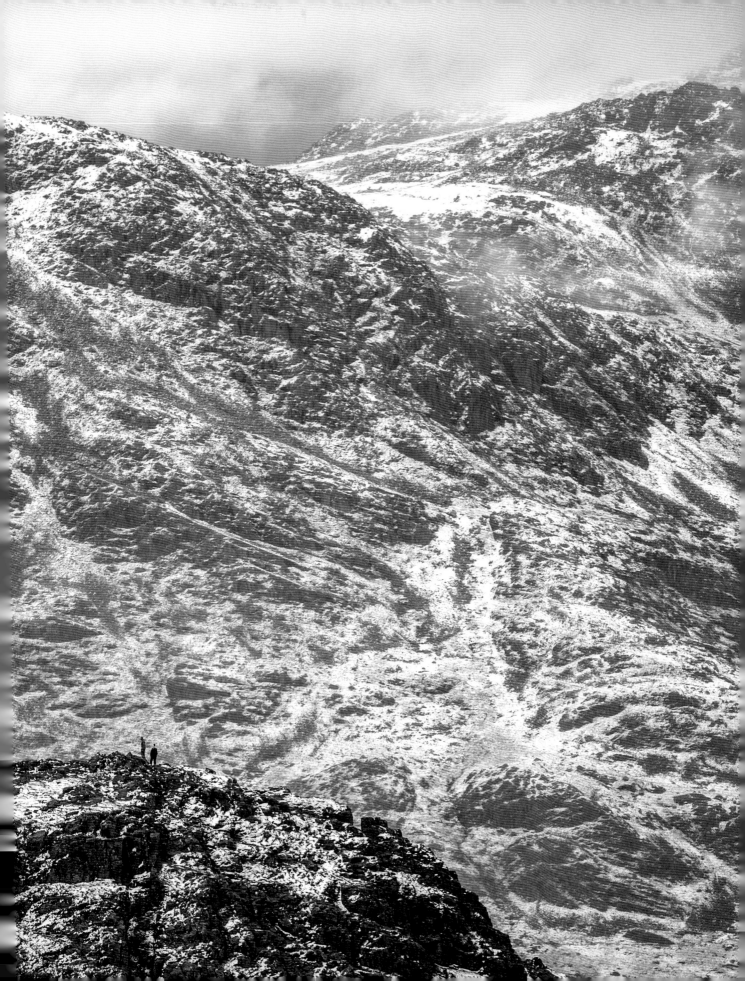

THE BARKLEY MARATHONS

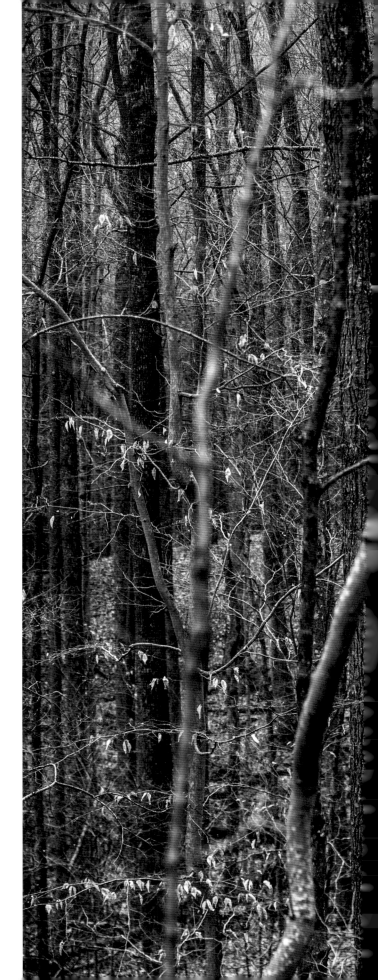

Bonkers and brilliant—this is a serious event with an eccentric twist that every ultra runner longs to conquer. With a race limit of 60 hours and a route you self-navigate, this is one for the thoroughbreds of adventure running. To date, only 15 people have ever finished. To enter, simply write to "Laz," and see if he'll invite you.

Do you want to finish every race you enter? If you like to run, conquer, and go home with a shiny medal, this event may not be for you. It is a unique and uniquely grueling run for those unique and uniquely bloody-minded people: ultra runners. Even among this hardy breed, only 15 people can brag of finishing the Barkley, two of whom completed it in an earlier, shorter iteration than that run today.

The wooded lands of Frozen Head State Park, near Wartburg in Tennessee, are the setting for this wacky and well-loved event, the brainchild of local running enthusiast Gary "Lazarus Lake" Cantrell. He designed the course after hearing the story of the 1977 escape of James Earl Ray from nearby Brushy Mountain State Penitentiary. Ray, sentenced to 99 years' imprisonment for the assassination of Martin Luther King, Jr., escaped Brushy and ran for 55 hours in the woods, covering, as it turned out, only ▶

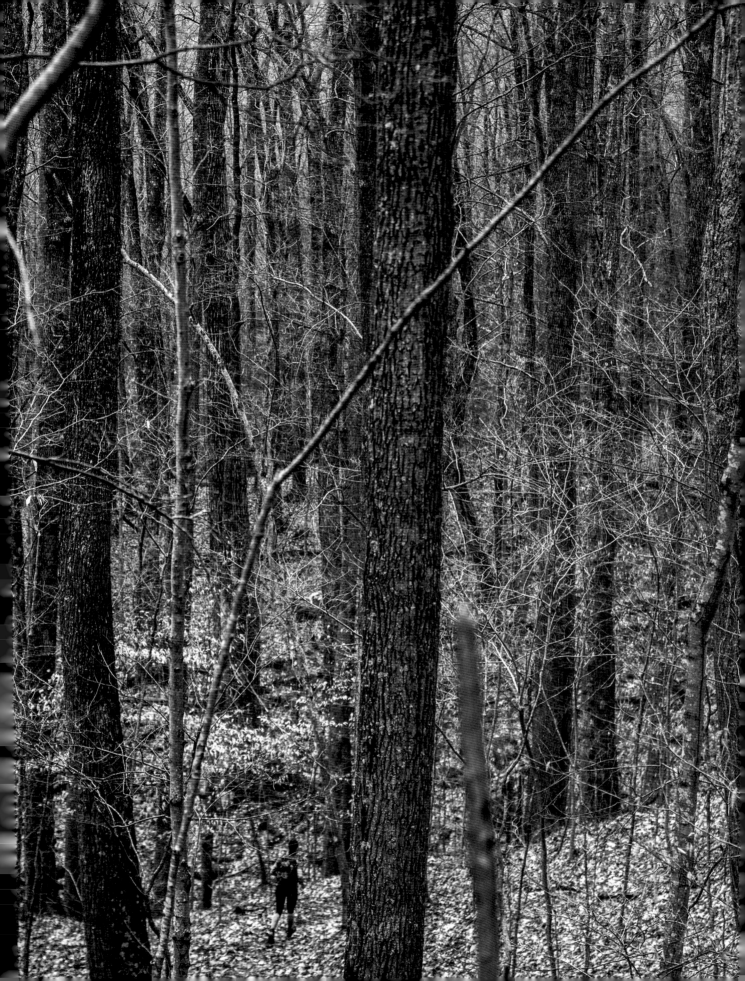

It is a unique and uniquely grueling run for those unique and uniquely bloody-minded people: ultra runners. Even among this hardy breed, only 15 people can brag of finishing the Barkley.

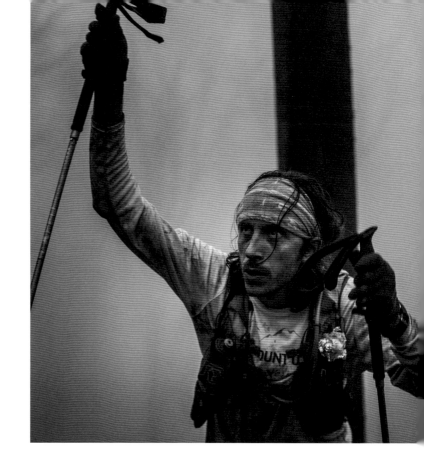

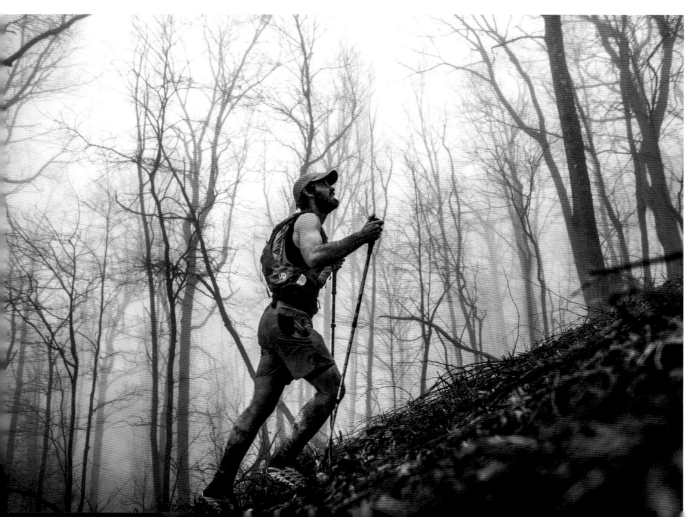

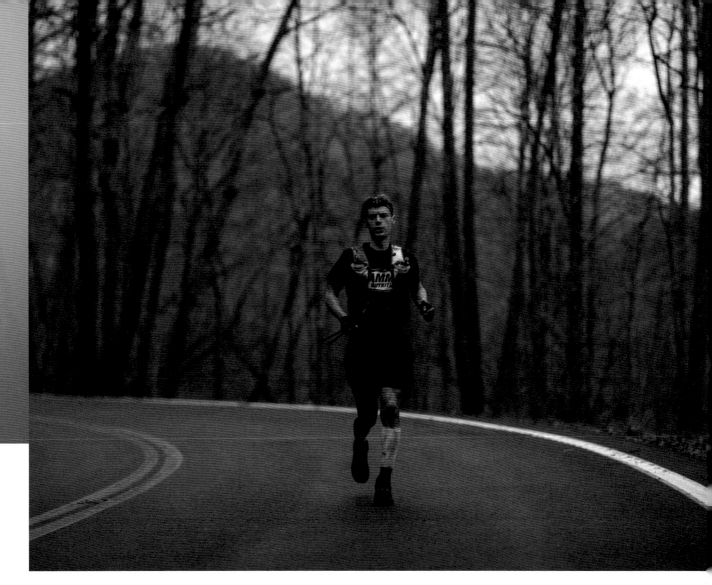

Almost all of the route that makes up a single loop of The Barkley Marathons trails through dense woodland, leaving participants to their own devices when tackling dense vegetation, slippery slopes, and the dark of night.

▶ 13 kilometers (8 miles). Cantrell is said to have joked, "I could do at least 100," mocking Ray's mileage, and the Barkley challenge was born. It is named for Cantrell's running companion Barry Barkley.

The course itself basically consists of a 32.2-kilometer (20-mile) loop over rough, uncleared terrain, five laps of which must be completed for a runner to be considered as having finished the full ultra. It is completely unmarked, and use of GPS technology is not permitted—runners must copy the one version of the map available at the start line and receive scanty directions. The path is traditionally marked by books located at various points, and participants must tear a page from each to prove they have completed the loop. The only aid stations are two points where water is available and, to make matters worse, some say the loop is in fact more than the stated 32.2 kilometers, approaching something like marathon distance.

With more than 18 kilometers (roughly 60,000 feet) of elevation gain over the full course, it's no wonder that more than half of the races held since 1986 have ended with no finishers at the 60-hour mark.

What else? Well, other eccentricities of the event include the mysterious entry procedure, the only readily available details of which are the registration fee of USD 1.60 and the requirement of writing an essay explaining why you should be allowed to participate. Those who are accepted to run—including one "human sacrifice," considered the person least likely to complete—receive a "letter of condolence" and first-timers are asked to bring a license plate from their home state or country to the event. Prior finishers submit a pack of Camel cigarettes to Cantrell, while veteran non-finishers must submit an additional "fee," usually an item of clothing picked out by, again, Cantrell. A one-hour warning of the race start is signaled ▶

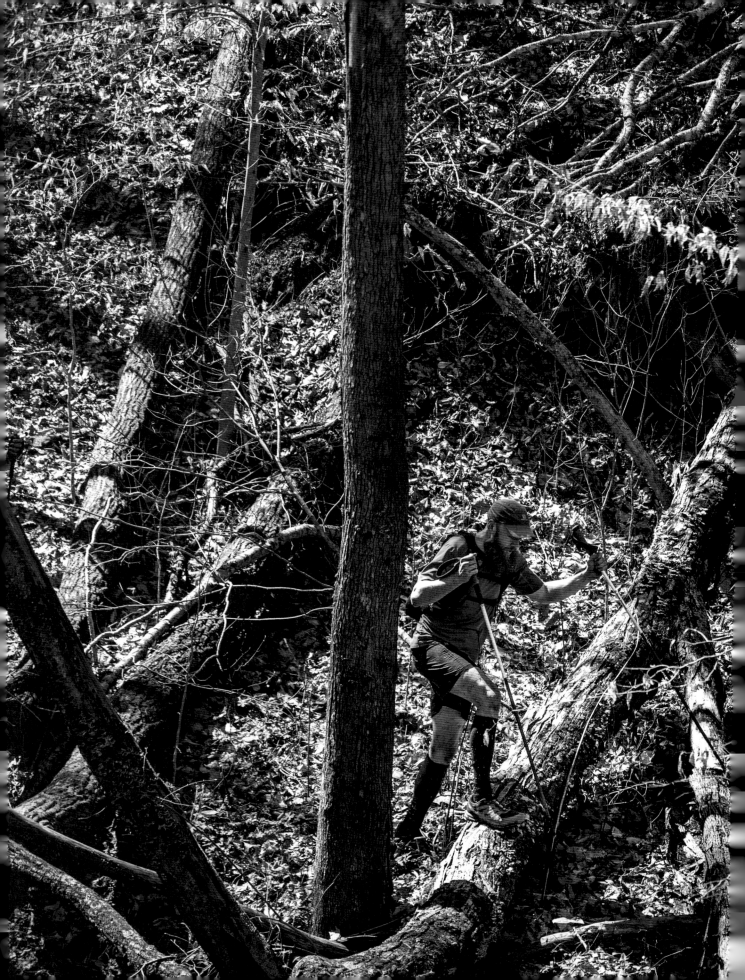

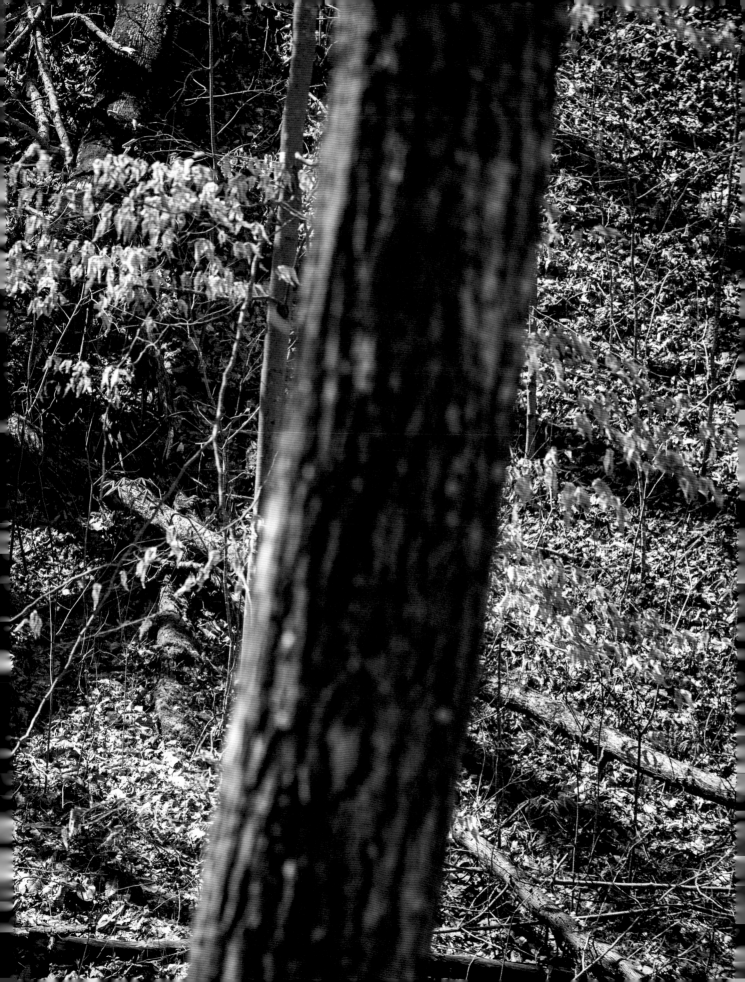

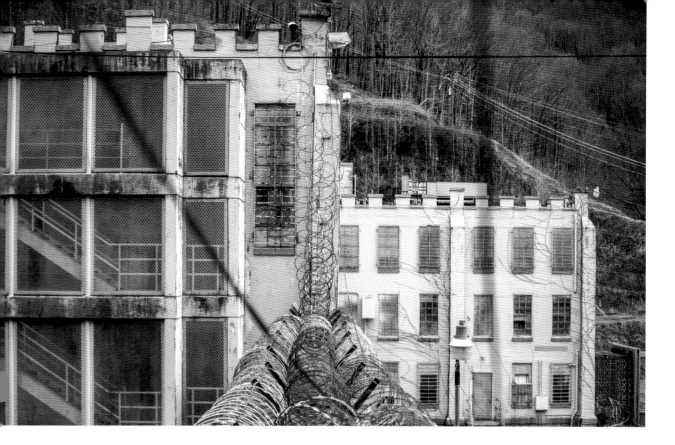

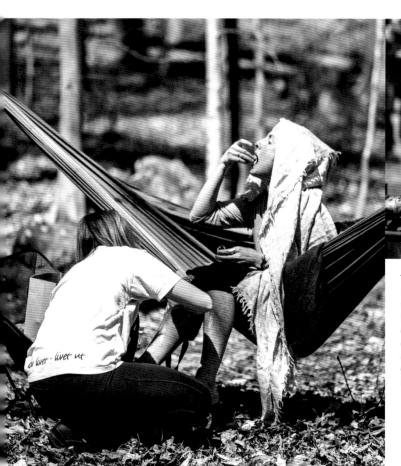

Top: the now-closed Brushy Mountain State Penitentiary, whose grounds the route passes through. Opposite: participants' crews await them at the race campground, with food supplies and medical aid. One of the park's gates near the campground marks the start and finish of the race.

▶ by the sound of a conch. Runners then set off to run two loops clockwise, two loops counterclockwise, and a fifth that is run in different directions by alternate runners (assuming you get that far—in 2012, 22 out of 35 entrants gave up during or after the first loop).

Despite its insane level of difficulty, the Barkley—the "race that eats its young"—has an avid following and places fill up quickly on the day registration opens. Cantrell, despite all evidence to the contrary, claims he wants runners to finish, stating, "Humans are made to endure physical challenges." There's no greater challenge out there. ■

Length: 96.6 or 160 km (60 or 100 mi)

Location: Frozen Head State Park, Tennessee, U. S.

Date: late March/early April

Type: trail/mountainous

Temperature Ø: 6–20 °C (43–68 °F)

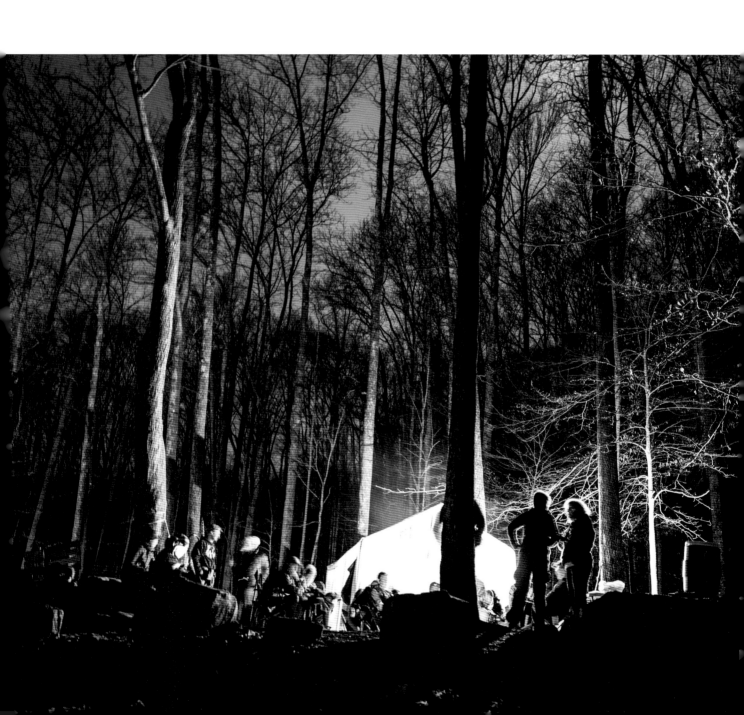

ÖTILLÖ SWIMRUN UTÖ—WORLD SERIES

Run, swim, repeat—that's the name of the game in a race that began in Sweden when four friends embarked on an island-hopping challenge across the Stockholm archipelago (*ö till ö* meaning "island to island" in Swedish). Now, less than two decades later, the sport of swimrunning has become a global sensation.

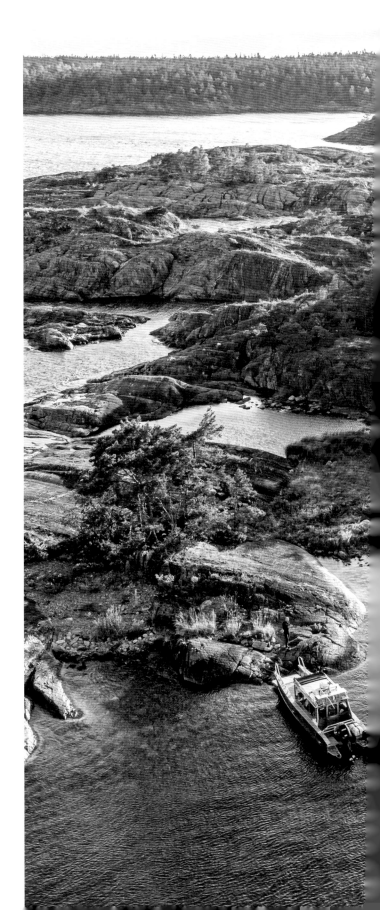

Like most good ideas, the ÖTILLÖ Swimrun was the result of a barroom bet. In 2002, four friends were drinking late into the night on the island of Utö (one of the many islands that make up the archipelago off the Baltic coast of Stockholm). A challenge was issued to race from Utö to the small town of Sandhamn, on the island of Sandön, 54 kilometers (34 miles) away as the crow flies. They would split into two teams and make their way across the 24 islands in between by swimming and trail running. The last team to make it to Sandhamn would pay for drinks. They set off the very next morning and reached Sandhamn more than 26 hours later, after 65 kilometers (40 miles) of trail running and 10 kilometers (6 miles) of open-water swimming.

Today, competitors still enter in teams of two, but the length of the race has been refined to a fixed course of 35 kilometers ▶

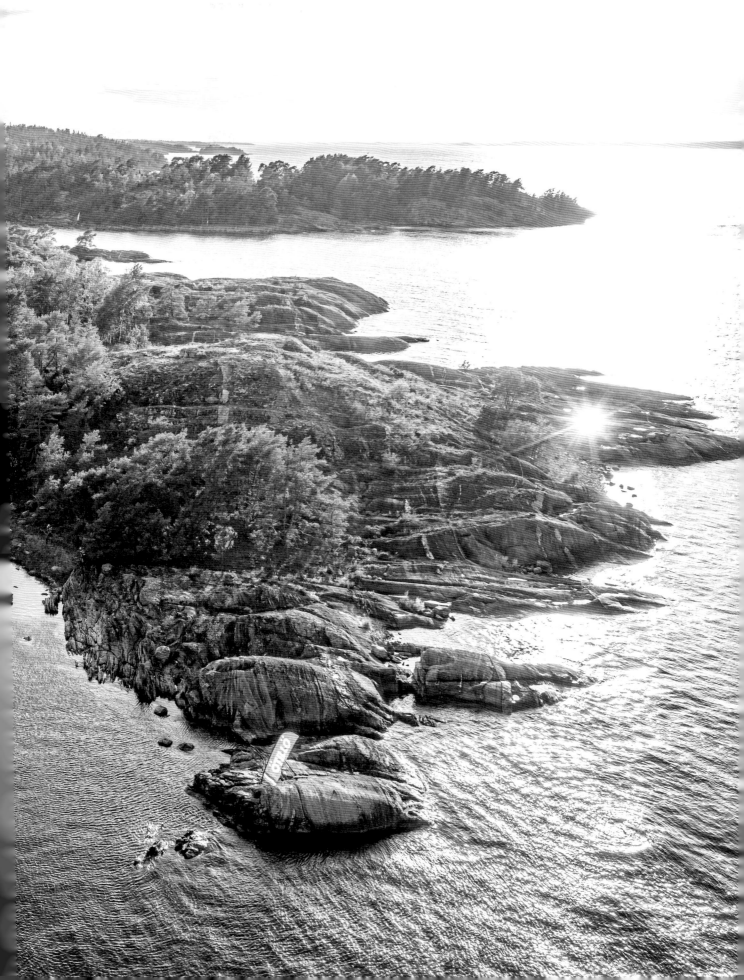

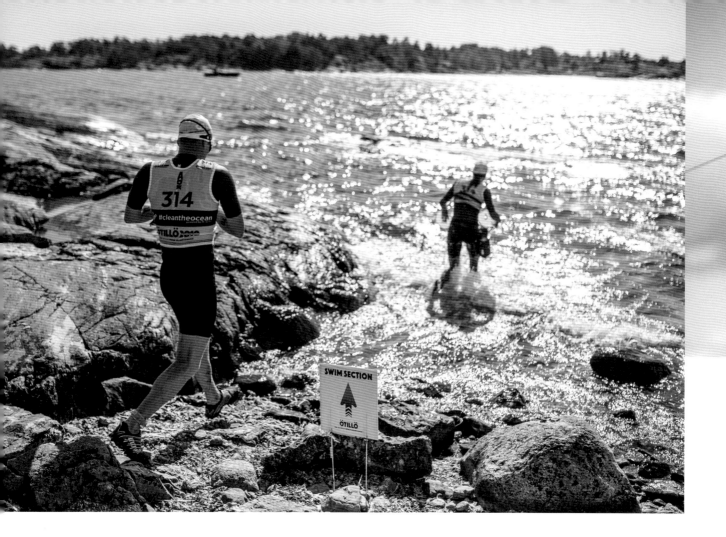

(21.7 miles) on land and 5.5 kilometers (3.5 miles) in the water. The course now runs in reverse, from Sandhamn to Utö, where it finishes at the same bar in which the original idea was hatched. Participants have from dawn until dusk to finish the race, with cut-off points placed at intervals along the course to eliminate those who are struggling or might not finish within seven and a half hours. The top teams cross the finish line in just over four hours, and with space for only 160 teams, the herd thins quickly.

The Baltic Sea can be notoriously difficult, with frigid and choppy waters. In one aquatic stretch, nicknamed the "pig swim," participants are battered by waves for a mile between the islands of Mörtö klob and Kvinnholmen, and strong currents make it nearly impossible to take a direct path between the entry and exit points. And yet many competitors are drawn to ÖTILLÖ for this very battle against the unknown; a common motto is, "Hope for the best but prepare for the worst."

Most of the islands traversed are roadless and uninhabited—part of the organizers' goal to foster a connection with nature. At every event, participants are encouraged to spend an hour collecting trash at the end of the day. Runners are rewarded with unspoiled terrain, pristine views, and probably the freshest air in Europe.

For the less ambitious, ÖTILLÖ also offers two shorter races in Utö: the 8.4 kilometer (5.2-mile) Experience, and the Sprint at just under 15 kilometers (9.3 miles). There are ÖTILLÖ events in seven other locations around the world, including Croatia and California.

The German 1,000 Lakes race is a speedy sand run that leads competitors to a finish at a sixteenth-century castle, and it's hard to imagine a more majestic course than the one on the Isles of Scilly, in southwest England. Since ÖTILLÖ was founded, the sport has become an international sensation. There are now 500 swimruns held globally with multiple governing bodies. Utö, though, remains the beacon.

And to think, it all started on a morning where four guys had a perfect excuse to stay in bed. ∎

Length: 41 km (25 mi)

Location: Stockholm archipelago

Date: September

Type: trail running, 35 km (21.7 mi), and open-water swimming, 5.5 km (3.4 mi)

Temperature Ø: 7–14 °C (45–57 °F)

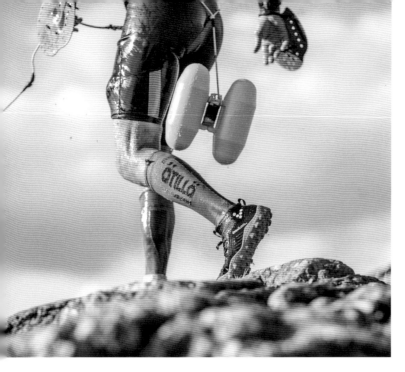

The Baltic Sea can be notoriously difficult, with frigid and choppy waters. In one aquatic stretch, nicknamed the "pig swim," participants are battered by waves for a mile between the islands of Mörtö klob and Kvinnholmen.

Most of the trail is on land, with sections of dirt road, single track, cliffs, and rocks, and a handful of short, sharp ascents. The open-water sections are relatively short, although some of them can be turbulent.

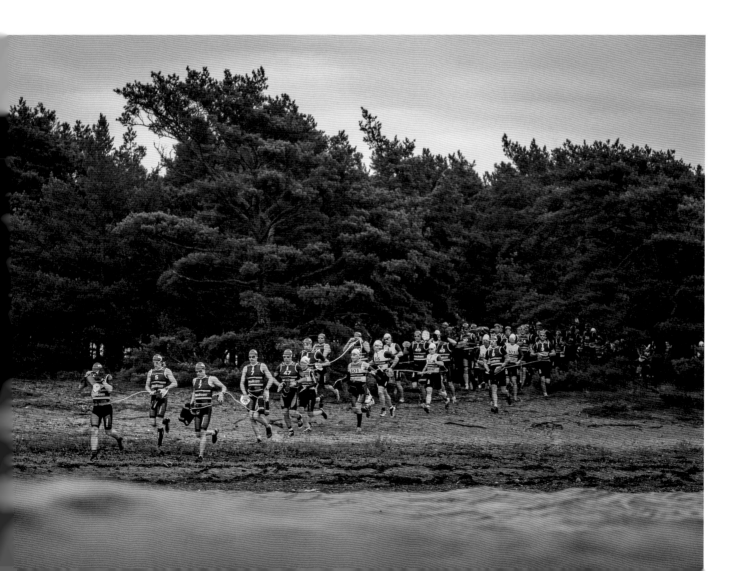

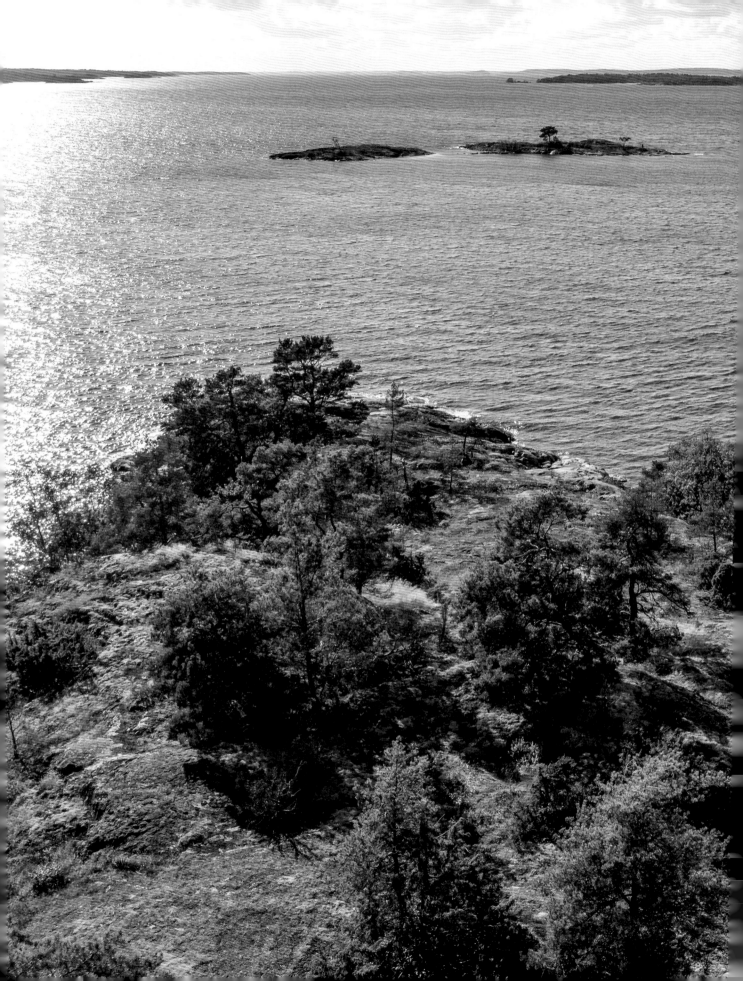

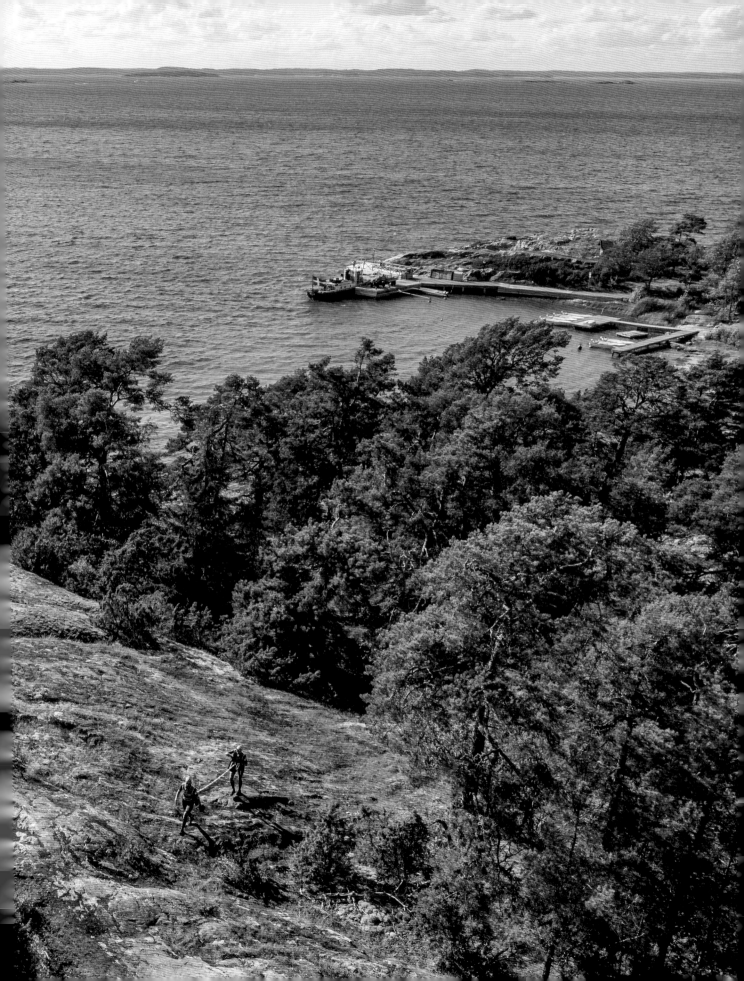

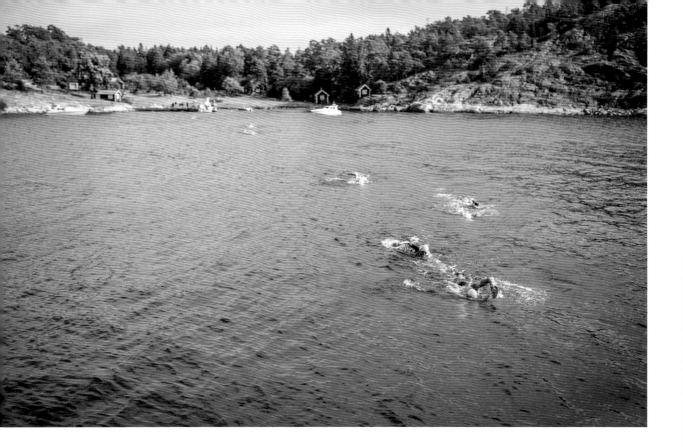

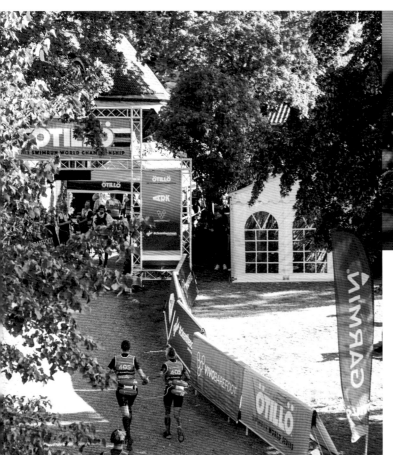

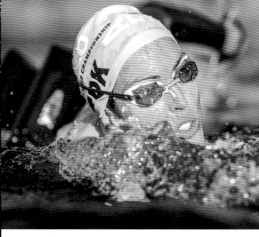

Many of the participants wear paddles and buoyancy aids for the swim sections, and some pairs run the entire race connected to one another with a short rope. Each pair must cross the finish line together.

Most of the islands traversed are roadless and uninhabited—part of the organizers' goal to foster a connection with nature. At every event, participants are encouraged to spend an hour collecting trash at the end of the day.

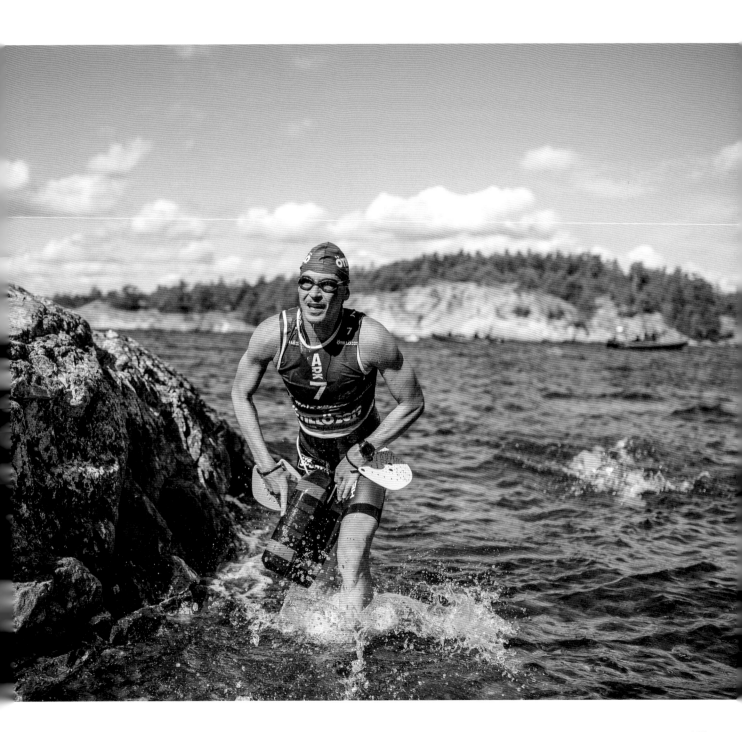

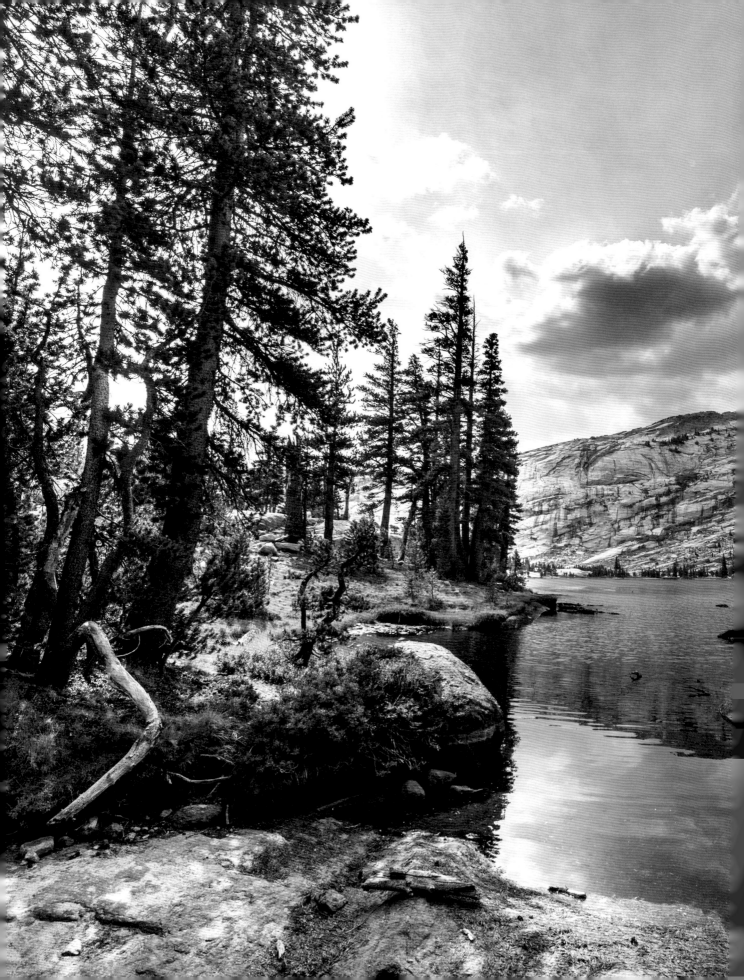

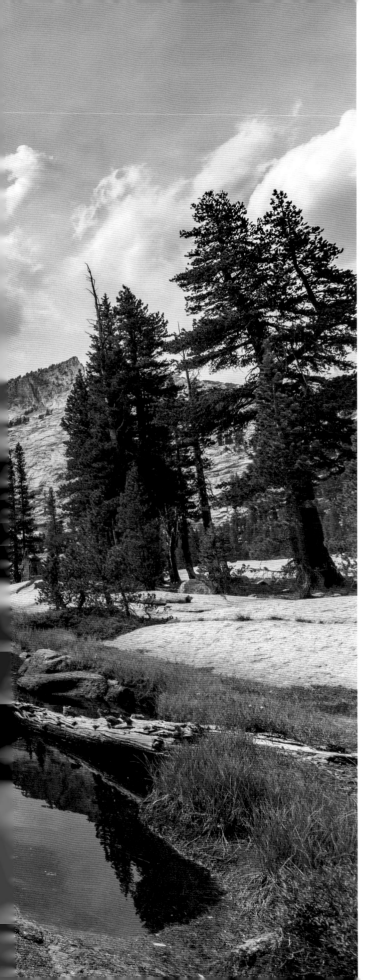

WESTERN STATES 100-MILE ENDURANCE RUN

Get your hands on the famous belt buckle—silver or bronze. All you have to do is run 160 kilometers (100 miles) of historic trail, climbing more than 5,500 meters (18,045 feet), and do so in less than 30 hours (under 24, if you want silver). This is one for the ultra-running bucket list.

Don't even think about it, even if you need a new belt buckle. The world's oldest 160-kilometer (100-mile) trail race is, as the training section of the event's website has it, "a very long way to run."

The 100-Mile Endurance Run is mostly raced along preserved, original portions of the Western States Trail, which runs from Salt Lake City, Utah, to Sacramento, California, crossing the Sierra Nevada Mountains along the way. The trail was historically used by Paiute and Washoe Indians, many of whom were displaced by the Gold Rushers of the late-nineteenth century—"'49ers" who followed it into California in search of wealth. Part of the run's route passes over a section designated a National Historic Trail, in use for more than 160 years.

The run itself has pedigree. It was first completed by Gordy Ainsleigh in 1974; a veteran of the Western States Trail Ride (the ▶

Course records are held by Jim Walmsley and Ellie Greenwood, in the men's and women's races, respectively; Walmsley completed the course in 2019 in an astounding 14 hours 9 minutes.

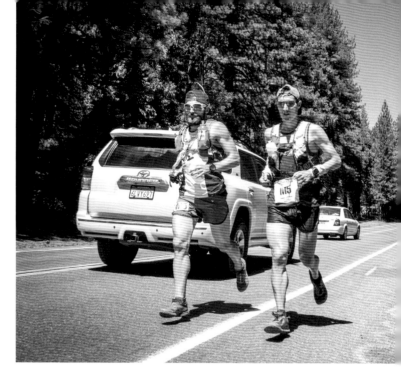

Above: while a short part of the route is on tarmac, the vast majority passes though remote and rugged territory. Opposite: crossing the American River with guide ropes stretched across the icy waters and personnel on hand to assist.

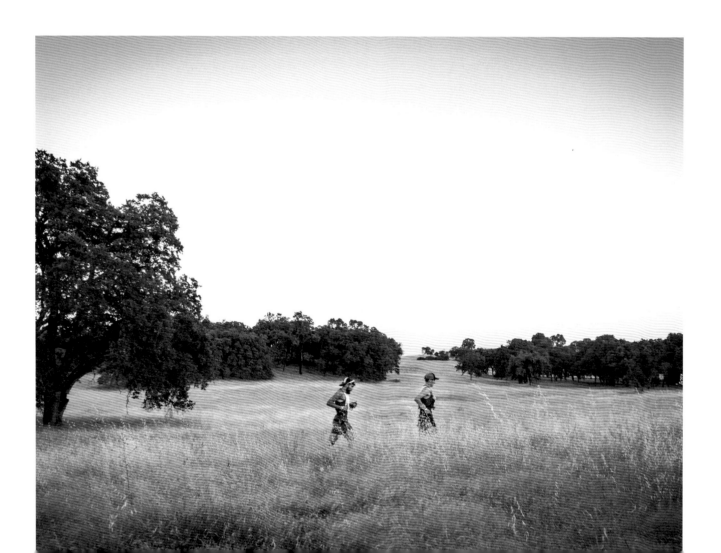

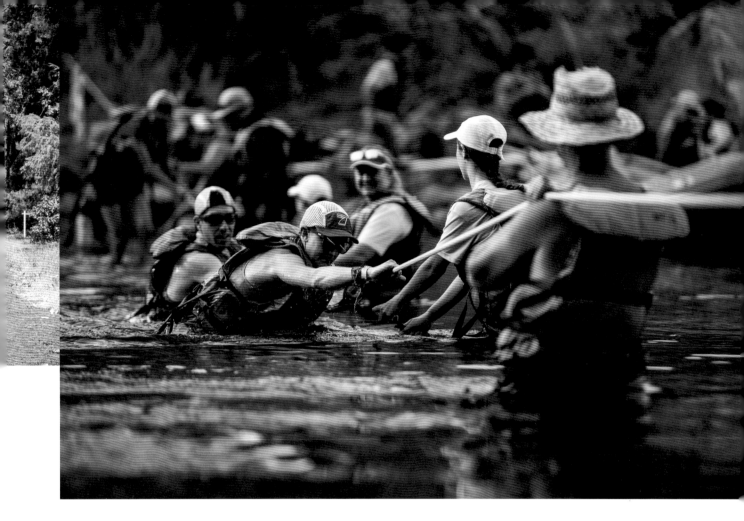

▶ Tevis Cup), Ainsleigh was attempting to complete the course within the same 24-hour time limit allowed to horses and riders, and he succeeded. Three years later, the first official version of the run took place, with only three finishers out of 16 entrants. Today, course records are held by Jim Walmsley and Ellie Greenwood, in the men's and women's races, respectively; Walmsley completed the course in 2019 in an astounding 14 hours 9 minutes.

This course is remote, wild, and rugged—breathtaking in its beauty, but unforgiving. The organizers of the race are at pains to emphasize the need for adequate preparation. You may find yourself racing in temperatures exceeding 43° Celsius (109° Fahrenheit), panting between the aid stations, or if you're particularly unlucky, running an amended "snow route," when cold conditions force the race down from the mountains.

Runners start out from Olympic Valley, California, ascending quickly towards Emigrant Pass (2,667 meters; 8,750 feet) and the Granite Chief Wilderness area in the beautiful Tahoe National Forest. This high-altitude section of the race is followed by yet more climb—to the top of Little Bald Mountain. Runners race on to pass the mining ghost town of Last Chance, before heading into the "canyons" (likely in the afternoon, as temperatures peak). Deadwood and El Dorado canyons drop 610 and 792 meters (2,000 and 2,600 feet), respectively, so this is a particularly punishing segment of the trail.

After a brief run on a paved section of the track, racers descend the American River Canyon to the Rucky Chucky river crossing, where they must ford the water using a guide rope (or rafts in high-water years). As night falls, there comes a slightly gentler section of the run, on the Auburn Lake Trails. At the lowest point of the trail overall, you encounter the No Hands concrete arch bridge. From here it's 2 kilometers (1.3 miles) to the finish line at Placer High School in Auburn, where cheering spectators will help you celebrate (and recover from) the run of a lifetime.

It's an astonishing race, both in terms of the course and the incredible feat of endurance necessary to complete it. As the race organizers have it: "When you can, run. When you can't run, walk. When you can't walk, walk anyway." That's all there is to it. ■

Length: 160 km (100 mi)

Location: Sierra Nevada, California, U. S.

Date: June

Type: trail

Temperature Ø: 15–32 °C (59–90 °F)

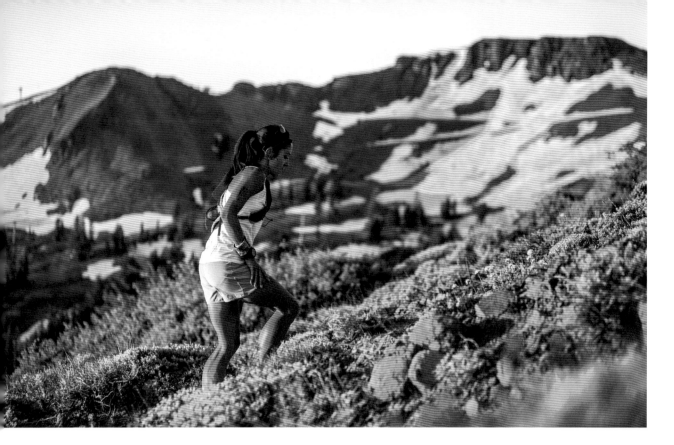

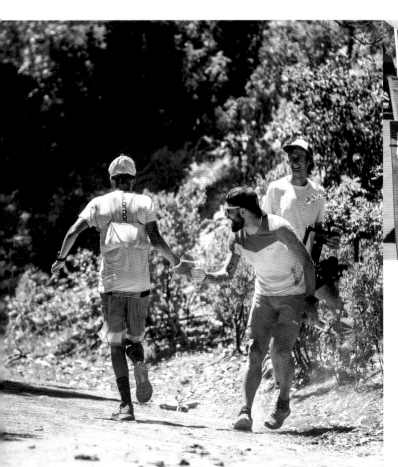

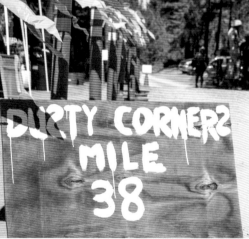

Running from 5 a. m. on the first day, a Saturday, participants in the race have to keep pace in mountainous terrain, on dirt tracks, and through woodland. Anyone crossing the line after 10.59 a. m. the following Sunday fails to qualify.

This course is remote, wild, and rugged—breathtaking in its beauty, but unforgiving. The organizers of the race are at pains to emphasize the need for adequate preparation. You may find yourself racing in temperatures exceeding 43° Celsius (109° Fahrenheit).

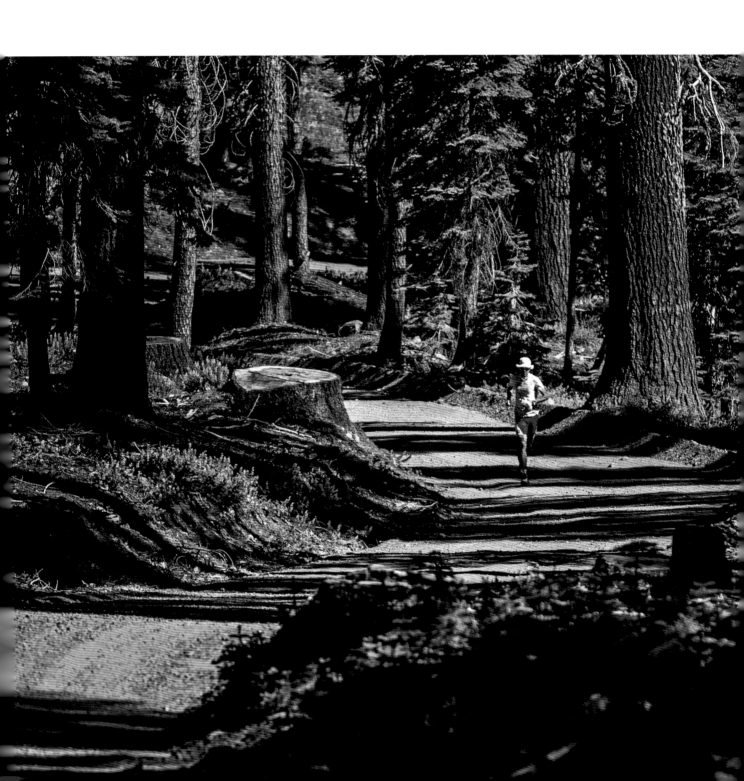

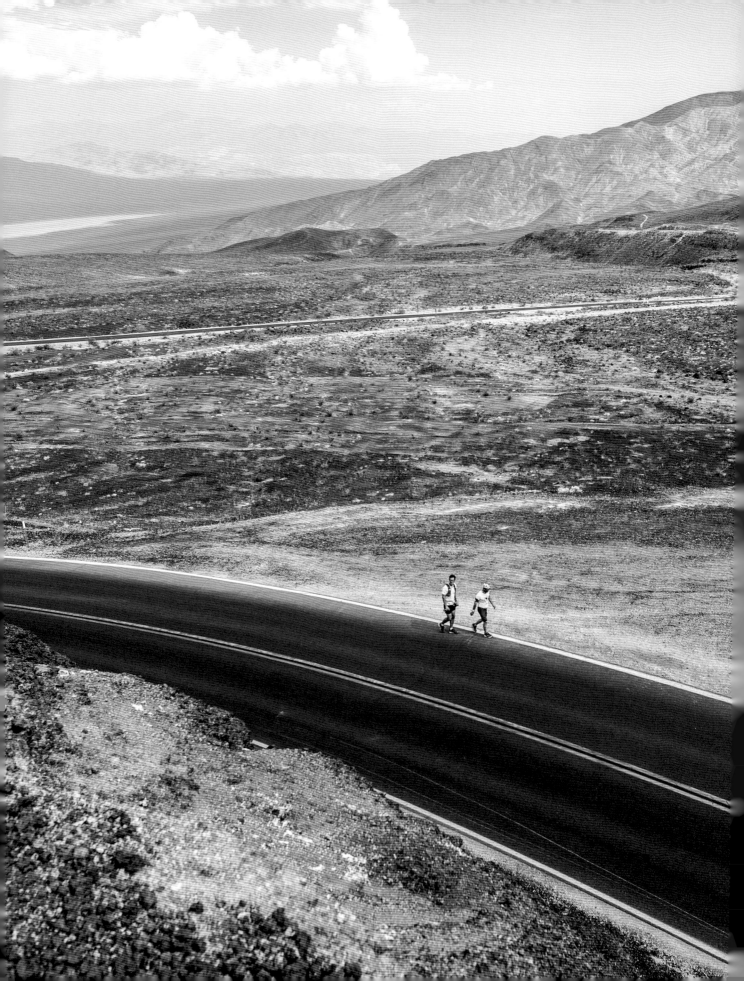

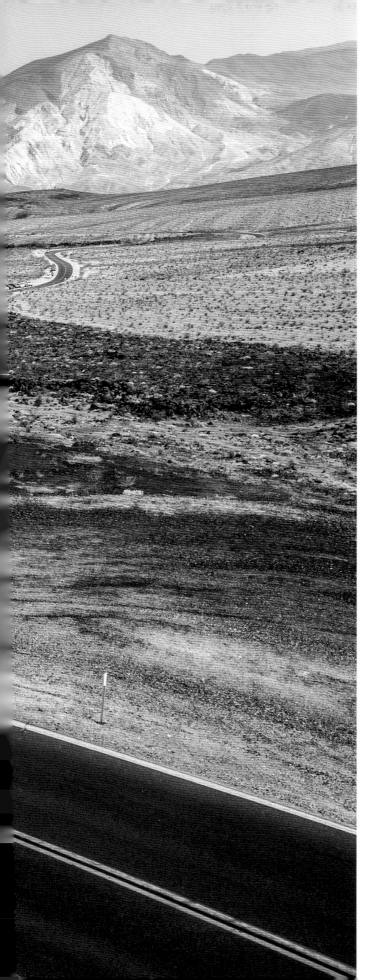

BADWATER 135

Man versus the sun. When your race medal, or belt buckle in this case, is branded with the motto *"Detur Digniori"* ("Let it be given to those most worthy"), it's a sign of the brutality to come. Taking place in a valley named Death, where not even plants are keen to survive, Badwater 135 is commonly known as the toughest footrace in the world.

If you're a fan of extreme sleep deprivation, exhaustion, outrageous heat, the risk of death, and what many class as the toughest ultra marathon in the world, try Badwater 135. You may have met your match.

This 217-kilometer (135-mile) nonstop race over three mountain ranges takes place in sweltering mid-summer heat. Starting at the lowest elevation in North America—the arid Badwater Basin, at 86 meters (282 feet) below sea level—and finishing at Whitney Portal, the trailhead to the highest point in the contiguous United States (Mount Whitney summit), the course has a cumulative ascent of more than 4,421 meters (14,505 feet) and runs through spots with names such as Furnace Creek, Devil's Cornfield, Devil's Golf Course and Lone Pine. Temperatures reach up to 55° Celsius (131° Fahrenheit) and, to top it all off, there is a 48-hour time limit for racers. It is a true test of even the hardiest athlete. ▶

This 217-kilometer (135-mile) nonstop race over three mountain ranges takes place in sweltering mid-summer heat. Temperatures reach up to 55° Celsius (131° Fahrenheit) and, to top it all off, there is a 48-hour time limit for racers. It is a true test of even the hardiest athlete.

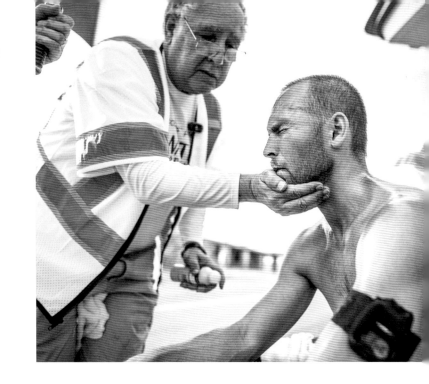

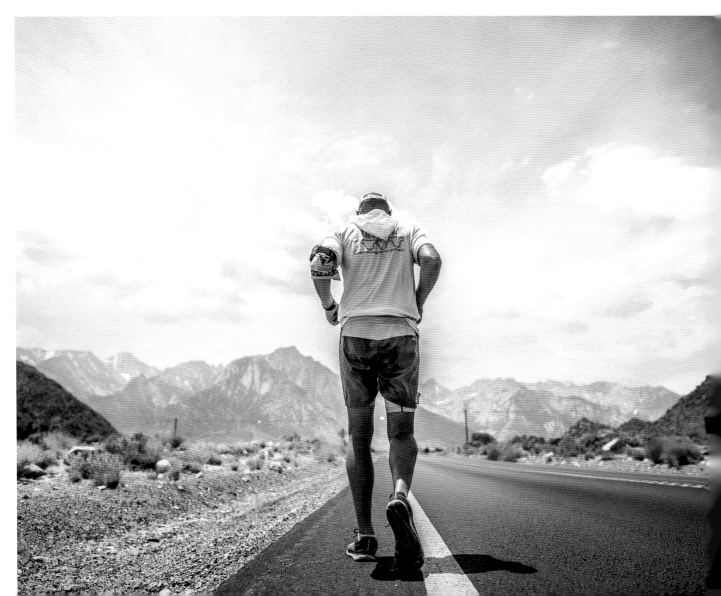

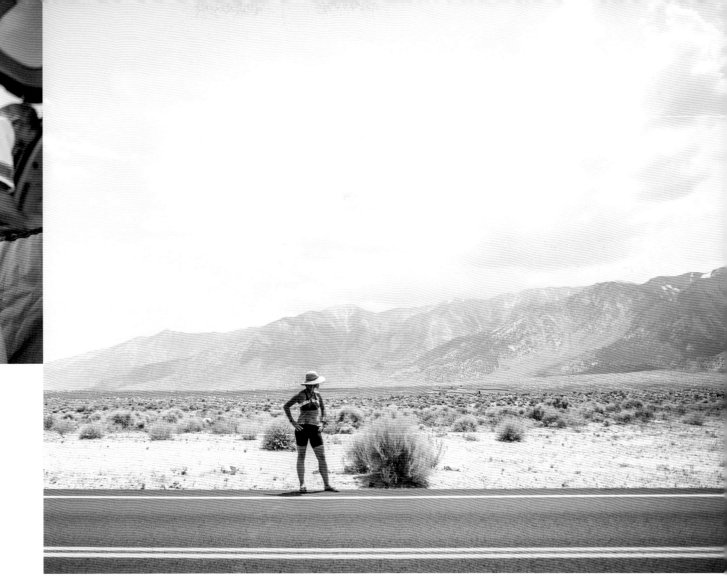

Runners taking part in this race face long spells alone, exposed to fierce sunlight, the wide-open landscape literally offering no end in sight. Intervention from the support team is kept to the bare minimum.

▶ Up to 100 endurance runners are admitted to the race each year, committed to the Badwater ethos of "exploring the inner and outer universes," and the entry requirements are stringent. For 2022, just one of the requirements for applicants is to have completed at least one 160-kilometer (100-mile) race in the 13 months prior to it, even if they have previously crossed the finish line at Badwater. And there are still many non-finishers.

Those who attempt the route follow in the footsteps of ultra-running pioneers committed to conquering this inhospitable stretch of land. Al Arnold, in 1977, was the first person to successfully run from Badwater Basin to Mount Whitney—he was inducted into the Badwater Hall of Fame in 2002, in recognition of this achievement and of his contribution to the history of the event. He himself had twice previously attempted the course, in 1974 and 1975: the first

run was cut short after 29 kilometers (18 miles), as Arnold was suffering from severe dehydration; a knee injury curtailed the second run. Arnold's record of just over 84 hours was only beaten in 1981, when Jay Birmingham completed the second-ever run over the route.

Richard Benyo and Tom Crawford organized the first official version of the race in 1987, with four runners competing (and completing) in that year, including the first woman to complete the course, Jeannie Ennis. The route was not "set" at this time and the rules were not as exhaustive as they are currently, with one competitor using cross-country skis to traverse the salt flats at Badwater.

Today, each runner is required to bring along a support team of two to four members, traveling in one motor vehicle. The roadside signs along the highway, warning of heat dangers even to drivers, give some indication of why—heat is the biggest ▶

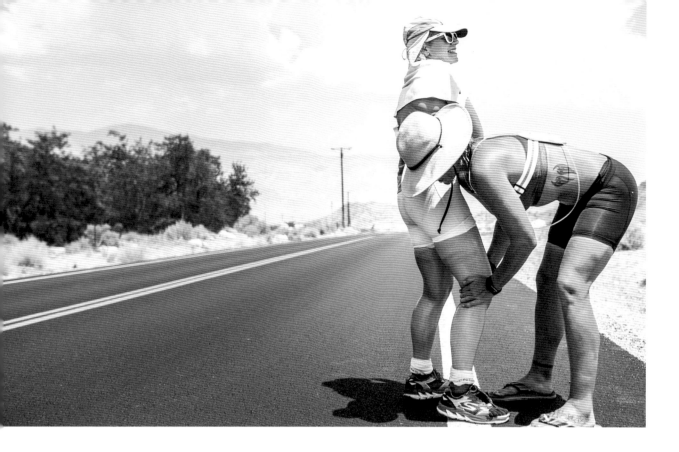

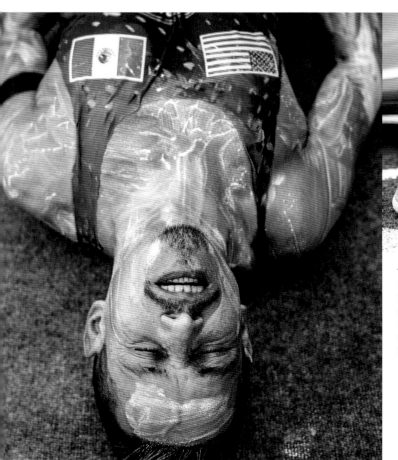

The hazards of taking part in this brutal race are many and the injuries frequent, and yet it has a surprisingly high hit rate, with as many as 80 percent of participants completing the course each year—a rare few in less than 24 hours.

► challenge for runners, and athletes taking on this race regularly suffer from delusions, fainting, and extreme dehydration. Many who have crewed and paced for the Badwater have noted the human ability to thermoregulate and cool through sweating being tested to the extreme in this race with the escalating heat putting strain on the gastrointestinal system in particular. Your body's ability to metabolize food and maintain its fluid balance is severely impaired, and so some calculation is required in order to plan your fluid and nutrient intake carefully and safely.

Needless to say, the race has pedigree and will continue to beat many who attempt it. Those who complete the course and receive the coveted Badwater 135 belt buckle, the Holy Grail of endurance running, can truly say they have conquered the elements and made an exceptional personal achievement. ■

Length: 217 km (135 mi)

Location: Death Valley, California, U. S.

Date: July

Type: road/mountainous

Temperature Ø: 30–50 °C (86–122 °F)

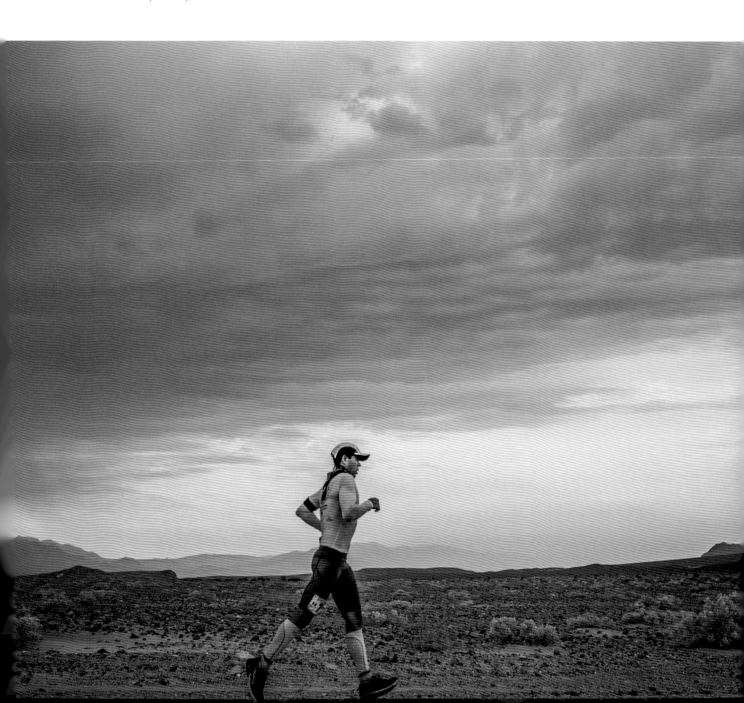

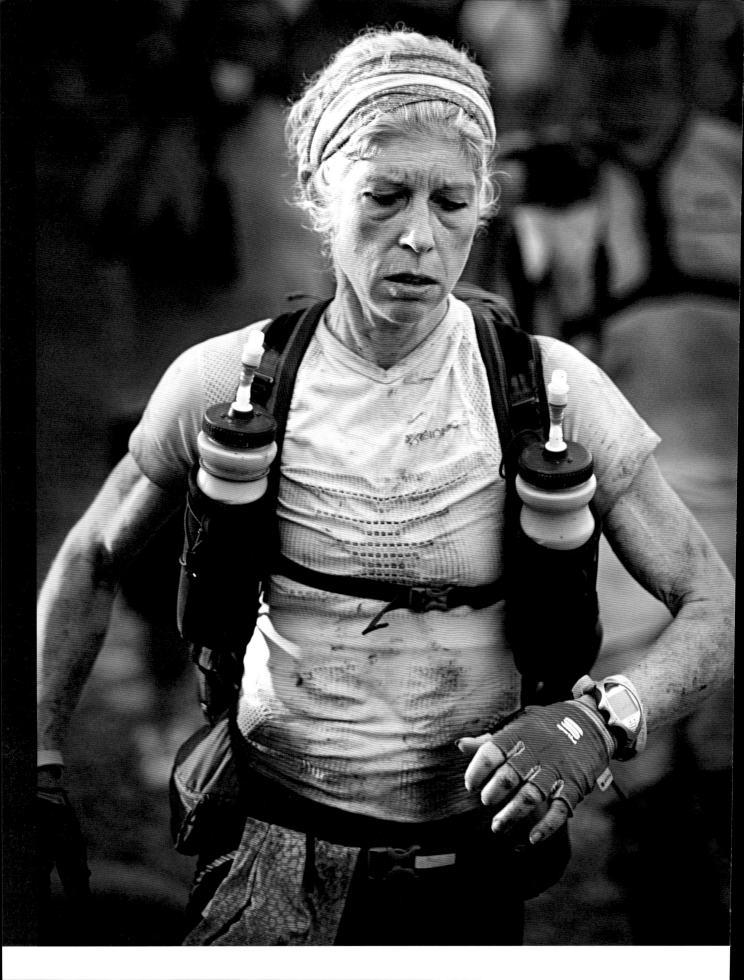

Covering Distance and Collecting Records with Mimi Anderson

When she was 36, Mimi Anderson couldn't last a minute on the treadmill. Less than 20 years later, she was holding three world records in endurance running.

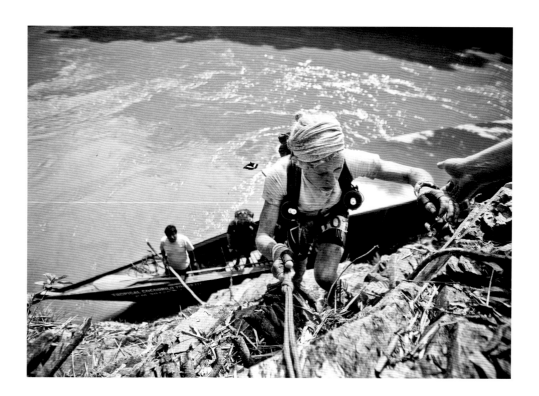

The most famous adage in mountaineering is the answer to why one would climb Mount Everest: "Because it's there." Ask Mimi Anderson why she runs and she'll tell you it's because she can. The British distance runner has covered more kilometers than most cars will in their lifetime. And, at 57, she's still going.

Anderson was a late bloomer. She didn't start running until she was 36 and a mother of three. At the time, she couldn't last for more than a minute on the treadmill. She had spent nearly half of her life battling anorexia, the result of a toxic relationship with her body triggered by a physically abusive nanny. "My legs are an area I never liked," Anderson says. "I've always wanted to have thinner legs, so that's why I started running."

After Anderson ran her first mile on the treadmill, running was no longer a vanity project. Her confidence was growing. She reveled in the bliss of setting a goal and achieving it. Running gave her space and freedom, and self-esteem. Some people work much

harder for these luxuries. Anderson worked harder too. She was running up to 10 kilometers (6.2 miles) on the treadmill when her friends suggested she join them on a 16-kilometer (10-mile) trail run near her home—it was Anderson's first outdoor run. "When I got to the end … I felt a million dollars," Anderson says, her voice expressing the euphoria of that day. "It was like my feet had been given a pair of wings and I could fly. I went around like the Cheshire cat. And that stays with you for days." The more ambitious her goals became, the more she saw food as fuel and not an enemy.

Less than 20 years after her first run, Anderson had become a multiple record holder. In 2008, she became the fastest woman to run the length of Great Britain, from John o' Groats in Scotland to Land's End in England (JOGLE), a distance of 1,407 kilometers (874.3 miles). In 2010, she broke the female record for distance running on a treadmill in a week: she ran 648 kilometers (402.6 miles) in seven days, on two hours' sleep a night. In 2011, she became ▶

▶ the fastest woman to run a double crossing of the Badwater 135 ultramarathon, which takes runners from California's sole-melting Death Valley to an altitude of 2,552 meters (8,373 feet). Anderson finished the round trip more than 21 hours' faster than the previous women's world-record holder. She has also run through deserts in Morocco, Libya, Namibia, and Chile.

The conditions for Anderson's most memorable race were the polar opposite. In 2007, she embarked for the Canadian Arctic to compete in the 6633 Ultra, which is essentially a human dogsled race without the dogs. The runners had nine days to cover 566 kilometers (352 miles) in a climate too tough for trees to grow. It is a self-sufficient, nonstop race, meaning sleep and survival are up to you. Many hallucinate. About two-thirds of the way into the race, Anderson felt a sinking feeling in her soul. Her father had been sick for some time. At that moment, she felt him die. "It feels as if you've been hit in the heart and it just went all the way down to my feet, and it came back up and I burst into tears," Anderson says. "I just remember looking up at the sky and saying, 'Dad, now is not a good time to die because if I cry, it's all going to freeze up.'" After the race, she tried to call her husband from an Arctic landline. Wrong number. She only knew one other number—her mother's. "Somebody out there was saying, 'You don't need to get hold of your husband, you actually need to get hold of your mother,'" Anderson says. Her mother confirmed that her father died within minutes of her moment of intuition. Anderson finished with a course record, nonetheless.

Anderson's most ambitious feat—perhaps the most ambitious feat of any female runner—came in the fall of 2017. She planned to run across America, from Los Angeles to New York City—a distance of 4,586 kilometers (2,850 miles). Her goal was to finish in 53 days. If she was successful, she would beat the 1979 record by more than two weeks. In running terms, that's about two marathons a day for nearly two months. In layman's terms, it's unfathomable. Anderson spent several years planning the route and getting money together to bring a small team to the U.S. On top of that, she raised money for two charities—Marie Curie, an organization that provides care and support for people with terminal illnesses and their families, and Free to Run, which uses adventure sports to help to empower women and girls, and develop their leadership skills, in regions of conflict.

Anderson's body, too, said *no more*. Forty days into her run, she was forced to see a doctor. For more than a week she had endured bone-grinding pain in her right knee. "My knee was going more and more in, sort of like a V," says Anderson. "That affected my back and I was leaning over to the left. I looked a real state." Morphine could only do so much. She had to make a choice: continue and risk knee-replacement surgery or drop out. After 3,568 kilometers (2,217 miles), Anderson's running shoes came to a halt and never touched American soil again.

Facing a lengthy absence from running, Anderson returned to England and entered a blue period. Her injury compounded the grief of not having finished the race across the U.S. Imagine a monk being robbed of meditation. She grew irritable and again found herself counting calories. "I do what my physio tells me to do,

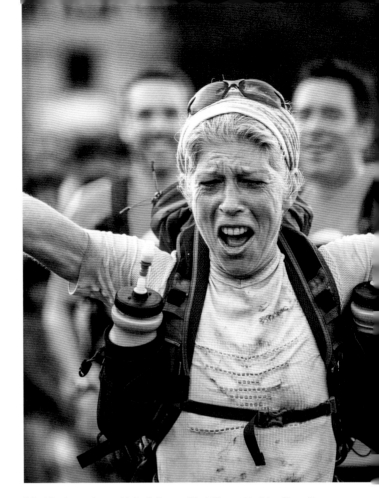

Mimi Anderson is a multiple Guinness World Record holder. She still holds the record for the fastest crossing of Ireland on foot, running from Malin Head to Mizen Head in 3 days 15 hours 36 minutes, in September 2012.

but my husband would always say, 'I wish you'd find something else because you're getting really moody and quite grumpy,'" Anderson says.

She found something else almost immediately, however. A year after her injury, 10 years after achieving her JOGLE world record, Anderson cycled from Land's End to John o' Groats. She finished in nine days. A year later she biked from Vancouver to the Mexican border. Most recently, she cycled 400 kilometers (249 miles) for charity on her turbo trainer. Next, she plans to bike with a friend across Southern Africa, from Namibia to Mozambique. During the most recent charity ride, Anderson watched episodes of the Netflix show *After Life*. Is cycling her afterlife, her life after running? "Five years ago, a friend said to me, 'What are you going to do if you can't run anymore?'" Anderson says. "I thought, I can always cycle if necessary." And if that's no longer possible? "I'll invent something." No need to yet. She has a 23-kilometer (14.3-mile) run planned for a week after we speak. ∎

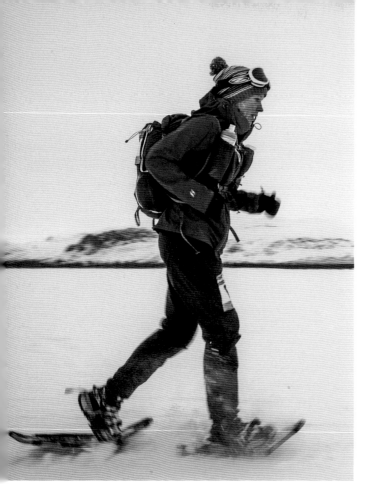

"When I got to the end ... I felt a million dollars. It was like my feet had been given a pair of wings and I could fly. I went around like the Cheshire cat. And that stays with you for days."

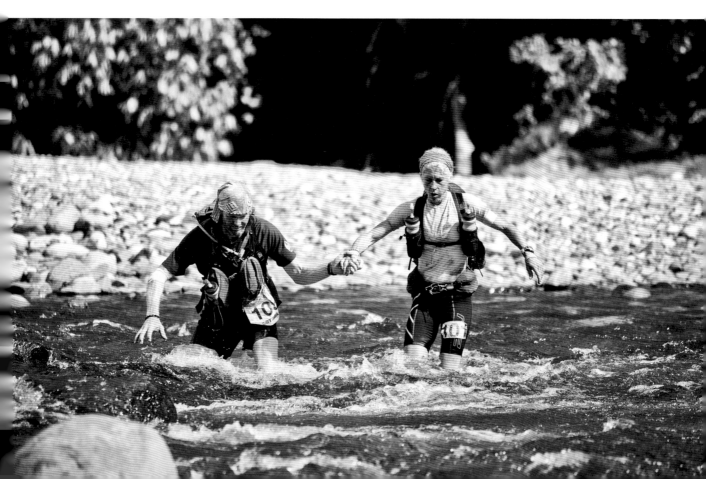

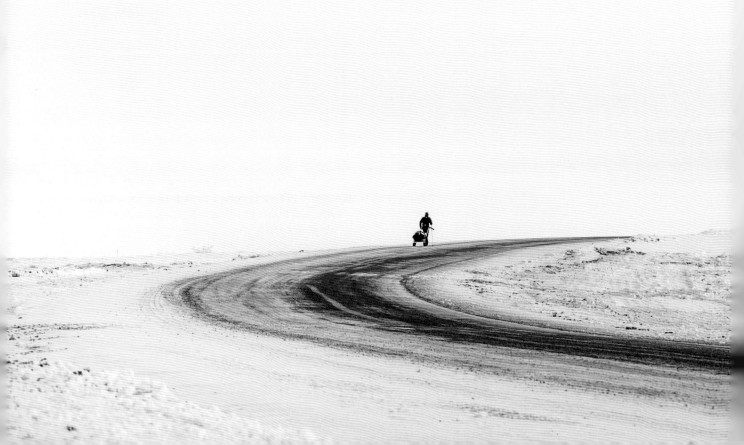

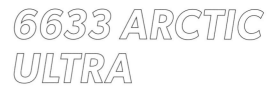

6633 ARCTIC ULTRA

Running long distances in the Yukon territory is brutal. The harder it is, the better it feels to finish. Dragging a sled 612 kilometers (380 miles) across terrain that includes ice roads in nine days, or 193 kilometers (120 miles) in three, is not always fun. The Yukon will either eat you up and spit you out, or you'll grow to respect it in ways you never imagined.

The 6633 Arctic Ultra is regarded, and respected, by many as the toughest footrace on the planet.

It is the brainchild of Welshman Martin Like, who created the race in 2007 and continues as its director today, assisted by his wife (and fellow ultra runner) Sue, and business partner Stuart Thornhill. The three share a passion for demanding running—for pushing themselves and other participants beyond the limits of what they thought possible; accordingly, this is a staggeringly difficult run, without support or stops. Each entrant must complete his or her chosen course carrying—or more accurately, pulling—all the supplies required for the duration. Assistance from anyone outside the official race support team is forbidden.

Two courses are available, both crossing the line of the Arctic Circle. The starting point is the Eagle Plains Hotel—an already ▶

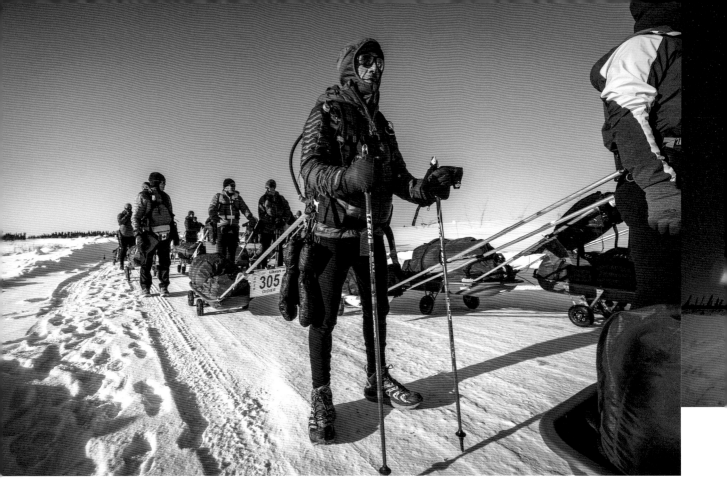

Above: participants assemble before the start of the race. On average, of the 20 or so runners who take part in the full course, more than half fail to complete it.

▶ remote location, 362 kilometers (225 miles) north of the Klondike Highway in northern Yukon. This "oasis" is the last stop for bed, food, and fuel before Fort McPherson, a First Nations hamlet nearly 193 kilometers (120 miles) north. This is the finish line for those running the shorter version of the race, but only checkpoint three out of eight for those attempting the full 612 kilometers (380 miles) to Tuktoyaktuk, a community in the Inuvialuit Settlement Region, on the banks of the Arctic Ocean.

On starting the race, with the beautiful Richardson Mountains in view, racers descend approximately 10 kilometers (6.2 miles) to a bridge at Eagle River, then begin the ascent—steep at first—to the emergency (occasionally used) airstrip on Dempster Highway. On reaching the first checkpoint, at 712 meters (2,336 feet) above sea level and right on the Arctic Circle, runners have already endured tough, hilly, notoriously windy terrain, but also some of the most beautiful and wildly remote scenery to be seen anywhere in the world.

Beyond the Arctic Circle, the mountainous course is consistently breathtaking, in every sense of the word. Hurricane Alley—a relatively open stretch running from the 50-kilometer (31-mile) point—is named for winds so strong that they can tip trucks over on the highway, and this is not even the hardest part of the race, with similarly extreme winds battering the ascent to Wright Pass, at 92 kilometers (57 miles).

Beyond Fort McPherson, where racers can shelter in the school hall, long sections of road, including a 121-kilometer (75-mile) section of ice road and the final 161-kilometer (100-mile) stretch of hard-packed forest trail, lead through some of the most desolate and remote, yet beautiful, landscape available to the ultra runner.

This is the extreme of extreme. Many attempt but few finish. ∎

Length: 193 or 612 km (120 or 380 mi)

Location: Yukon and Northwest Territories, Canada

Date: February

Type: trail/ice

Temperature Ø: -40–-25 °C (-40–-13 °F)

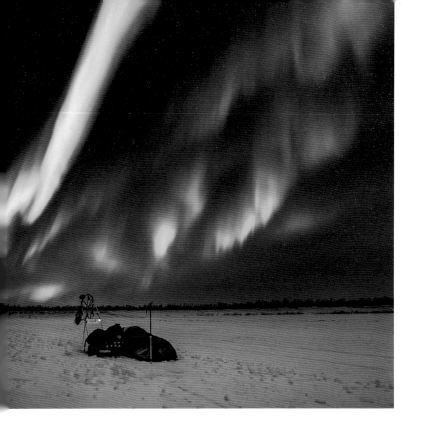

Beyond the Arctic Circle, the mountainous course is consistently breathtaking, in every sense of the word. Hurricane Alley is named for winds so strong that they can tip trucks over on the highway.

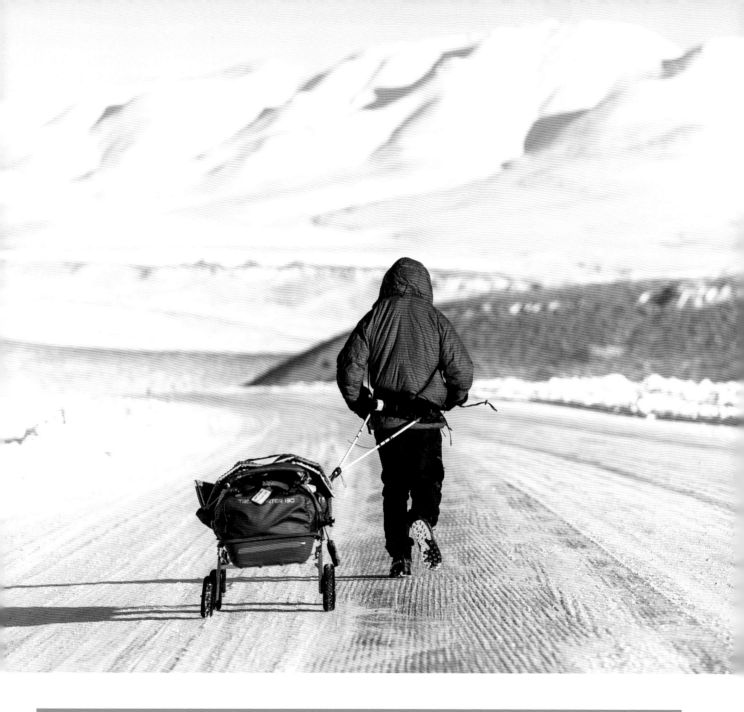

Beyond Fort McPherson, long sections of road, including a 121-kilometer (75-mile) section of ice road and the final 161-kilometer (100-mile) stretch of hard-packed forest trail, lead through some of the most desolate and remote, yet beautiful, landscape available to the ultra runner.

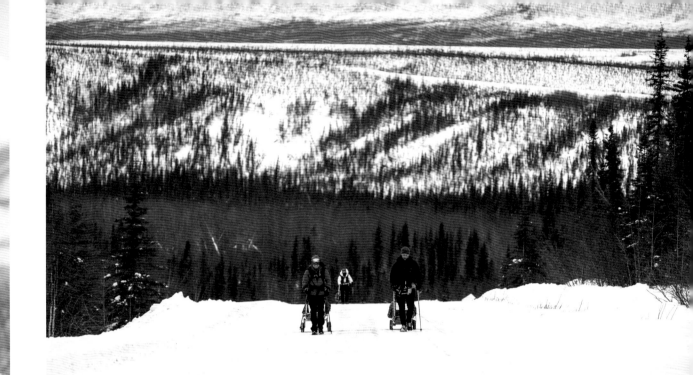

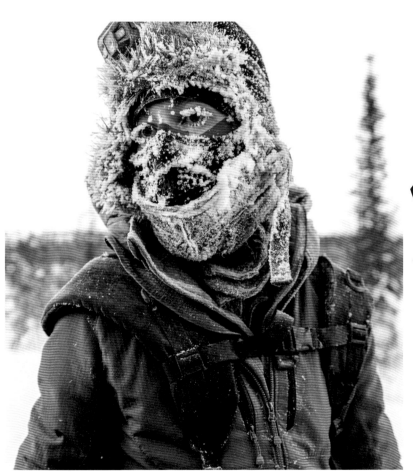

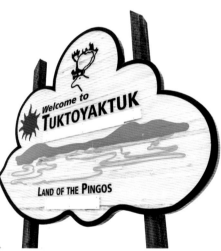

Above: destination Tuktoyaktuk!
Fewer than 50 race participants
have ever completed the full
course across the frozen Arctic
landscape. In 2018, Romanian
Tiberiu Uşeriu, set a new record
of completing the event in
172 hours 50 minutes.

Sights to Behold: Inspiring Runs Through History and Heritage

This collection of routes captures some of the most spectacular architectural, historical, and natural heritage in the world. From ancient Buddhist temples to the Bosphorus Bridge, and with stunning scenery along the way, these are for the runners who look up en route.

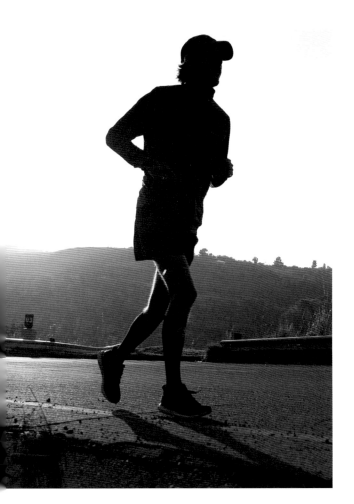

Opposite: the vibrant city of Antigua, with its colonial Spanish architecture, nestles on a plain that stretches out from the foothills of the Acatenango volcano. It's one of three volcanoes close to the city—two of them being active.

Antigua

In southern Guatemala lies the little gem of Antigua Guatemala city, also Antigua, known for its Spanish-influenced architecture. Its beauty has seen it awarded official Unesco World Heritage site status.

Run here and you won't be disappointed. The cobbled streets around Antigua make the run a little tricky, but you're rewarded with the Acatenango volcano as your stunning backdrop.

Weave in and out of the colorful archways, absorbing the local culture. It's easy to extend your cobbled 5-kilometer (3.1-mile) run to a full marathon distance if you venture out beyond the hills that circle the city. Be sure to take a backpack with water, as once you're out in the mountains, you'll need it! For an energy kick be sure to sample the finest coffee of Latin America. For a mid-run snack … Well, you're in the birthplace of chocolate, so it would be a shame not to taste it.

If you're feeling extra-ambitious, you could even take part in the Ultramaratón Guatemala—an official trail race 100 kilometers (62 miles) long.

Angkor Wat

This is an official Unesco World Heritage site, the largest religious monument in the world, and Cambodia's most famous landmark— you won't want to miss it.

Built in the twelfth century, this Buddhist temple complex covers an incredible 162.6 hectares (401.8 acres) of land, so you'll have plenty of routes to take, with every turn uncovering a new breathtaking view. Be sure to check out the 18-kilometer (11-mile) loop that takes you past the top three temple sites of this area: Angkor Wat, Bayon, and Ta Prohm.

Running this route at sunrise is advised: not only do the humidity and heat get pretty intense here during the rest of the day, but the sun rises behind the main temple, which is an incredible moment ▶

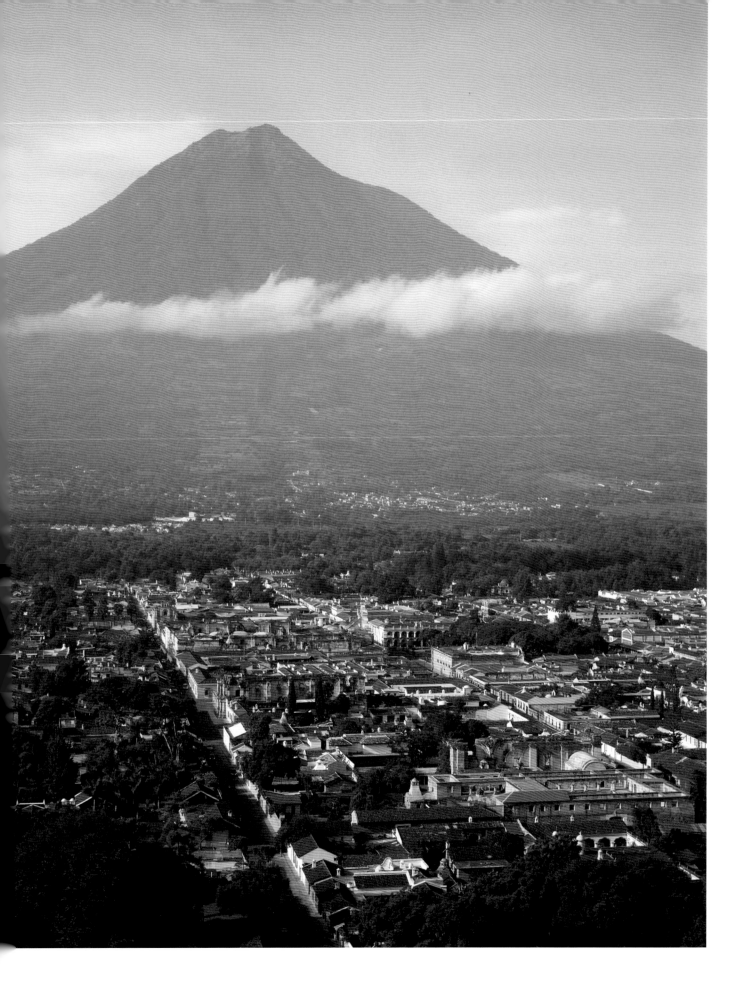

▶ to witness. As this is a sacred and religious site, shoulders and legs should be covered at all times, so running early also minimizes the risk of overheating and dehydration!

Maseru

Running anywhere in Lesotho is magical, but the barren lands of the Maseru region in the northwest are truly stunning. Backpackers and cyclists often spend weeks hiking and sleeping in shepherds' huts in order to experience the landscape.

Lesotho is a gem in Southern Africa. It is safe, accessible, and beautiful. For running on roads or trails, the country offers opportunities to train with heat and altitude. If you fly into the capital, Maseru, and walk in any direction, it won't be long before the mountains become your friends. There are cows, sheep, goats, pigs, and lots and lots of long, straight roads sweeping up and around the rocky valleys.

The high-altitude, landlocked kingdom is encircled by South Africa, and is crisscrossed by a network of rivers and mountain ranges, including the impressive peak of Thabana Ntlenyana (3,482 meters; 11,424 feet). On the Thaba Bosiu plateau, near Maseru, are ruins dating from the nineteenth-century reign of King Moshoeshoe I. Thaba Bosiu is overlooked by the iconic 1,532-meter (5,026-foot) peak Mount Qiloane, an enduring symbol of the nation's Basotho people. This is runnable from Maseru's airport.

Great Glen Way

The Great Glen Way is a trail that includes a number of Scotland's most important cultural and historic sights. A 125-kilometer (77.7-mile) route with plenty of ups, it takes you from the Old Fort at Fort William, which sits at the foot of Ben Nevis, to the historic city of Inverness, with its nearby Bronze Age cemetery, the Clava Cairns. Along the way, you'll have the chance to visit thirteenth-century Inverlochy Castle—the location for a battle both in 1431 and in 1645, during the English Civil War—the Spean Bridge Commando Memorial, and the Clansman Center, a living museum that gives you a taste of seventeenth-century life in the Highlands. With the ▶

Below: the Thaba Bosiu plateau, Lesotho, an area known for its sandstone escarpments, which form a natural "fortress" nearly 120 meters (394 feet) high above the surrounding plain. Opposite, top: the towers of Angkor Wat rise above the verdant Cambodian landscape.

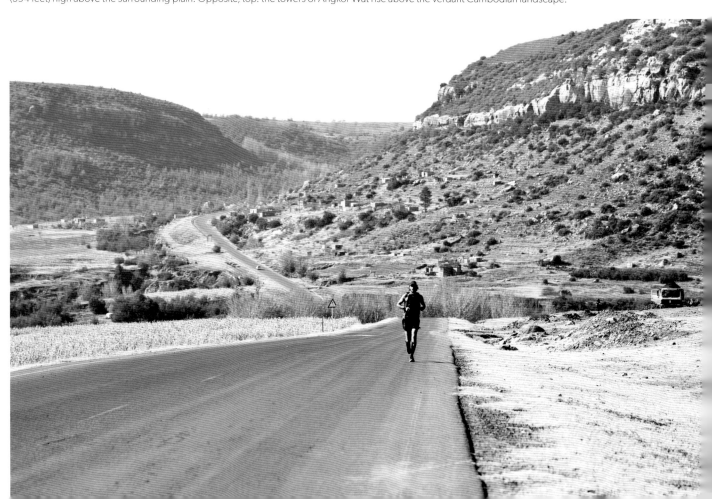

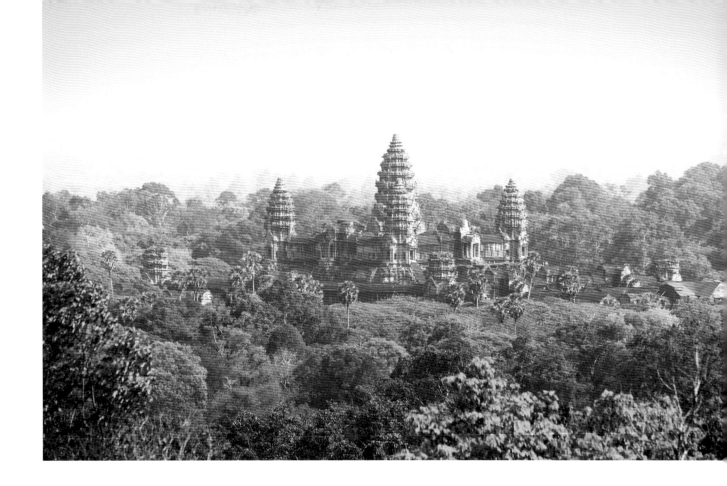

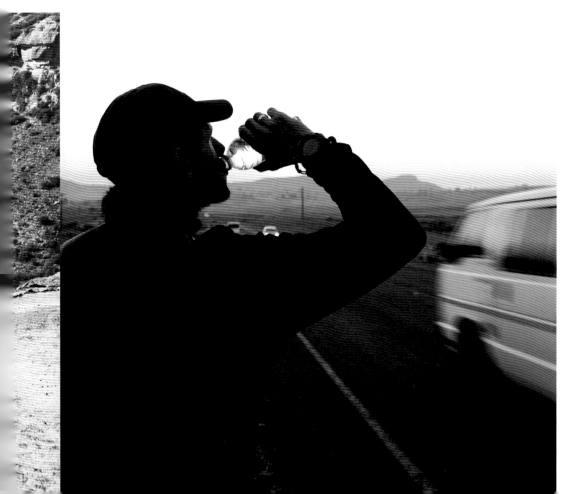

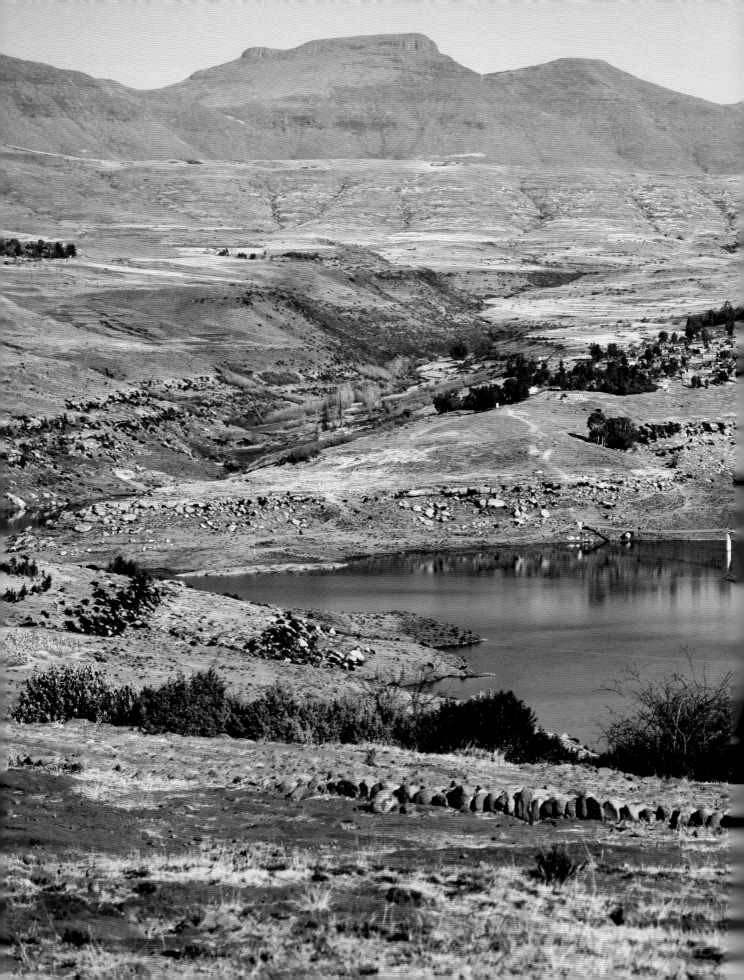

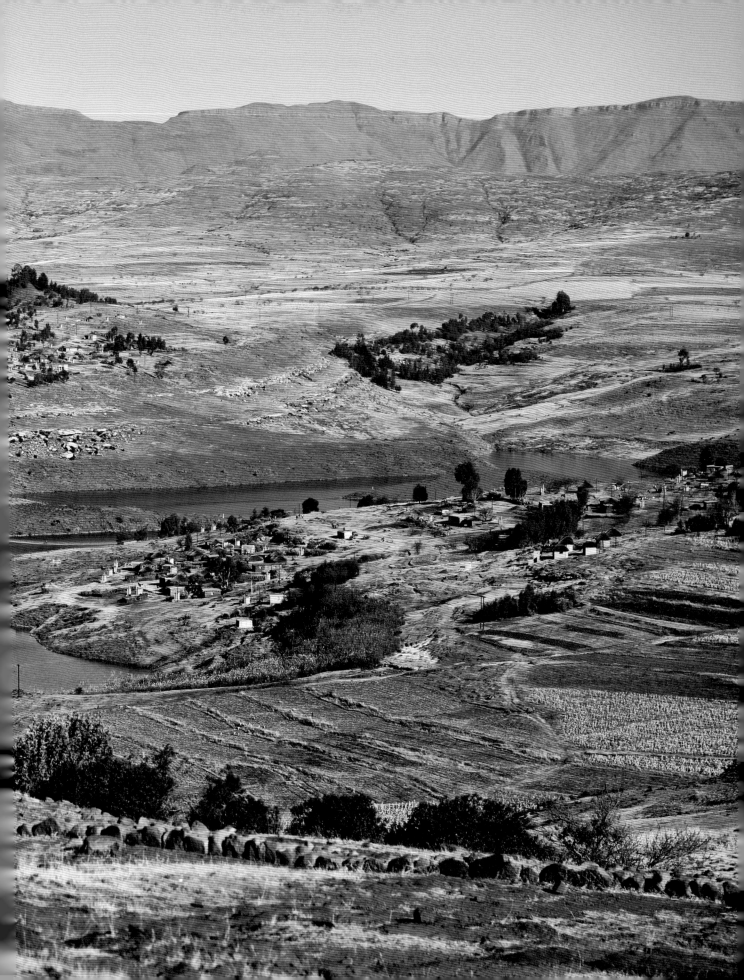

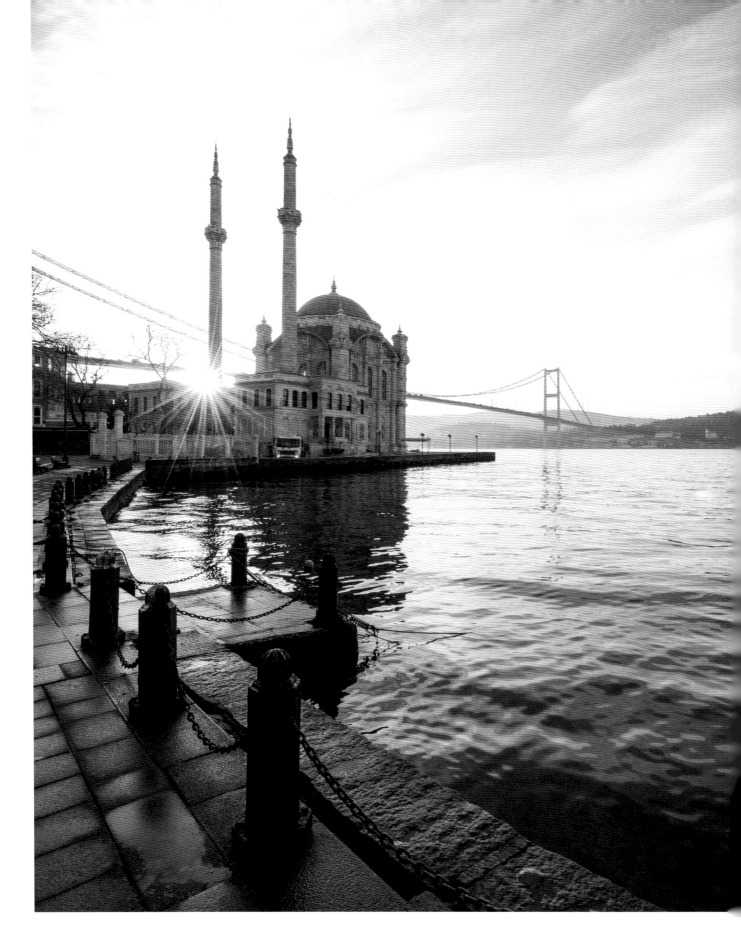

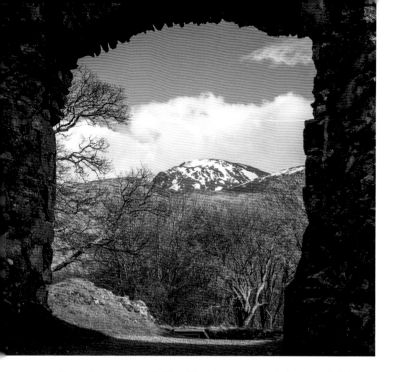

Above: the snowy peak of Ben Nevis as seen through the ruins of Old Inverlochy Castle. Opposite: Ortaköy Mosque, on the shores of the Bosphorus, Istanbul, with the Bosphorus Bridge in the background.

▶ option of camping anywhere you wish, this trail is also ideal for any ultra runner who likes to combine a bit of wilderness with their heritage, with the route leading you the lengths of Loch Lochy and Loch Oich, as well as the forests above Loch Ness. You're even allowed fires in many places; just be sure to bring insect repellent and a mosquito head net in summer.

You'll pass many a walker, hiker, camper, and runner on your way. Be sure to say hello: the Scottish are a friendly bunch and will not hesitate to help you with directions.

Istanbul

Run in the magical meeting place of Asia and Europe, where natural and cultural beauties combine. From its bustling bazaars, to the famous Blue Mosque and the Hagia Sophia, this city will present new wonders at every turn, and offers great running options if you're there for a short break.

If you're staying in the old town, early-morning runs down to the waterfront will be accompanied by the call to prayer and you'll be rewarded with the sight of the Golden Horn and Bosphorus Bridge. Look out for welcoming waves from the locals, too.

The waterfront is the best place to run in Istanbul, but for something with a climb, head to Çamlıca Hill, and for woods and trails, the expansive Belgrad Forest is just a short drive north of the city. If you have time to spare, hop over to Büyükada Island, which is accessible by ferry; there is a 11.8-kilometer (7.3-mile) loop around it.

Heritage Runs: The Basics

Antigua
Guatemala
Route:
Antigua old town
Distance:
varies

Angkor Wat
Siem Reap, Cambodia
Route:
Angkor Wat–Bayon–Ta Prohm
Distance:
18 km (11 mi)

Maseru
Lesotho
Route:
Maseru airport–Thaba Bosiu
Distance:
25 km (15.5 mi)

Great Glen Way
Scottish Highlands, U. K.
Route:
Fort William–Inverness
Distance:
125 km (77.7 mi)

Istanbul
Turkey
Route:
waterfront; Çamlıca Hill;
Belgrad Forest; Büyükada Island
Distance:
varies

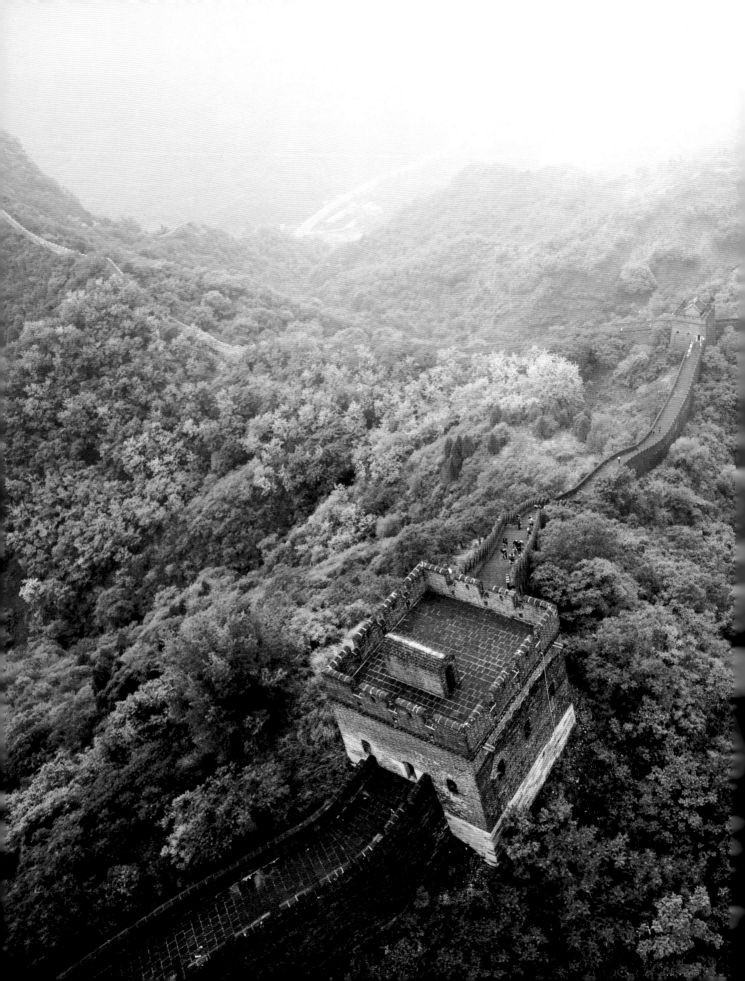

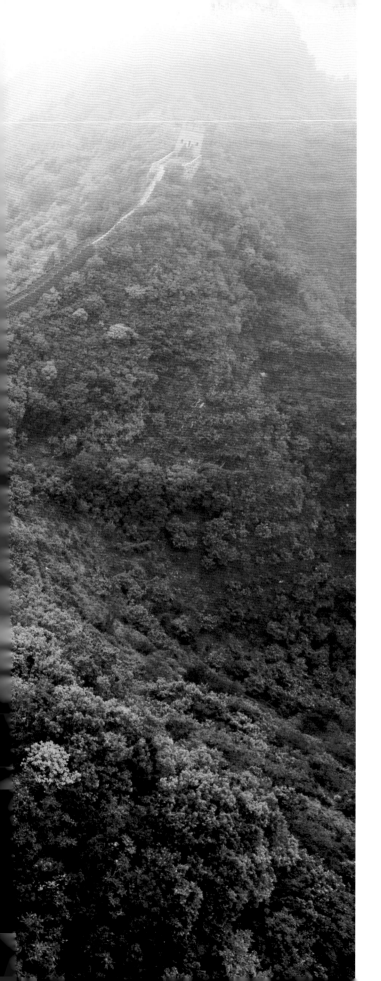

GREAT WALL MARATHON

If visiting Beijing and experiencing the culture isn't enough, go a "step" further. Run a grueling marathon along the magnificent Great Wall of China! This special race offers a unique perspective, taking participants through rural villages and China's lush countryside, all while running along or next to the Great Wall.

A sell-out event that has welcomed more than 25,000 runners since its launch in 1999, this run is monumental in every sense of the word. It is not only one of the world's most popular marathons (participants from 68 nations took part in 2019) but, arguably, one of the most demanding, with more than 5,000 steps of the Great Wall to climb. Runners follow a route along a highway, rough tracks, and, of course, the ancient wall itself. While parts of the course have been restored, much remains in its original state, meaning that runners have to scramble over loose and missing stones and crumbling, overgrown areas of the wall, navigating extreme sections of ascent and descent. If you're looking for a challenge steeped in history—with an emphasis on "steep"—look no further.

Entrants are young and old, a mixed bunch far removed from the team of 350 Danish athletes who first attempted a Great Wall ▶

It is not only one of the world's most popular marathons (participants from 68 nations took part in 2019) but, arguably, one of the most demanding, with more than 5,000 steps of the Great Wall to climb.

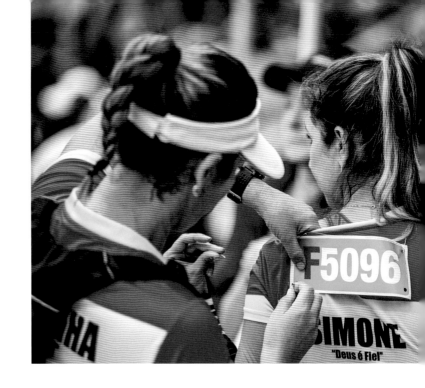

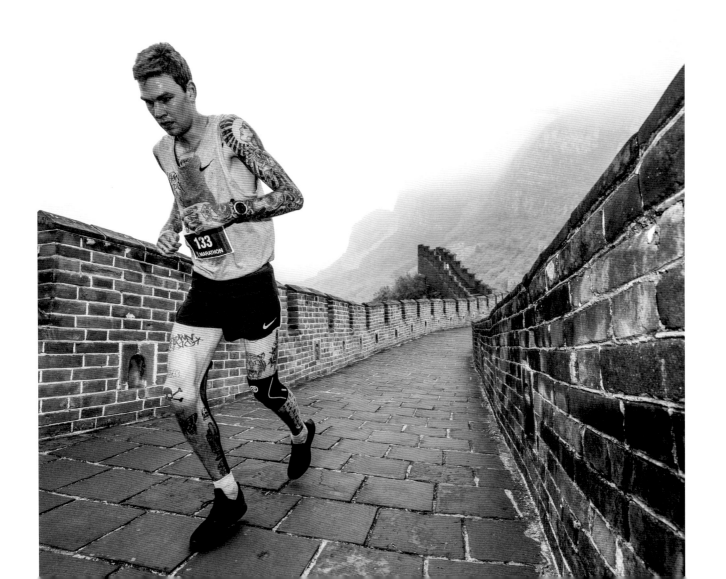

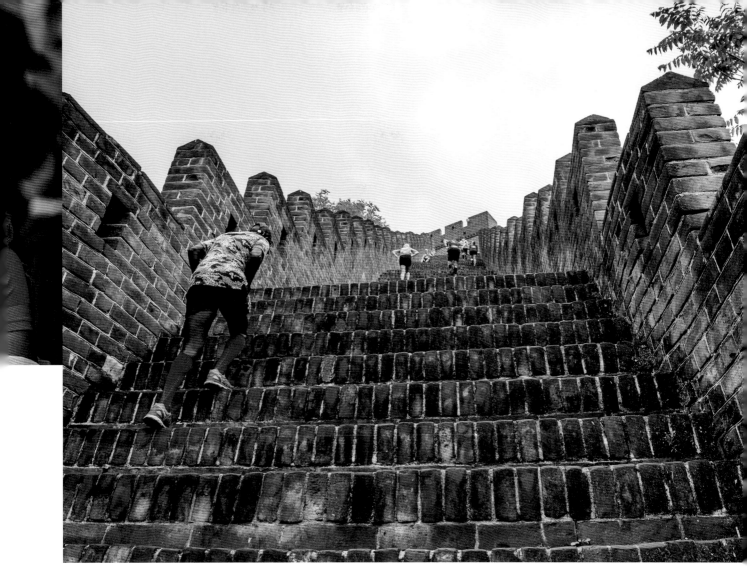

The race is uphill from the start, with the first of the 5,164 steps kicking in at about 5 kilometers (3 miles). From this point, the course follows a 3-kilometer (1.8-mile) stretch of the Great Wall, including 1 kilometer (0.6 miles) around the magnificent Huangyaguan fortress itself.

▶ marathon in 1999 (some things remain constant, however—Dane Henrik Brandt has taken part in every race in the marathon's 20-year history!). They can choose from three distances, all of which start and end in the Yin and Yang Square of the Huangyaguan fortress section of the wall. Participants in the full marathon pass through this square twice over the course of the race, looping over a section of the wall itself twice also and enjoying the breathtaking views of the lush, green landscape, with the wall appearing as a single vein ahead and behind. The course's lower section, through farmland and small villages, often has a festive atmosphere, with local onlookers cheering on participants; don't take too long admiring the view or taking selfies with supporters, though—there's an eight-hour time limit and a flight to catch. Those steps won't climb themselves.

Be aware that, as an international runner looking to take part, you must sign up for a tour package, as only Chinese nationals are eligible for an entry package that covers just the race. These six- or seven-day packages include transport, accommodation, and sightseeing, and will enable you to make the most of racing in this exciting historic region. ■

Length: 8.5, 21.1, or 42.2 km (5.3, 13.1, or 26.2 mi)

Location: Huairou District, China

Date: May

Type: trail/steps

Temperature Ø: 16–35 °C (61–95 °F)

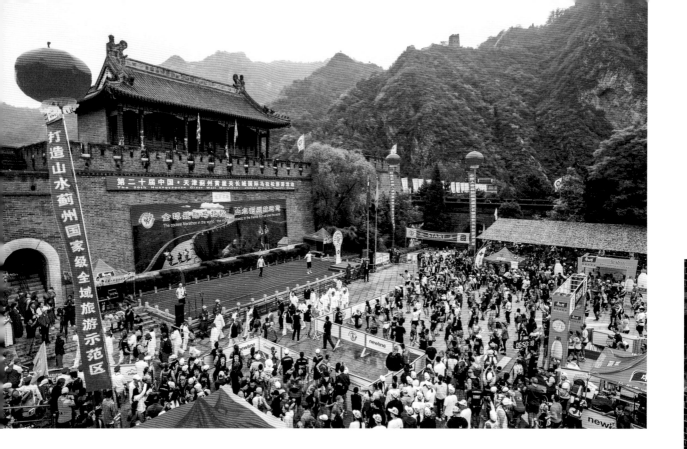

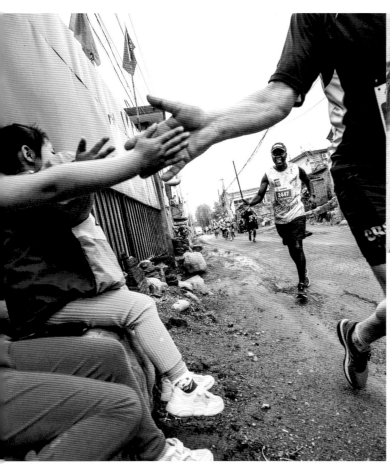

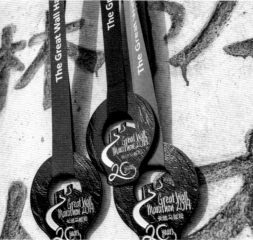

All races follow a loop that starts and ends at Yin and Yang Square and results are posted up in the square as the races unfold. All runners will receive a medal after crossing the finish line—with a green ribbon for the fun run, a red one for the half-marathon, and black for the full marathon.

The course's lower section, through farmland and small villages, often has a festive atmosphere, with local onlookers cheering on participants; don't take too long admiring the view or taking selfies with supporters, though—there's an eight-hour time limit.

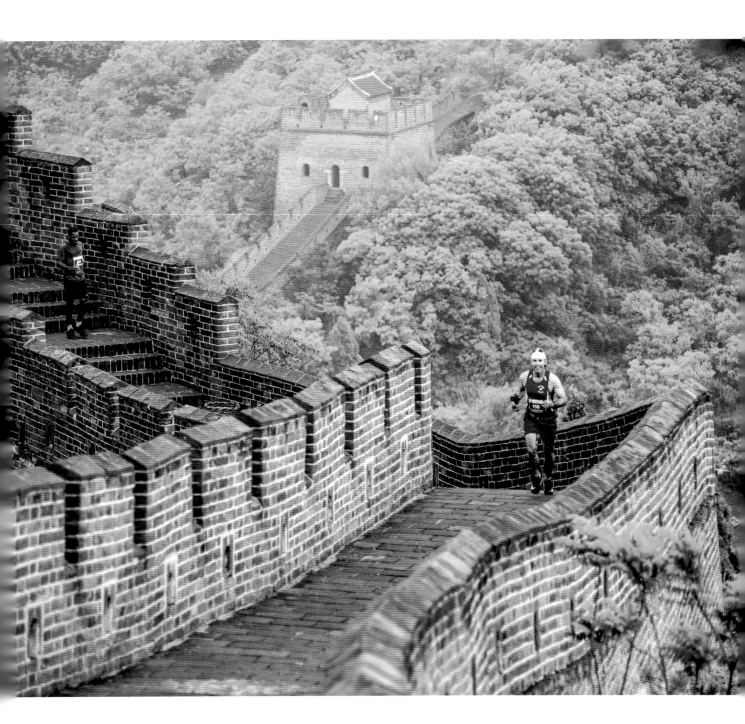

BAGAN TEMPLE MARATHON

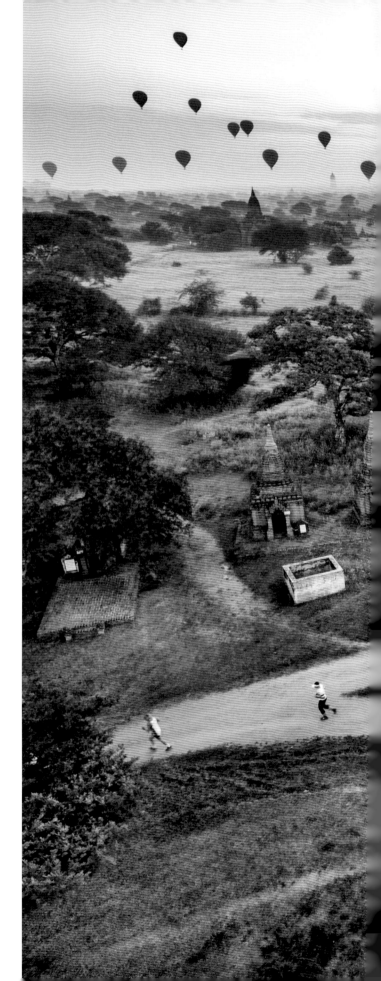

Run 42.2 kilometers (26.2 miles) and see more than 2,000 temples along the way. From being greeted by hordes of high-fiving local kids along the way, to letting your mind wander off into history, it's easy to forget you're in a race. The Bagan Temple Marathon takes you through, past, and around some of Myanmar's most sacred monuments.

Rarely in a race, or indeed in life, will you start your day in a building more than 1,000 years old. Built during the reign of King Htilominlo, in the early-thirteenth century, the temple that takes this monarch's name is both the start and finish line for the Bagan Temple Marathon. This historic structure sets the tone for a run of beauty, history, and culture, taking place in a breathtaking and relatively little-visited landscape.

Bagan, in central Myanmar, is a Unesco World Heritage site—an ancient city on a verdant plain that is cut through by the Ayeyarwady River. More than 3,500 recorded monuments—mostly temples and stupas—survive and are evidence of the glory of the Bagan kingdom, at its height between the eleventh and thirteenth centuries. Buddhist frescoes, carvings, and sculptures can all still be seen in these highly decorative structures. As you begin your run, ▶

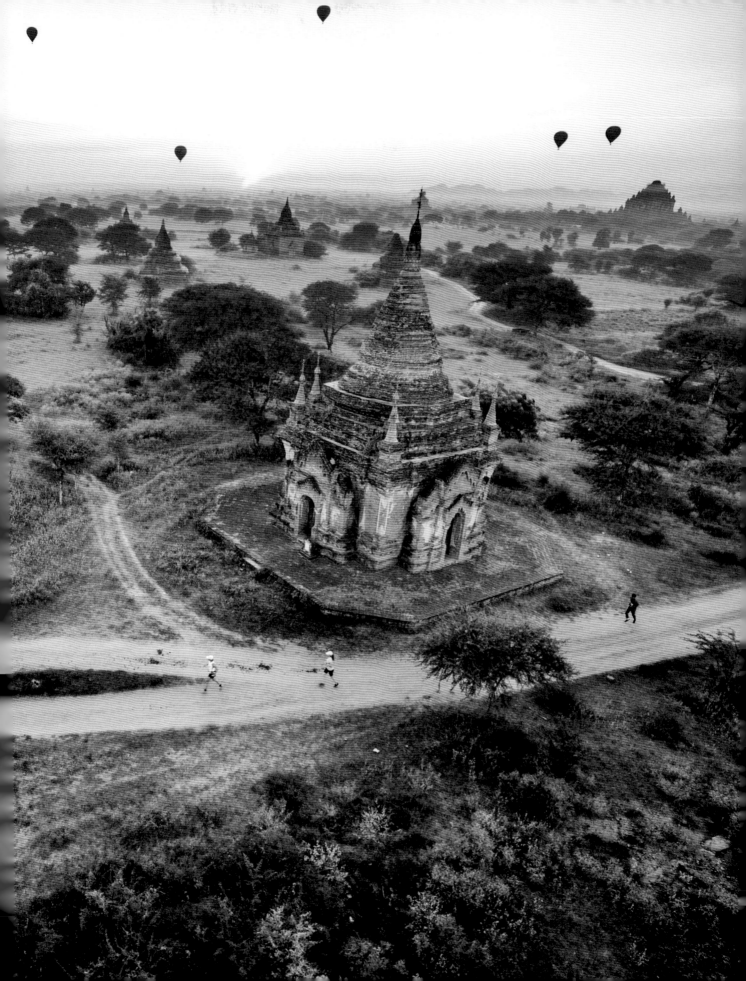

Be extra-prepared for mass attacks of high-fiving children decked out in their festive clothing waiting to say hello. It's a place where you'll forget about running and be lost in the new and unknown, marveling at every spectacle.

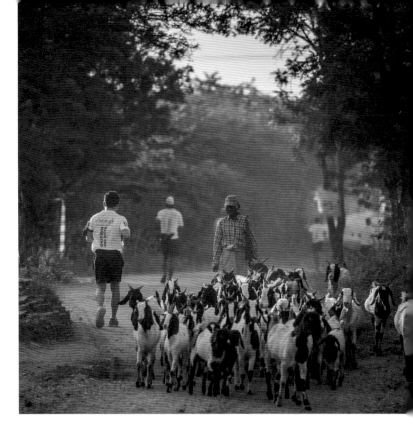

Village life continues for locals as the race courses through fields dotted with stupas. In every village, children wait eagerly to greet the runners passing through; some participants might even encounter a local drover with his herd of goats.

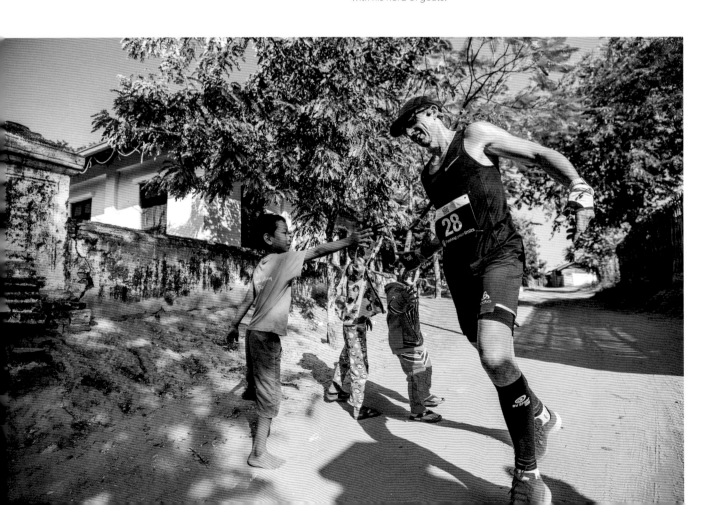

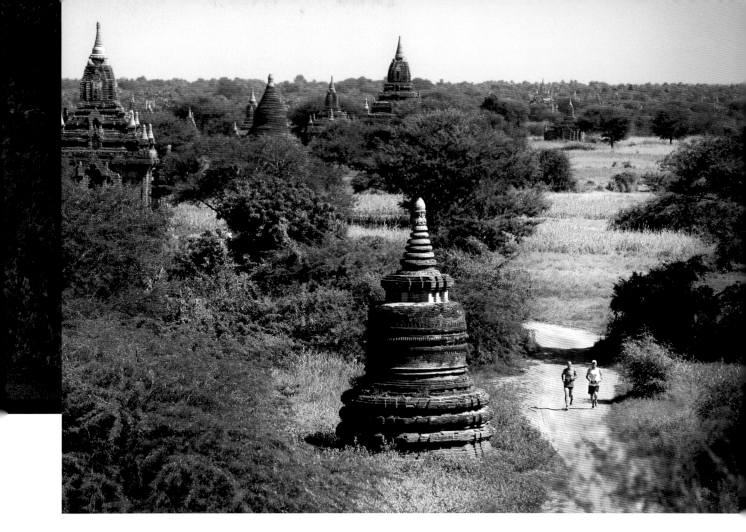

▶ you may experience one of the clear, beautiful sunrises of this region, the tops of pagodas bathed in deep purple and orange light and casting long, drawn-out shadows toward the horizon.

The hot and dusty conditions mean that, despite there being no mountains or ravines to navigate, this is nevertheless a challenging run. The weather in November is hot and humid, with temperatures reaching highs of approximately 30° Celsius (86° Fahrenheit)—this is not a marathon for those who favor fancy dress. Light and breathable apparel is advised. The sun is the only adversary on a course otherwise distinguished by beautiful scenery, friendly locals, and a truly mystical atmosphere—be sure to prepare, so that you can enjoy the experience to its fullest.

Sights shared by all runners—even those on the 10-kilometer (6.2-mile) course—include the 51-meter-tall (167-foot) Ananda Temple, while the twelfth-century Dhammayazika Pagoda, whose three brick terraces are decorated with terracotta tiles telling stories from the lives of the Buddha, comes just before those doing the half-marathon and marathon split. For those taking on the longest distance, running on the main tracks ends after just 10 kilometers into the course race. All marathoners turn off the normal roads and head into what feels like a different realm. They will pass ox carts laden with grain, traveling steadily on the sandy tracks, as farmers tend to their fields of rice and peanuts. Be extra-prepared for mass

attacks of high-fiving children decked out in their festive clothing waiting to say hello. It's a place where you'll forget about running and be lost in the new and unknown, marveling at every spectacle.

At the halfway point, runners enter the beautiful village of Nyaungdo, where they are back on dirt trails for a short span. Tuyin Taung Pagoda can be seen to the right as you proceed on these trails to the dam. Built in 1059, by King Anawrahta, this glittering golden monument is said to enshrine a relic of the Buddha.

Past the 30-kilometer (18.6-mile) mark, you may be cheered on by the residents of East Pwazaw as you enter the last stretch of the race; it may be a tiny village, but the voices here are mighty and sure to give you the boost of energy needed to get back to the finish. ∎

Length: 10, 21.1, or 42.2 km (6.2, 13.1, or 26.2 mi)

Location: Bagan, Myanmar

Date: November

Type: trail/mountainous

Temperature Ø: up to 30 °C (86 °F)

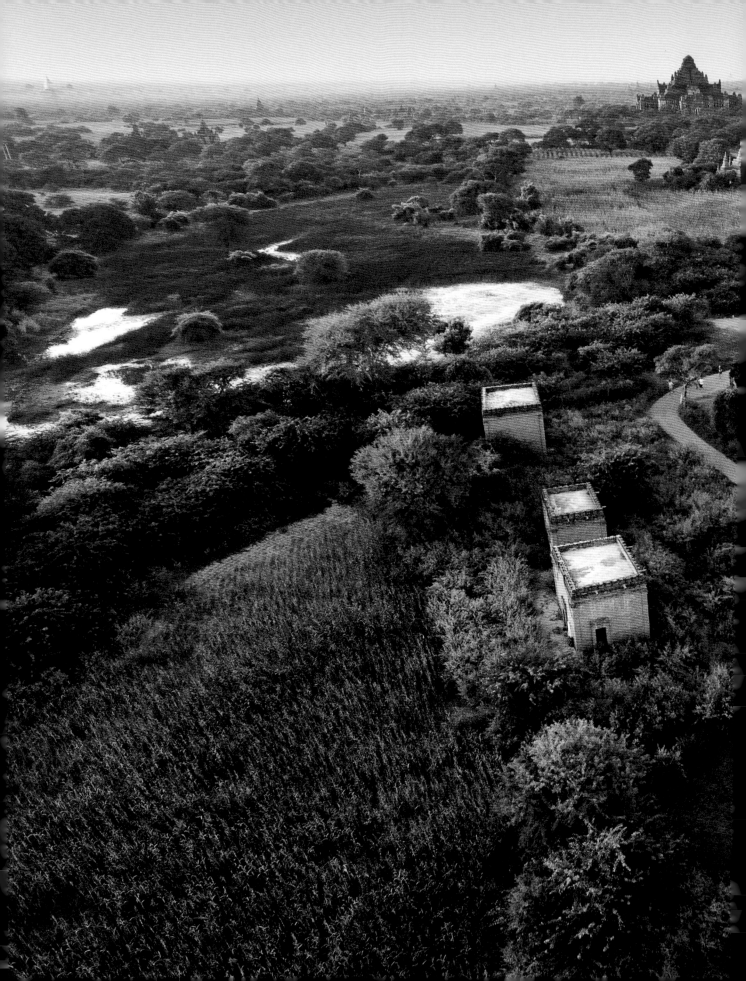

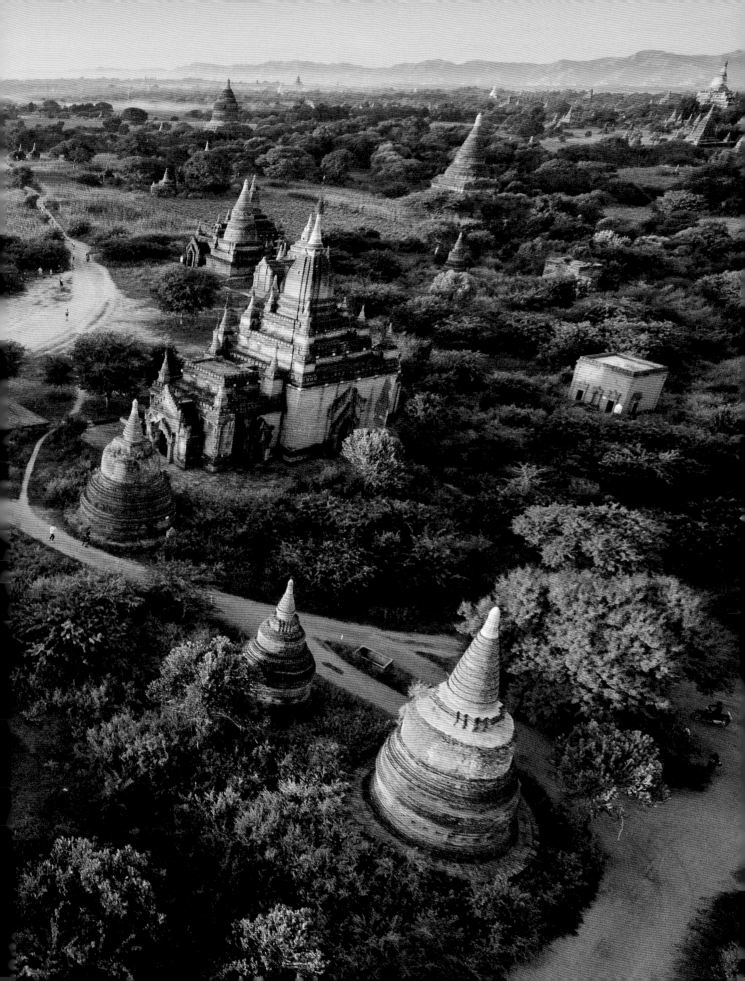

The sun is the only adversary on a course otherwise distinguished by beautiful scenery, friendly locals, and a truly mystical atmosphere—be sure to prepare, so that you can enjoy the experience to its fullest.

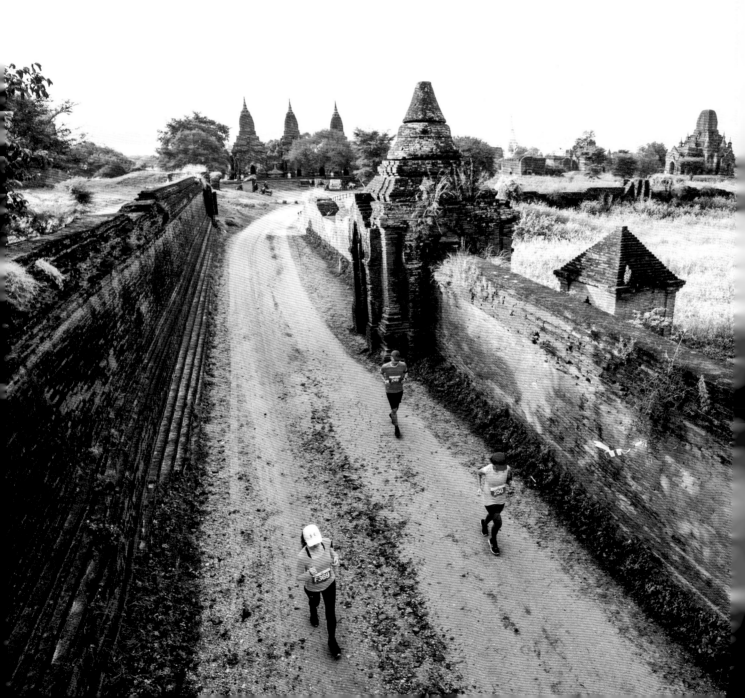

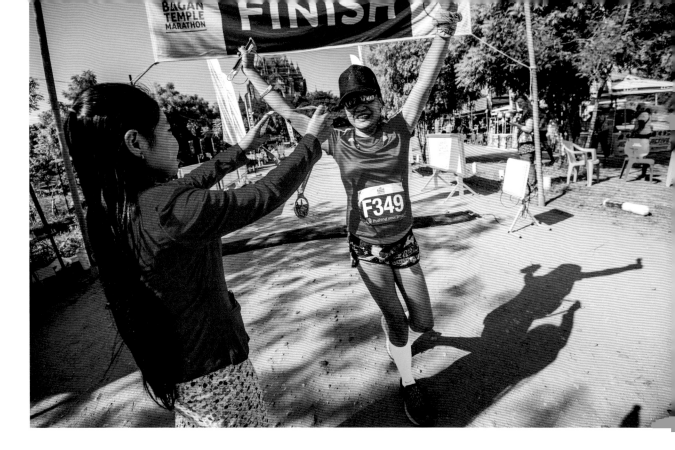

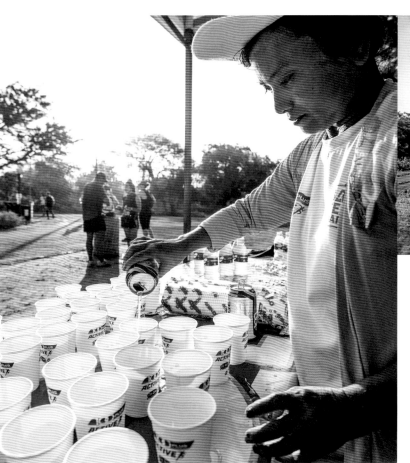

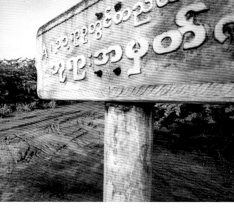

Above: as runners cross the finish line they are rewarded with a medal and cold refreshments. Previous page: both the marathon and half-marathon trail past six temples in total—Dhammayazika Pagoda can be seen on the horizon.

ULTRA X JORDAN

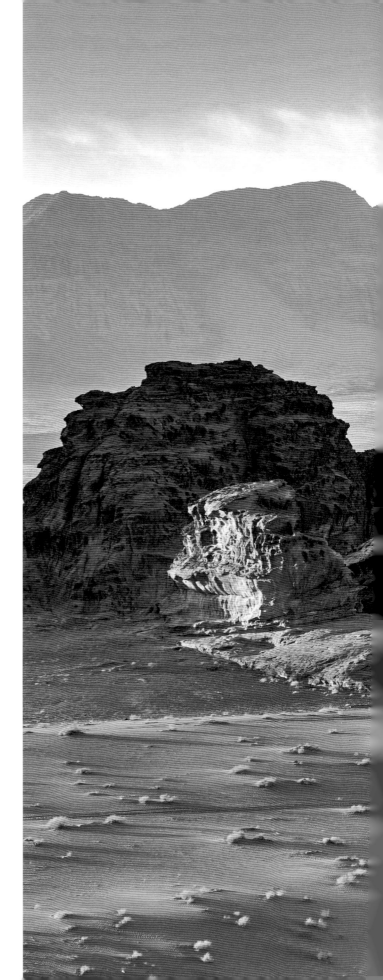

With 2,522 meters (8,274 feet) of elevation over 250 kilometers (155 miles) of desert, this could be a run that sounds too brutal to attempt. In fact, the temperatures are surprisingly bearable, and the desert is far from an abandoned wilderness. The rock formations towering into the sky will make you want to stop for photos every five minutes.

Let Jordan surprise you, punish you, and enrich your soul. More than 250 kilometers (155 miles) of running, with highs of 34° Celsius (94° Fahrenheit), over five days, in a truly beautiful desert setting—this is an all-time favourite for many runners.

Ultra X Jordan, previously known as the Wadi Rum Ultra, takes place in southern Jordan, to the east of Aqaba. Petroglyphs and inscriptions here are evidence of human habitation of the region stretching back into prehistory, though it is best known to present-day Western travelers for its connection with T. E. Lawrence, aka Lawrence of Arabia. Much of David Lean's 1962 film of that name was filmed on location here, and one of the dramatic rock formations of the region is named the Seven Pillars of Wisdom, after Lawrence's memoir. Wadi Rum itself is the largest wadi (dry watercourse) in the country, and is a dramatic setting for this race. Known as the ▶

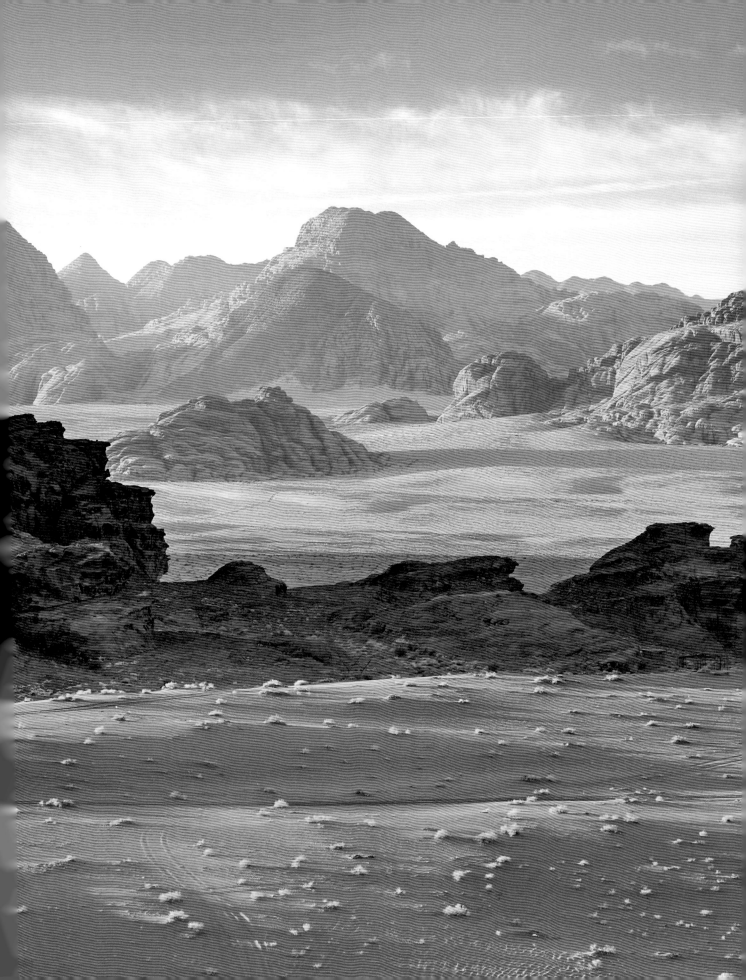

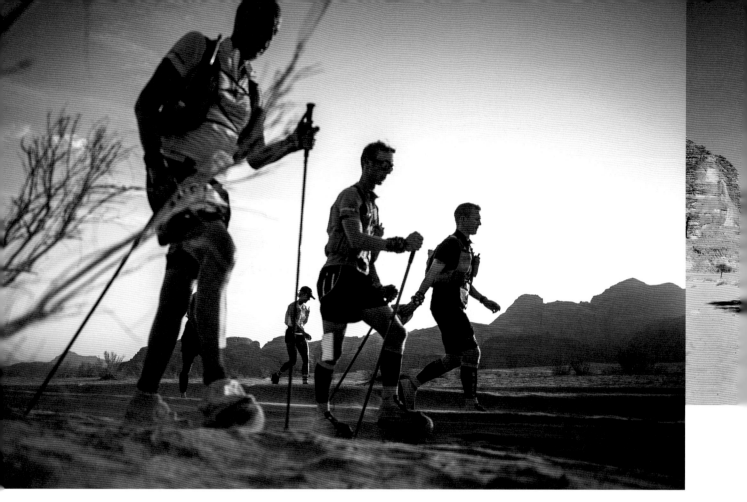

The Wadi Rum's "Valley of the Moon" nickname comes from the fact that the landscape is characterized by unique towering rock formations, that have been sculpted by erosion over many thousands of years. It's a barren desert terrain with little vegetation.

▶ Valley of the Moon, it is part of a unique landscape of sand dunes, historic sites, and other incredible wadis.

The ultra itself brings the challenges of a tough distance run combined with some level of relief and comfort, so that it is enjoyable rather than simply endurable. The nighttime campsites are staffed by medical-team members (who are also present along the course) as well as physiotherapists, and hot water is available. Your bags and supplies are also transported between the camps each day, so that there is no need to carry a week's worth of supplies on your back while you run.

An egalitarian race ethos means that competitors at all levels of experience are welcome, with walking as well as running expected. Entrants arrive in Amman two days ahead of the race start and take part in a welcome session, safety briefings, and kit checks, before being transferred to the Wadi Rum desert and their first campsite. From Monday to Friday, runners will camp in the desert at night and run across the landscape by day, with stages varying between 30 and 80 kilometers (19 and 50 miles) in length; Wednesday is the "long stage," starting and (for some) ending by the light of the moon.

Friday evening sees the big finish-line celebrations, including a barbecue round the campfire and a prize-giving and awards ceremony with local entertainment.

All good things, sadly, must come to an end, and Saturday sees participants transferred back to Amman, though not before they spend a couple of hours exploring the ancient city of Petra, a Unesco World Heritage site. It is this combination of physical challenge and new experiences in remarkable places that characterizes both this race and the wider series of which it is a part—the Ultra X. It's a good balance. ∎

Length: 250 km (155 mi)

Location: Wadi Rum, Jordan

Date: October

Type: trail/multi-stage

Temperature Ø: 24–34 °C (75.2–93.2 °F)

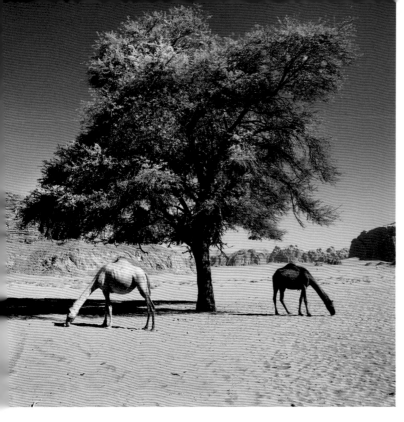

Wadi Rum itself is the largest wadi (dry watercourse) in the country, and is a dramatic setting for this race. Known as the Valley of the Moon, it is part of a unique landscape of sand dunes, historic sites, and other incredible wadis.

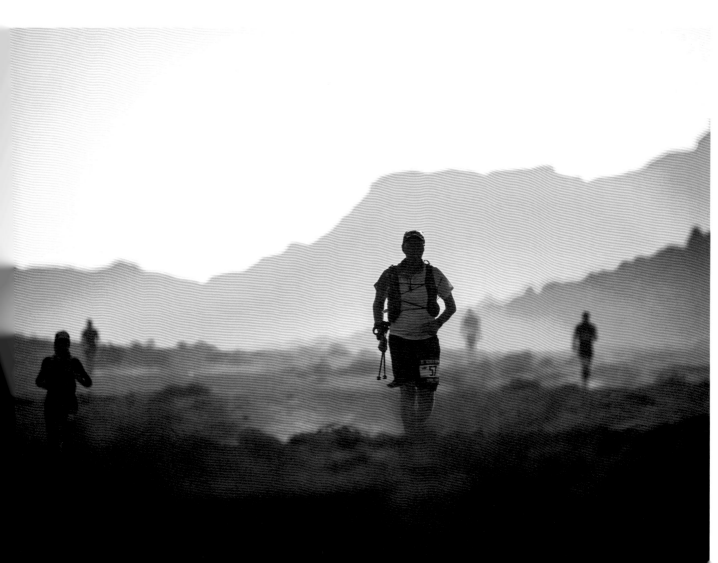

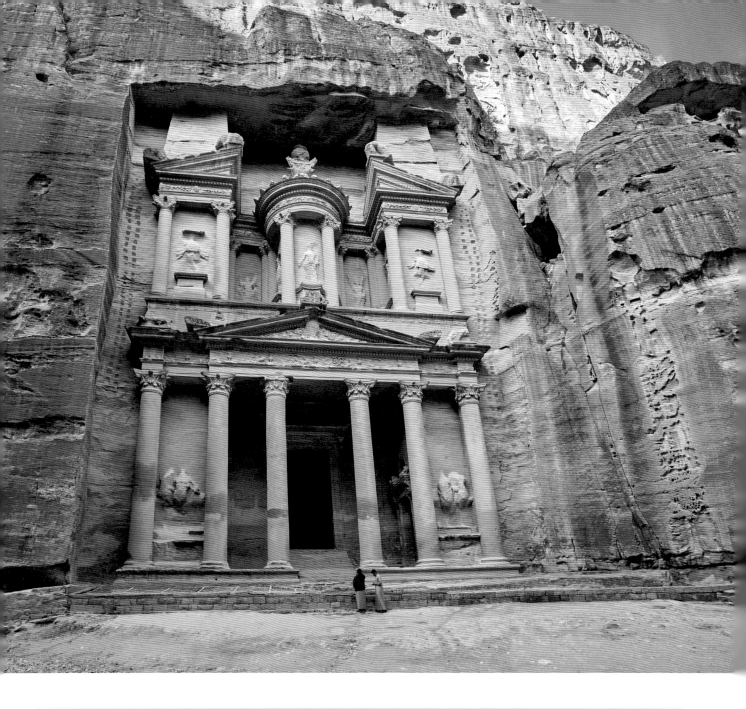

It is this combination of physical challenge and new experiences in remarkable places that characterizes both this race and the wider series of which it is a part—the Ultra X.

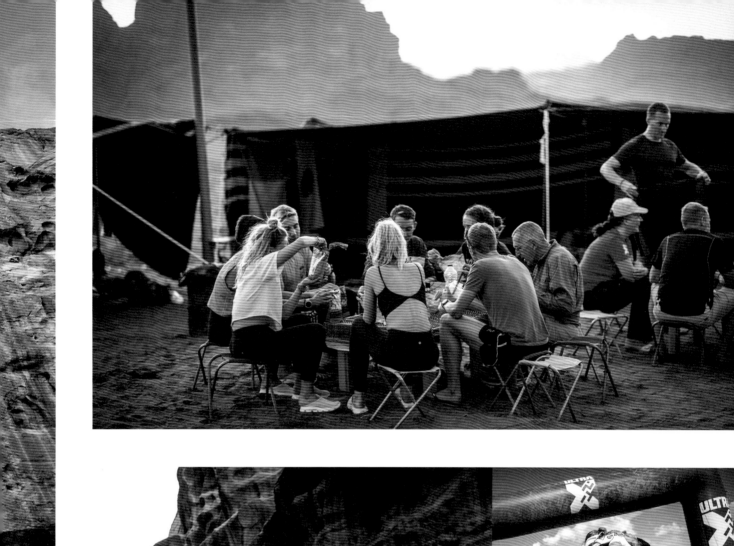

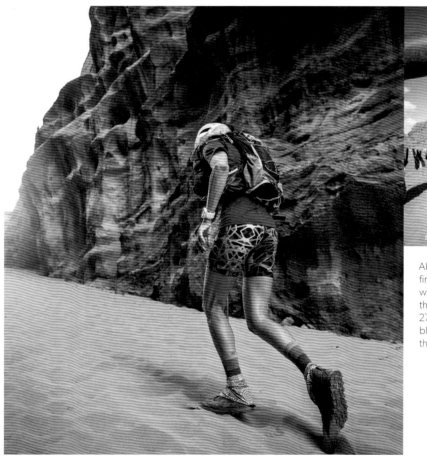

Above: when participants cross the finish line, each receives a medal with a colored ribbon to denote their finishing time—black for under 27 hours; white for under 30 hours; blue for over 30 hours. Opposite: the al-Khazneh, or Treasury, at Petra.

The Call of the Wild: Remote Runs in Spectacular Nature

If you're looking for a rugged and remote setting for your run, head to the lava fields of Iceland or the mountainous wilds of New Zealand. Hike along the trails of the Scottish Highlands, and explore the depths of Charyn Canyon. These dramatic locations offer untouched natural beauty in abundance.

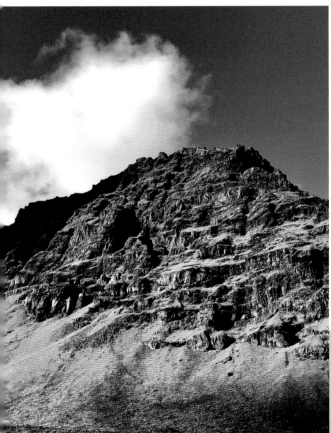

Above and opposite: almost 80 percent of Iceland is uninhabited, which makes it an ideal destination for trail running. Numerous gravel tracks crisscross the island, through fertile lowlands with rugged, rocky outcrops, many just 20 kilometers (12 miles) or so from the capital.

Iceland

A dream destination for runners around the globe, Iceland offers a wealth of running options, be it around the capital Reykjavík or out along the barren, volcanic coastline, with nothing but the birds and the breeze alongside you. This is the most sparsely populated country in Europe—you'll have no problem escaping from civilization.

For proper, hard-core running, your best bet is to pack a bag with a tent and some warm clothes and food, and just run in any direction from Reykjavík city center. You could even run from the airport. Better still, hire a car for a week and spend days upon days exploring the endless waterfalls, geysers, and hot springs.

Pick the time of year wisely. Iceland's weather offers spectacular effects. From January to April, and again from late August to mid-April, the clear skies and pitch-black nighttime darkness bring the green aurora of the northern lights. During the remaining months, the weather will be kinder and less harsh, but by no means hot. ▶

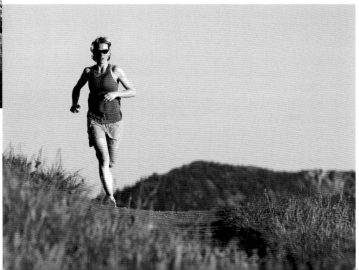

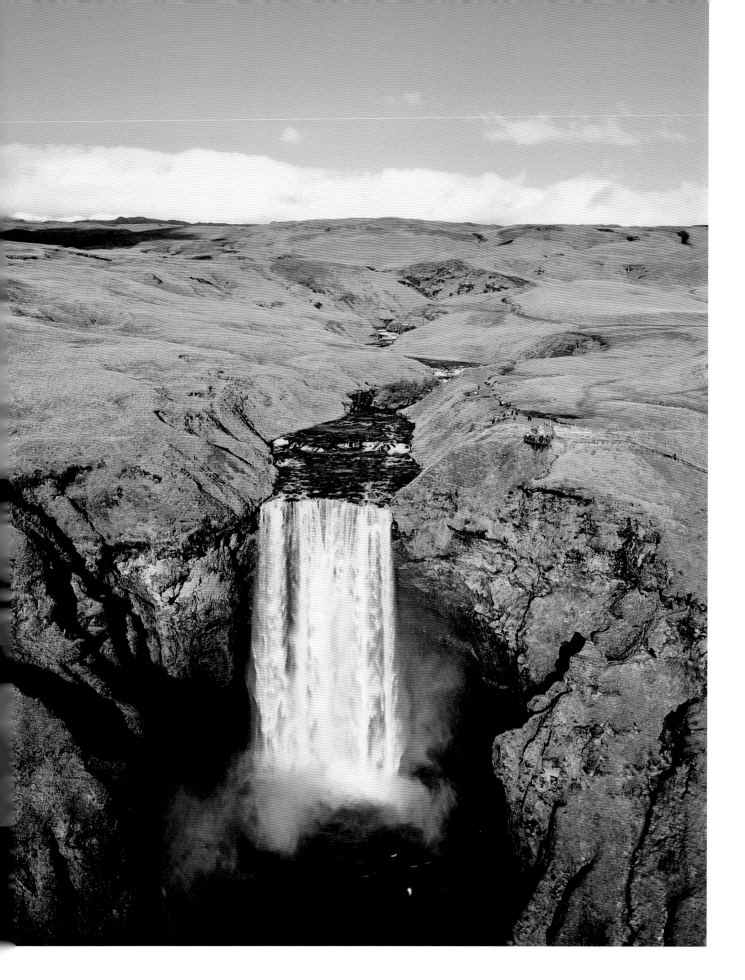

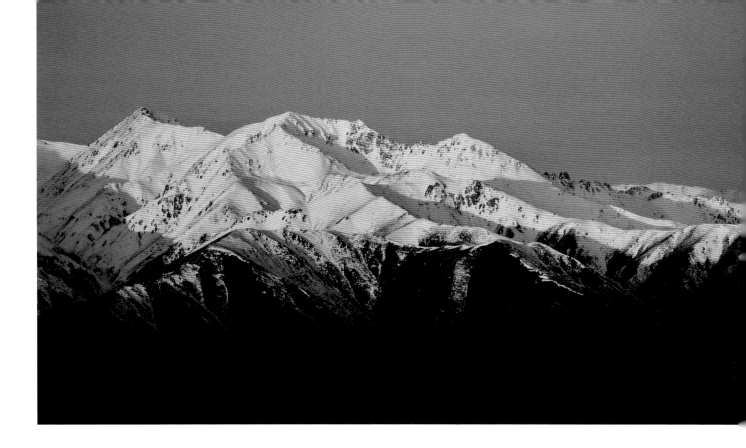

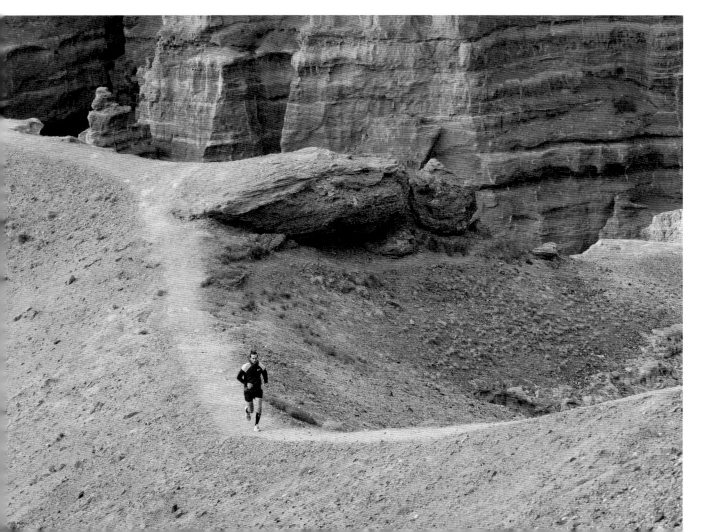

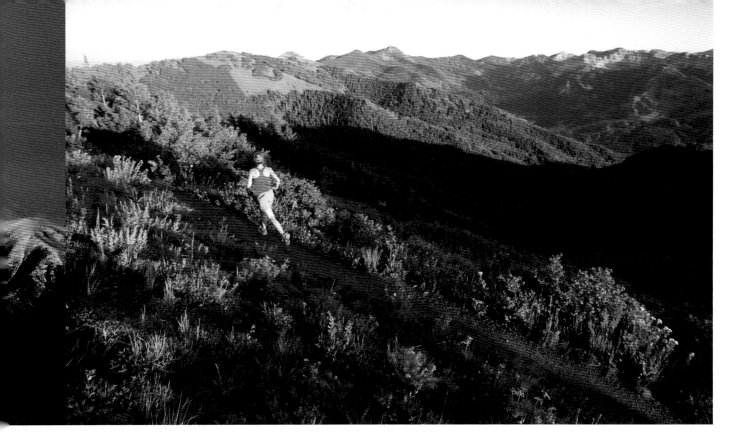

Above: there are many designated trails in and around the verdant Big Cottonwood Canyon, each graded according to ability.
Opposite: Charyn Canyon, where trail running is less established; the most obvious trail is in a spot known as the Valley of Castles.

▶ If you want an epic challenge, try running from north to south, or around the island. A single paved road circumnavigates the country, totaling 1,332 kilometers (821 miles). Perhaps drive, park the car, and disappear off into the northwestern landscape, where you're likely to see more stars than ever before.

Big Cottonwood Canyon

A day trip from Salt Lake City, Utah, to this awe-inspiring canyon in the Wasatch mountain range is a must. There are miles of trails, perfect for running and camping, with plenty of them a considerable challenge. They can be linked together to make your run as long or as short as you'd like.

A great classic in the canyon is the well-known Iron Cowboy triathlon route. The run totals 18 kilometers (11.2 miles), with 1,000 meters (3,281 feet) of ascent. Be sure to prepare—it's difficult, to say the least. The best way to experience such mammoth trails is to run with a filter bottle and access water from the rivers and streams along the way; otherwise, a large water bladder is a necessity. If that's not enough, try the trails around Lake Blanche, Mineral Fork, Donut Falls, Dog Lake, Desolation Lake, Silver Lake, and of course, Lakes Mary, Catherine, and Martha. The possibilities are endless.

Charyn Canyon

Kazakhstan is often overlooked, despite its wealth of running routes. A multi-day trip to Charyn Canyon is recommended—run any distance you like here, you'll likely run out before the canyon does.

The easiest way to get to and from the isolated canyon is to hire a local taxi from the large city of Almaty, about 200 kilometers (124 miles) away. This is not overly expensive and you can also arrange a date and time for pick-up once you have been dropped off. (Just make sure you have phone signal in case they let you down.) Alternatively, go for a long day trip; drivers are often keen to stay parked up and wait for you.

Running on top of, around, or through the canyon makes you feel tiny in a world of pink and orange rock. The canyon is barren, rugged, massive, and you'll be largely alone in nature. Be sure to take plenty of water, a tent, and some snacks. If you are staying overnight, explore during sunrise or sunset, when the cliffs are streaked in gold and amber as the light melts in and out of the canyon. By night, endless starry skies spread out above you.

It's important to note that, while the river may look incredibly inviting on a warm summer's day, it is fast flowing and swimming here is not recommended.

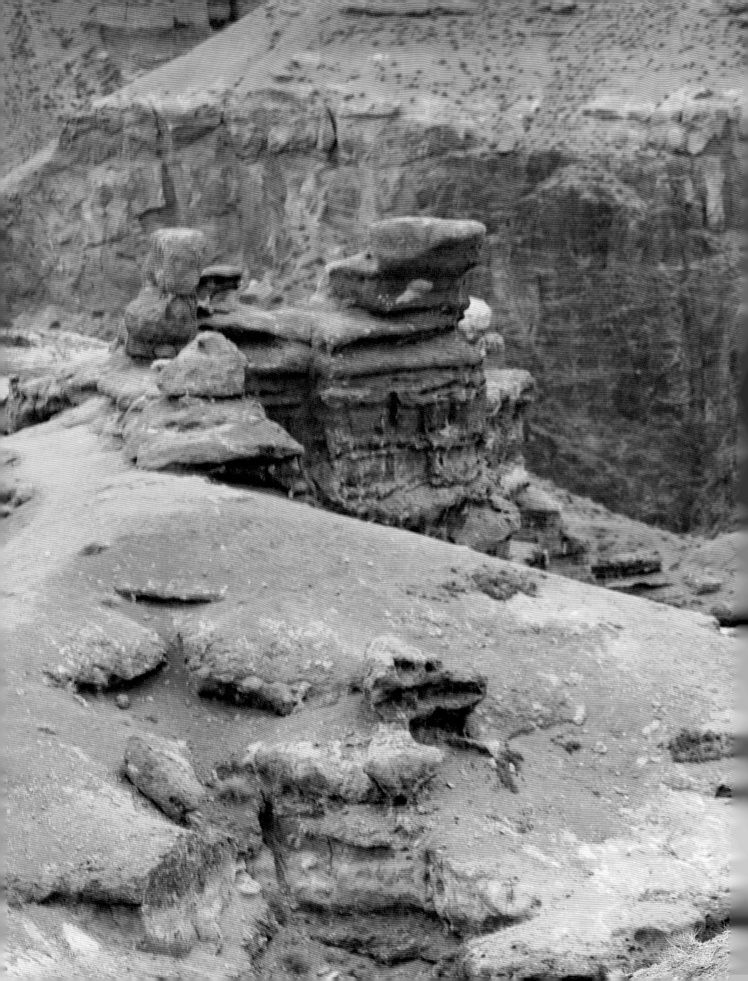

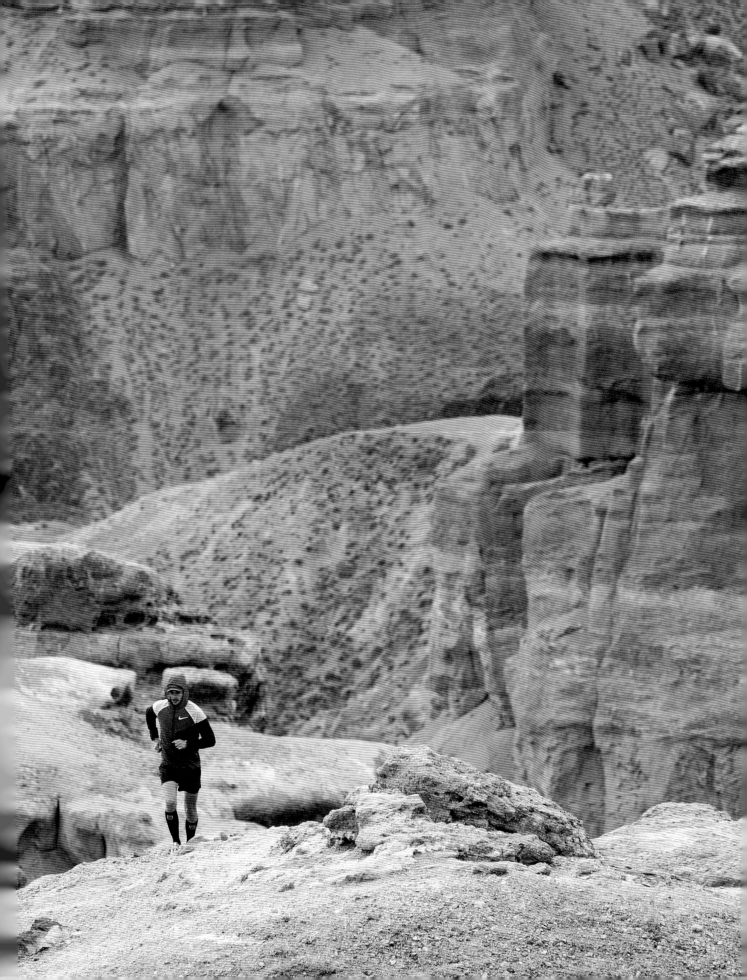

New Zealand

New Zealand is the home of many mountainous movie sets; steer clear of the cities and stick to the wilds for truly special running, with views that will take your breath away.

This landscape, with its sprawling mountain ranges, pristine forest paths, seaside roads, and snow-covered tracks, has drawn trail runners from all over the world for many years, and is increasing in popularity. One glorious middle-distance run can showcase the variety of climate and terrain on offer. And according to the World Health Organization, New Zealand also has some of the cleanest air in the world, adding to the already long list of reasons to head here and start exploring for yourself.

One of the best trails lies in the Wanaka region—the famously scenic Skyline Track—in the southwest of the country. Hiking here would take more than 10 hours (running, ideally less), but you're likely to be keen to stop for photos.

The mountains of New Zealand may remind runners of the Alps, but the beaches are unlike anything else on the planet. Try heading to the South Island town of Punakaiki, which is between Westport and Greymouth and has deserted beaches all along this stretch.

Jasper National Park

The largest national park in the Canadian Rockies, Jasper spans over 11,000 square kilometers (4,247 square miles). The scenery will blow your mind—this area is part of Unesco's Canadian Rocky Mountain Parks World Heritage site. From deep woodlands and clear blue lakes to glaciers and snowcapped mountains, some of the most spectacular vistas in Canada are found here.

The 233-kilometer (145-mile) route between the town of Jasper and Lake Louise is considered one of the most scenic drives in the world and the whole stretch can be run on paved surfaces. For smaller routes, choose one of the many trails east of Jasper such as Valley of the Five Lakes (4.5 kilometers; 2.8 miles), Jasper Discovery Trail (10 kilometers; 6.2 miles), or Saturday Night Lake Loop (24.3 kilometers; 15 miles).

This one is for the adventure seekers and those who admire and appreciate Earth's beautiful landscapes.

Below: Milford Sound, New Zealand—runners reaching here after taking the Milford Track from Lake Te Anau pass through temperate rain forest and pretty meadows along the way. Opposite: looking toward Spirit Island from a Maligne Valley trail, Jasper National Park.

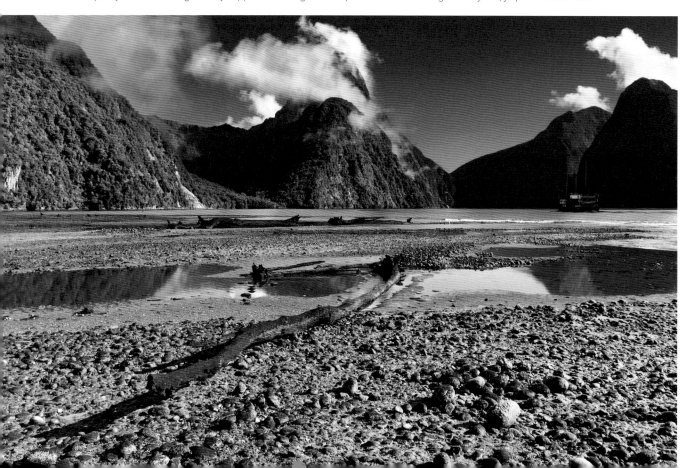

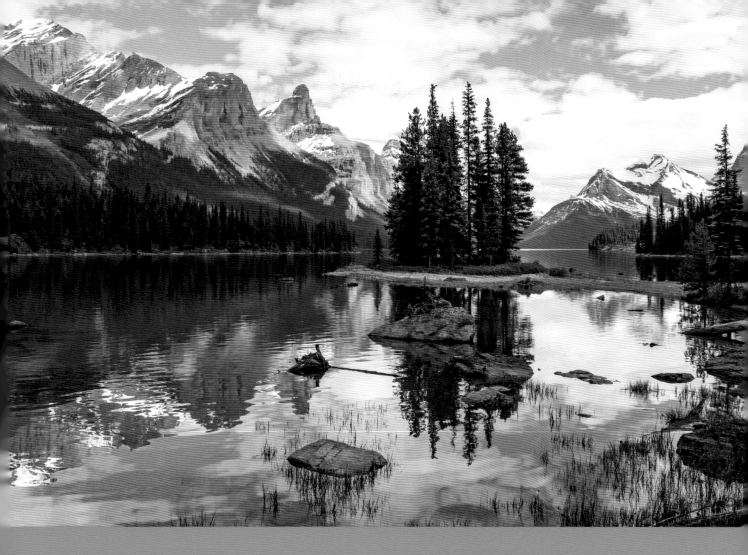

Wild Runs: The Basics

Iceland
Route:
Reykjavík; round country
Distance:
varies; 1,332 km (821 mi)

Big Cottonwood Canyon
Utah, U. S.
Route:
Iron Cowboy triathlon
Distance:
18 km (11.2 mi)

Charyn Canyon
Almaty Region, Kazakhstan
Route:
Charyn Canyon
Distance:
varies

New Zealand
Route:
Skyline Track; Punakaiki
Distance:
23 km (14.2 mi); varies

Jasper National Park
Alberta, Canada
Route:
Jasper–Lake Louise;
Saturday Night Lake Loop;
Jasper Discovery Trail;
Valley of the Five Lakes
Distance:
233 km (145 mi);
24.3 km (15 mi);
10 km (6.2 mi);
4.5 km (2.8 mi)

BIG FIVE MARATHON

With blue skies above and dusty orange dirt trails below, you'll spend 42.2 kilometers (26.2 miles) with your eyes glued to the scenery around you. This marathon offers the chance to run through the habitat of the most magnificent animals in the world. It's a holiday, safari, and run all rolled into one.

You may never want to run a normal marathon again after the wonders of running alongside the animals of the African savanna. The adrenaline and endorphins released by marathon running are profound, but this adventure race ramps it all up a notch.

Taking place on the Entabeni Game Reserve, in Limpopo province, South Africa, this race can only be entered by taking up a place on one of the multi-night packages offered by the organizers (unless you are a South African national, in which case race-only entry is possible). These trips combine the euphoria of marathon running with the holiday of a lifetime—accommodation is provided, in camping grounds and luxurious lodges on the private reserve, and days are devoted to bush walks and exhilarating game drives under the eyes of the magnificent Entabeni monolith. Entabeni is a Big Five reserve, meaning that runners have the opportunity to ▶

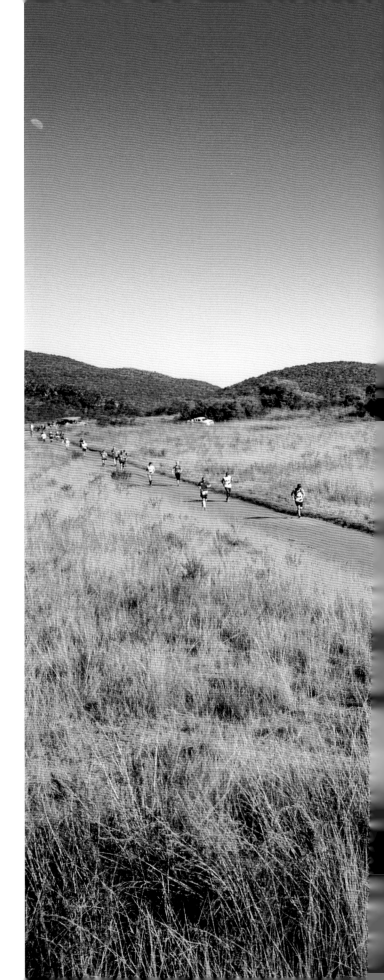

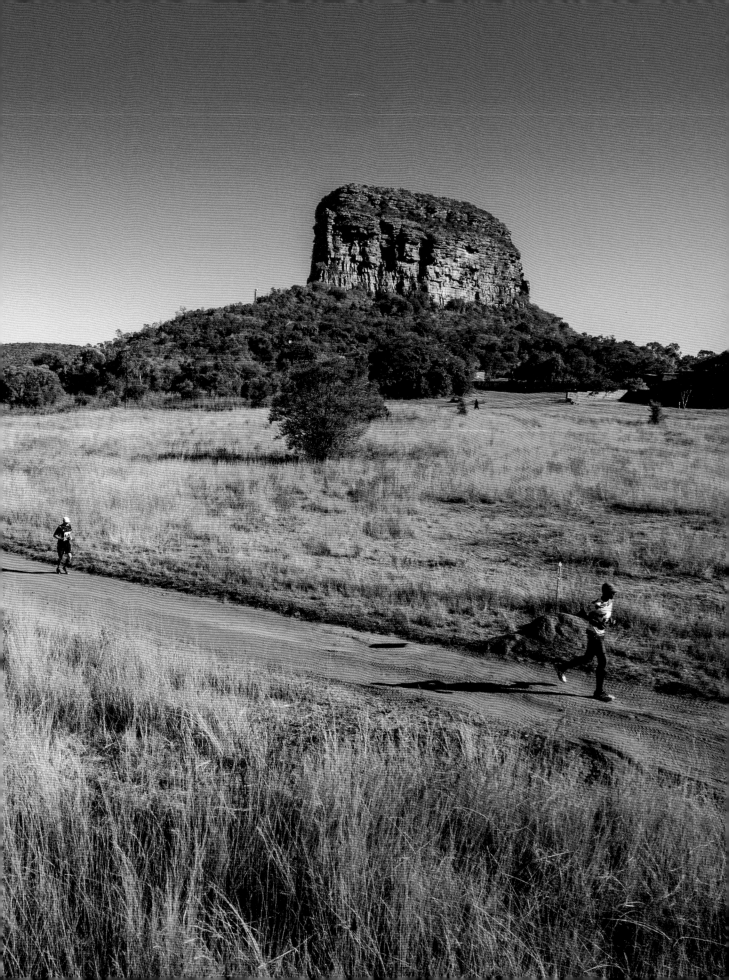

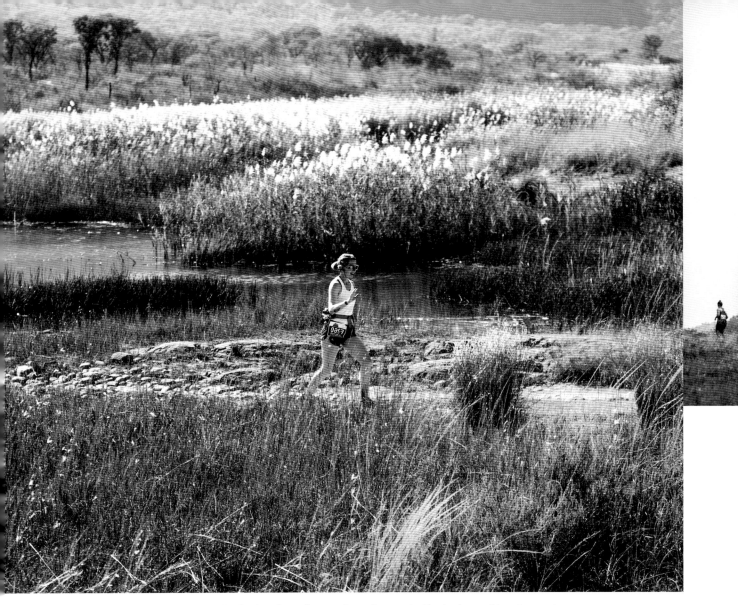

Above: crossing the grass-swept savanna in the Entabeni Game Reserve. Opposite, top: the Entabeni monolith, an impressive natural landmark that's visible for miles. Opposite, bottom: runners at the start of the race at Lakeside Lodge.

▶ spot iconic African animals: the lion, leopard, rhinoceros, elephant and Cape buffalo, alongside many other species. No fences, enclosures, or rivers separate you from the wildlife.

The course itself is a loop of trail and bush running, starting and finishing at a reserve lodge. Challenges include stretches of loose trail with potholes, sand tracks, and an extraordinarily steep descent at Yellow Wood Valley. The movement of free-ranging animals means that there is also the chance of sudden route changes, as the organizers quickly accommodate the natural residents of the park. The terrain isn't easy, but with your mind wandering and your eyes open to the breathtaking savanna, the race is one to cherish rather than endure. The end will come, and so slower running can be embraced. Along the way you can enjoy the camaraderie of your fellow runners, the blue skies, and the mesmerizing sight of some of the world's greatest creatures. It is a race like no other. ■

Length: 21.1 or 42.2 km (13.1 or 26.2 mi)

Location: Entabeni Game Reserve, South Africa

Date: June

Type: trail/bush

Temperature Ø: 15–25 °C (59–77 °F)

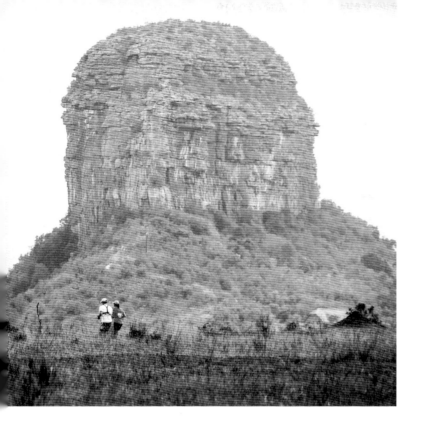

Entabeni is a Big Five reserve, meaning that runners have the opportunity to spot iconic African animals: the lion, leopard, rhinoceros, elephant and Cape buffalo, alongside many other species.

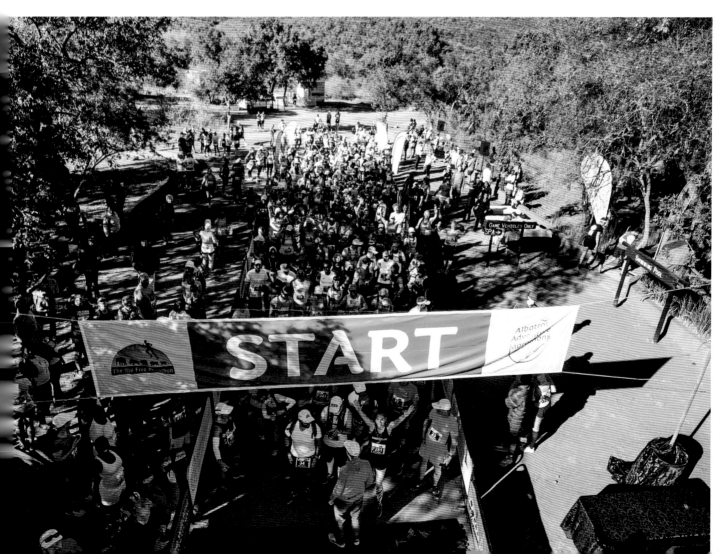

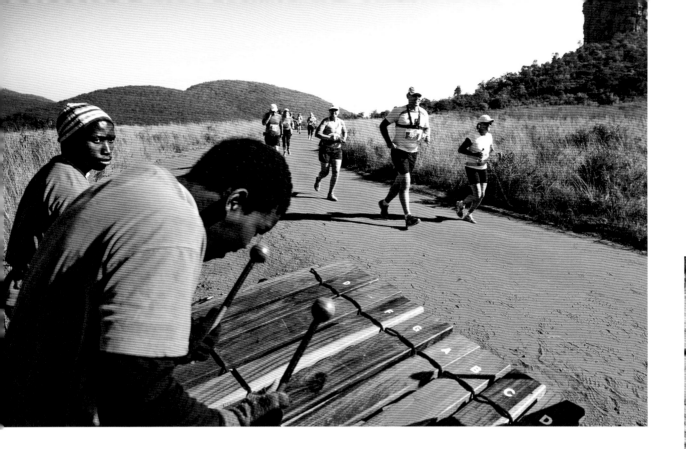

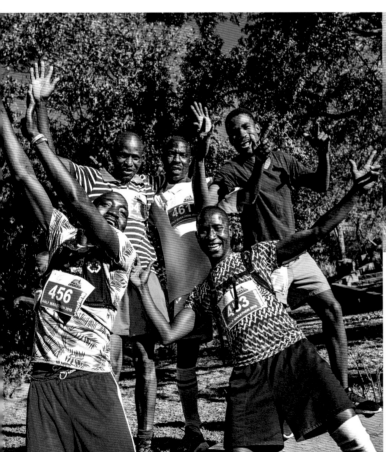

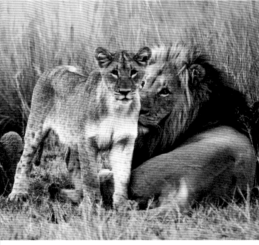

Top and opposite: dirt roads made of red sand make up the route through the plateau section of the marathon, but most of the looping track is uneven, with loose rocks and potholes.

The course itself is a loop of trail and bush running, starting and finishing at a reserve lodge. Challenges include stretches of loose trail with potholes, sand tracks, and a steep descent at Yellow Wood Valley.

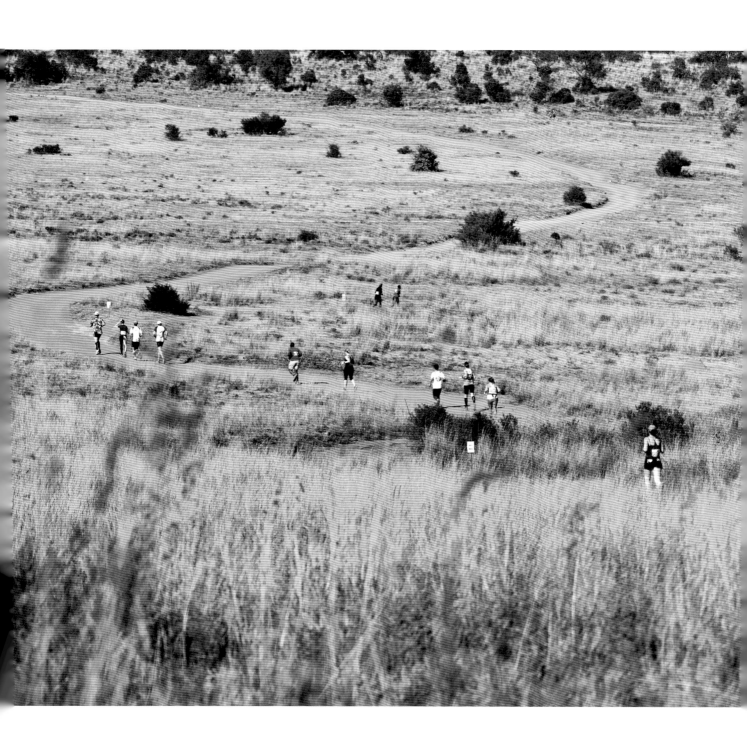

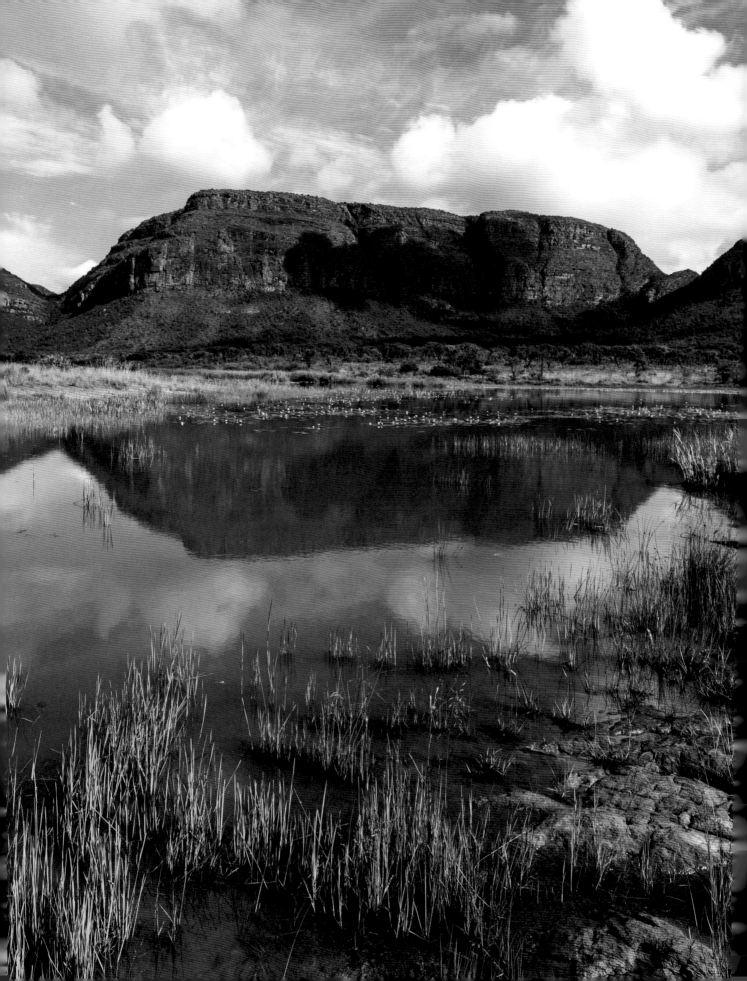

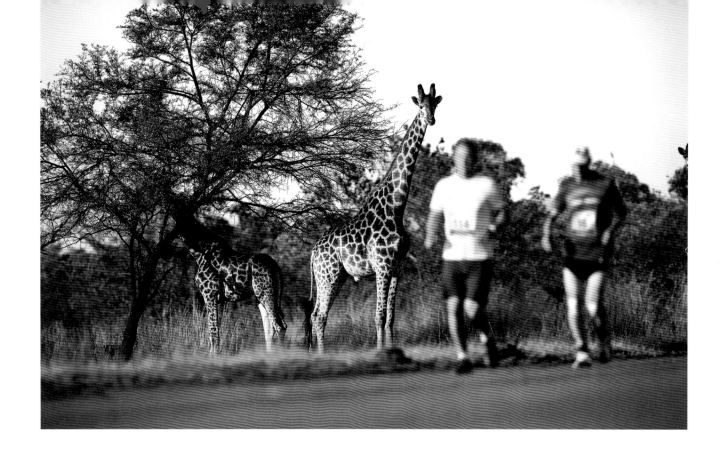

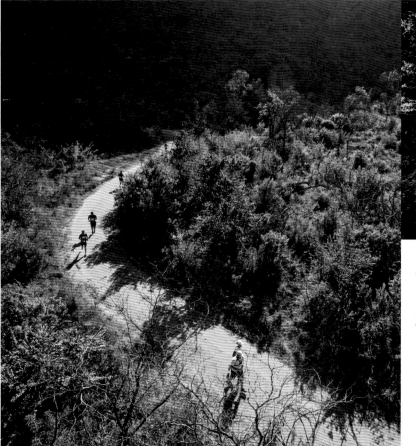

Signs warn of danger and potential encounters with wild lions. The risk is greatest just after descending through the Yellow Wood Valley section of the route—a sharp descent of some 3 kilometers (1.8 miles).

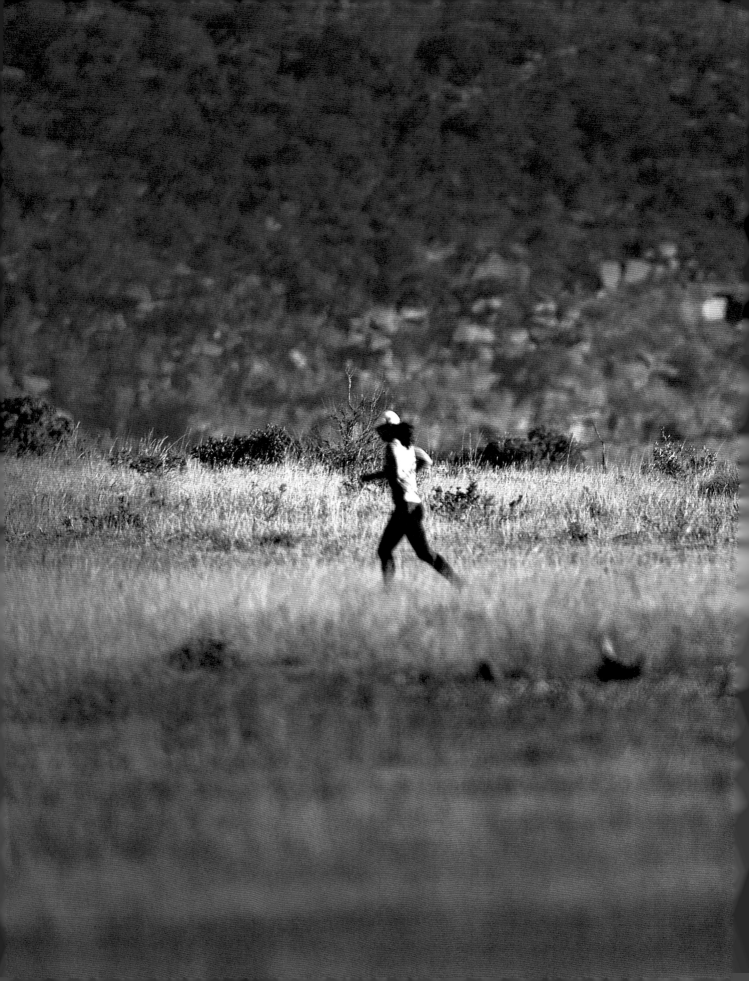

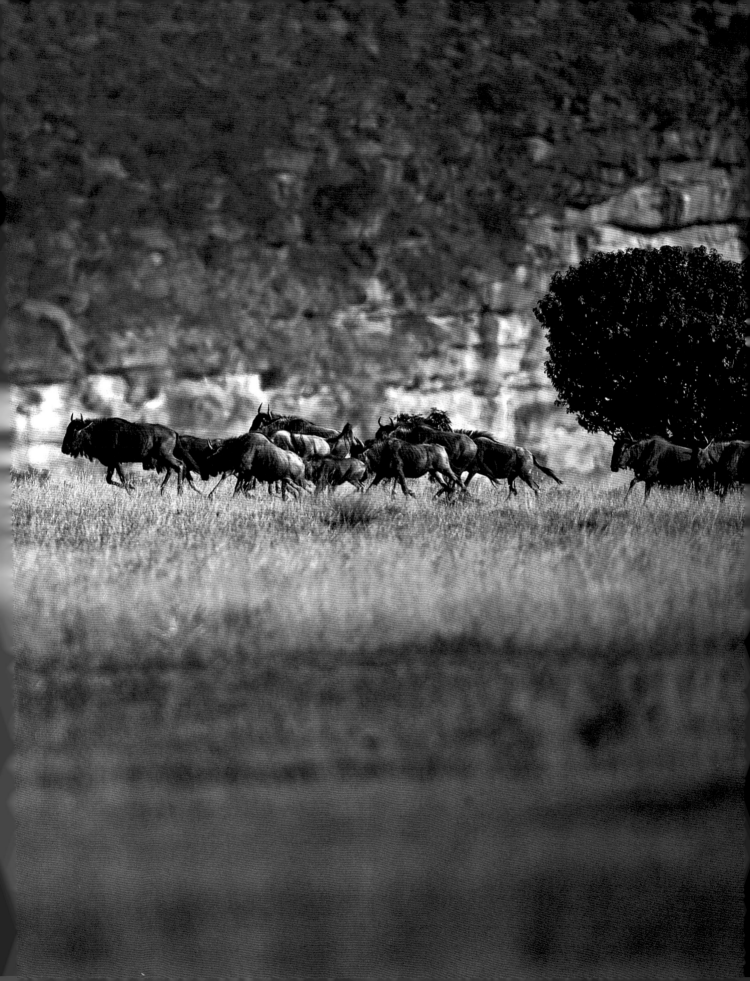

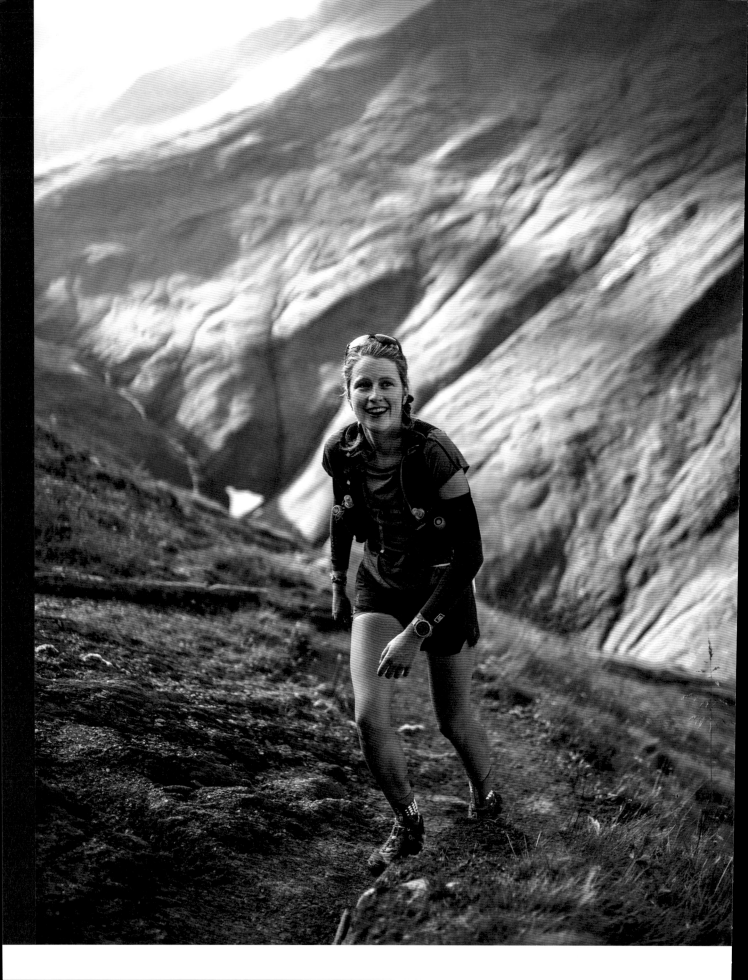

Reaching Peak Performance with The Marmots

Professional trail runners Katie Schide and Germain Grangier spend so much time in the mountains they're known as "the marmots."

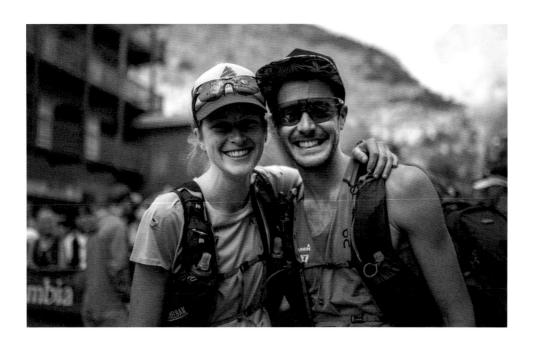

"We try to move through the mountains as quickly as possible," says Katie Schide when describing what she and Germain Grangier do for a living. Her nonchalance masks the punishing reality of what is essentially mountain parkour at an ultramarathon distance on terrain more suited to mountain goats than humans. As running becomes even more popular, and its variations increasingly audacious, it's no wonder the number of such races has grown tenfold over the past decade. Not that the hype can be credited for the rise of the sport's first power couple—Schide and Grangier were doing this long before it was cool.

Schide grew up in Maine, the most rural state in the U.S. A multi-sport athlete in high school, she discovered trail running in New Hampshire's White Mountains, where she retreated for the summer vacations between her geology studies in Vermont. At 19, during her inaugural season as a member of a local trail crew, she attempted her first White Mountain Hut Traverse, a ragged route that connects eight huts along the region's spine. She completed the 80-kilometer trek (50-mile) in 24 hours, just fast enough to have her name included in the finishers' log. "I always ran to stay

in shape for other sports, but I soon realized I could combine my running fitness with my love for long, fast hiking days in the mountains," Schide says. She has spent long, fast days in the mountains ever since. In the summer of 2019, she had another go at the Hut Traverse. This time, she cut her original time in half and finished as the fastest woman ever to complete the course.

What happened in the decade between working in the huts and traversing them at record speed? For starters she met Grangier, her partner and coach. Born in the Alps, he was on skis before he could walk. Eventually, he took up competitive mountain biking. For him, the more time spent outside, the better. "If you have kids, take them running, biking, swimming, climbing, whatever," he says. "They will push boundaries and fail—a lot. At school, failure is lame, but in sport, failure is a degree. If you want to grow, put shoes on your feet, go outside, and repeat." He combined his education in failure with a geology degree, which crystallized in him an "at oneness" with the environment. "I constantly try to understand the history of the mountains around me," he says. "It adds another sense of meaning to my runs." ▶

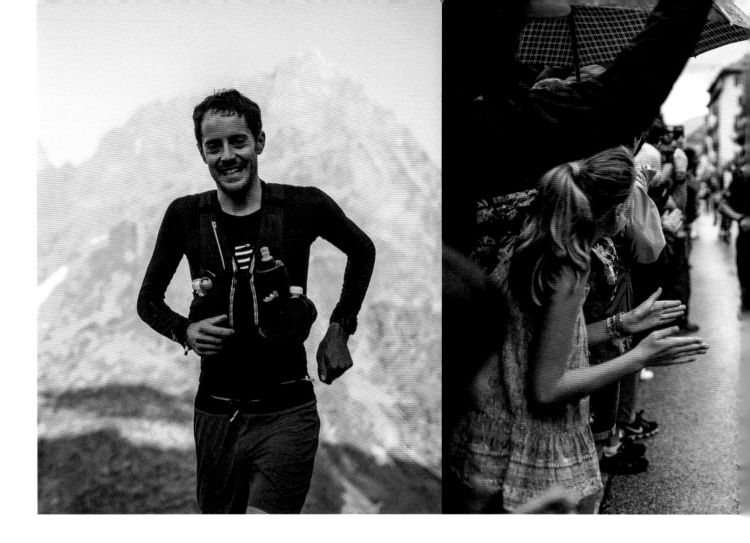

► When Schide and Grangier met at a trail race in Italy, they encouraged each other to start training upwards of 30 hours a week. "We come up with new ideas for routes, races, and training together and can build off of each other's excitement," Schide says. "We see each other working toward a goal, and it inspires us to keep moving forward and support one another. There is always someone who 100 percent understands what you are doing and is there to be your biggest cheerleader." Since 2017, Schide and Grangier have cheered each other on to titles at some of the most grueling races in Europe and North America.

Their summer project is running the glacier Haute Route from Zermatt in Switzerland to Chamonix in France—essentially the Matterhorn to Mont Blanc. The approximately 160-kilometer (99-mile) route will draw them over 10 of the 12 highest peaks in the Alps, with roughly 15,000 meters (50,000 feet) of elevation gain. "The most challenging part will be the technical climbing, glacier travel, route finding, and altitude," Schide says. With favorable conditions, they expect to finish within 40 to 50 hours (or about seven bowls of instant noodles in mountain-running parlance). "The goal is not for a specific time, more to share a huge adventure and see what our bodies are capable of," she explains.

Course records and gold medals are just a bonus on top of the real accomplishment. "For us, running is more a way to be fully present in one place," Schide says. "We are both geologists by training, so we are always aware of our surroundings and the history of the landscapes around us." Despite maintaining a lively social-media presence and a career supported by sponsorships, Schide and Grangier strive to keep things simple. "You can learn a lot about yourself when you have the opportunity to be alone with your thoughts for many hours a day," Schide says. "I love that there aren't any Strava segments in these parts. That way I'm always the queen of the mountain."

Together, Schide and Grangier are known as "the marmots," a name borrowed from the giant alpine squirrels with which they share the mountains. "We love watching them run around with their big bellies, jumping between rocks and whistling to each other," Schide says with a smile. "They are silly, but also extremely athletic animals that always make us laugh." On Instagram, the couple often share jokes about Schide's yearning for snacks and how annoying it is when Grangier is photographed during the 1 percent of a race he slows down to walk. Interspersed with the humor are flashes of introspection. In one caption, Grangier writes, "Recently someone asked me, what can we wish for your future? Honestly, I'm pretty happy with what I have. My body works, my relatives are healthy, I have a place to live. Every day, I'm outside with [Katie]. I'm living a dream. It would be crazy to ask for more. I feel lucky." ∎

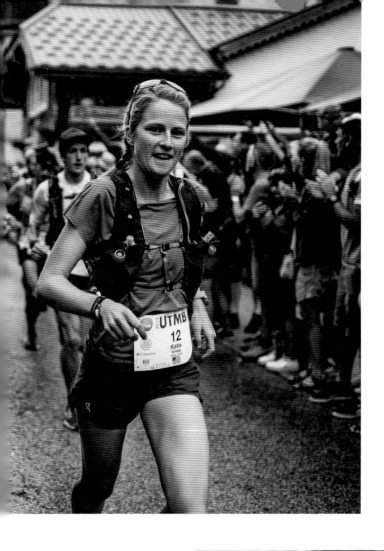

"If you have kids, take them running, biking, swimming, climbing, whatever. They will push boundaries and fail—a lot. At school, failure is lame, but in sport, failure is a degree. If you want to grow, put shoes on your feet, go outside, and repeat."

Above: Schide competing in the Ultra-Trail du Mont-Blanc (UTMB) in August 2019. She finished in sixth place—an incredible achievement considering it was her first attempt at a 160-kilometer (100-mile) event. It was also a first for Grangier, who placed ninth in the men's race.

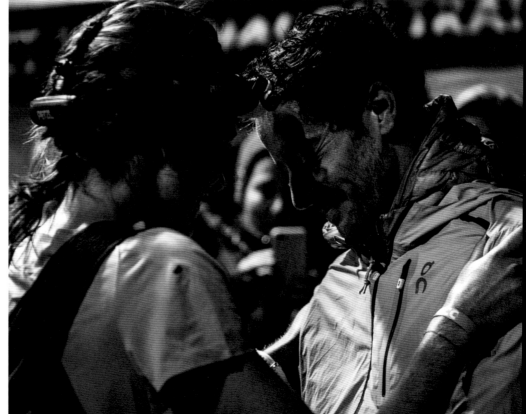

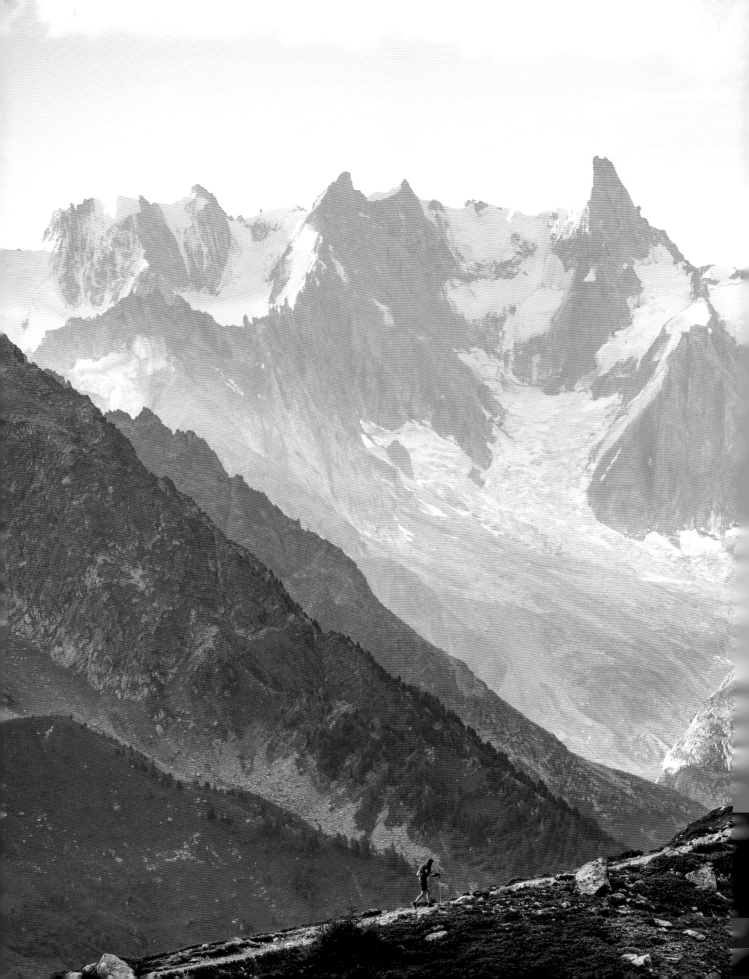

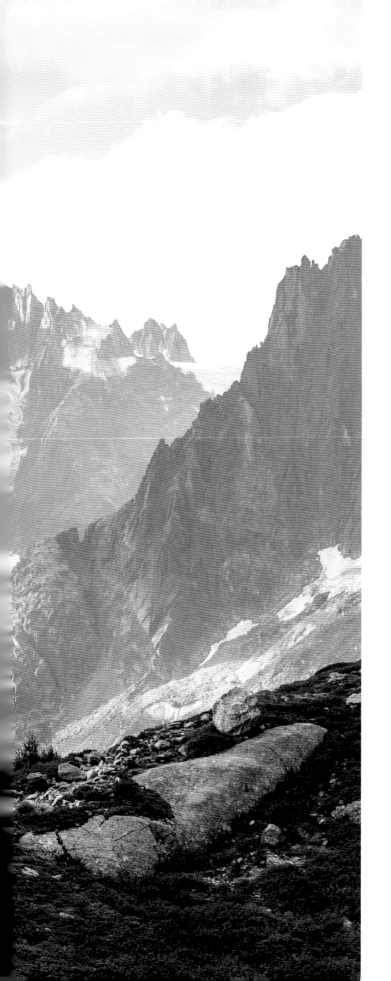

ULTRA-TRAIL DU MONT-BLANC

One of the toughest ultras in the world. Runners are expected to have a strong level of experience and be ready to handle the often extreme weather of the French Alps. Leaving Chamonix at 6 a. m., participants race through Italy and Switzerland before returning to one of the best finish lines in trail running.

The Ultra-Trail du Mont-Blanc (UTMB) is a single-stage mountain ultra marathon, part of a week-long trail-running event of the same name, which incorporates seven races of different degrees of difficulty. The ultra itself is part of the famous Ultra-Trail World Tour family of races; recognized from 2013, this group of 100+- kilometer (62+- mile) trail runs forms the gold standard of the sport, with events held across the globe. It is not for the fainthearted.

With a race cut-off time of 46 hours 30 minutes, and 171 kilometers (106 miles) of alpine trail to run, expect serious hills—the total elevation gain of the course is more than 10,000 meters (nearly 32,808 feet). Although the precise route varies slightly every year, runners broadly follow the path of the breathtaking Tour du Mont-Blanc through France, Italy, and Switzerland. From punishing ascents to immediate, quad-burning descents down steep narrow trails, ▶

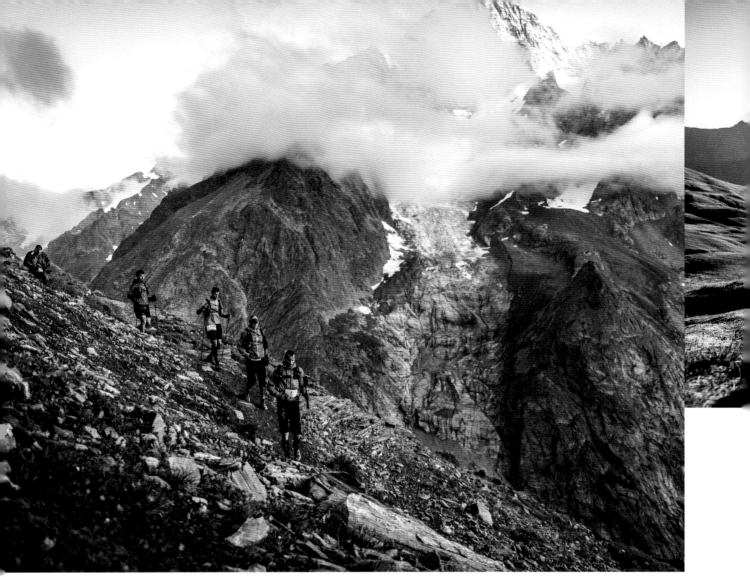

The UTMB route follows the Tour du Mont-Blanc hiking path—literally a massive loop around the tallest mountain in the Alps—which usually takes seasoned hikers seven to nine days to complete. The best runners complete the course in about 20 hours.

▶ with the occasional deadly drop on either side, you'll want to look at the view, but it's probably best to keep an eye on your footing too.

The starting line is in Chamonix, at 1,035 meters (3,395 feet) altitude. The first "major" peak, occurring roughly a quarter of the way into the race, is the Croix du Bonhomme (2,479 meters; 8,133 feet). Runners enter Italy on the Col de la Seigne, approximately 15 kilometers (9.5 miles) on, at an altitude of 2,516 meters (8,255 feet). Col du Grand Ferret (2,537 meters; 8,323 feet) is the highest point of the course and marks the entrance to Switzerland, at roughly the 100-kilometer (62-mile) mark. Even beyond this, however, there are hills to climb, including Les Tseppes (1,932 meters; 6,339 feet), before the final descent back into France and on to the race finish at Chamonix. There are aid stations and checkpoints along the way, but the race operates on a principle of "semi-autonomy," with

runners expected to take responsibility for their own wellbeing and safety between these stations.

The UTMB point system, according to which hopeful entrants must qualify, ensures safety during the race. Beyond this, strict bag checks are carried out to confirm that each racer has the mandatory kit—clothing, equipment, and documents—required for survival in the Alps, with the extremely variable weather emphasized: you might race one year in scorching sunlight and the next in freezing fog and downpours. Many runners, despite the strict entry criteria, do not finish. Those who do have probably run through two nights, over 32 to 46 hours, to complete the course, although elite athletes may complete the loop in slightly more than 20.

Still, while it might be one of the hardest races out there, it is also one of the most beautiful. By day, night, sun, and storms, this ▶

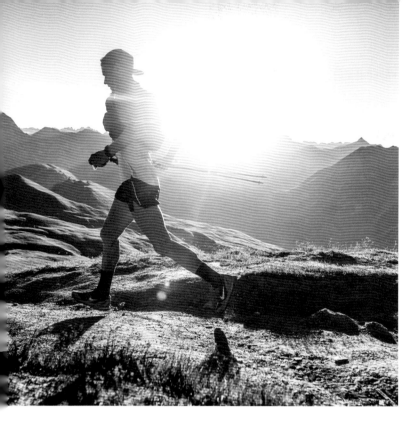

With 171 kilometers (106 miles) of alpine trail to run, expect serious hills. Although the precise route varies slightly every year, runners broadly follow the path of the breathtaking Tour du Mont-Blanc through France, Italy, and Switzerland.

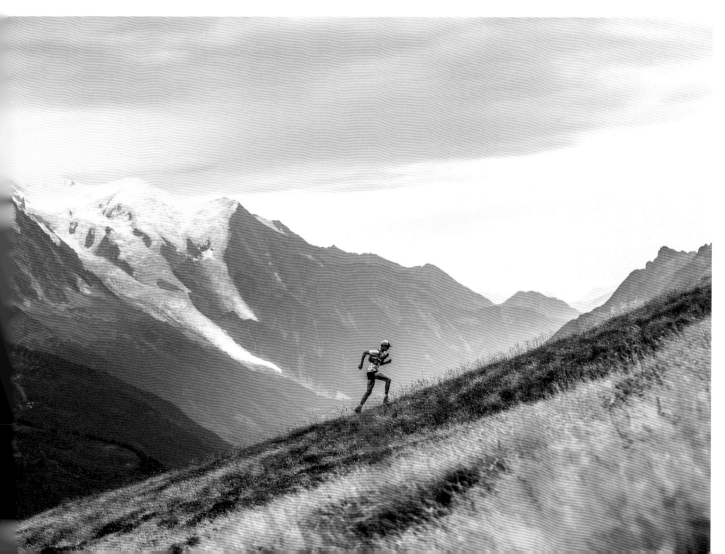

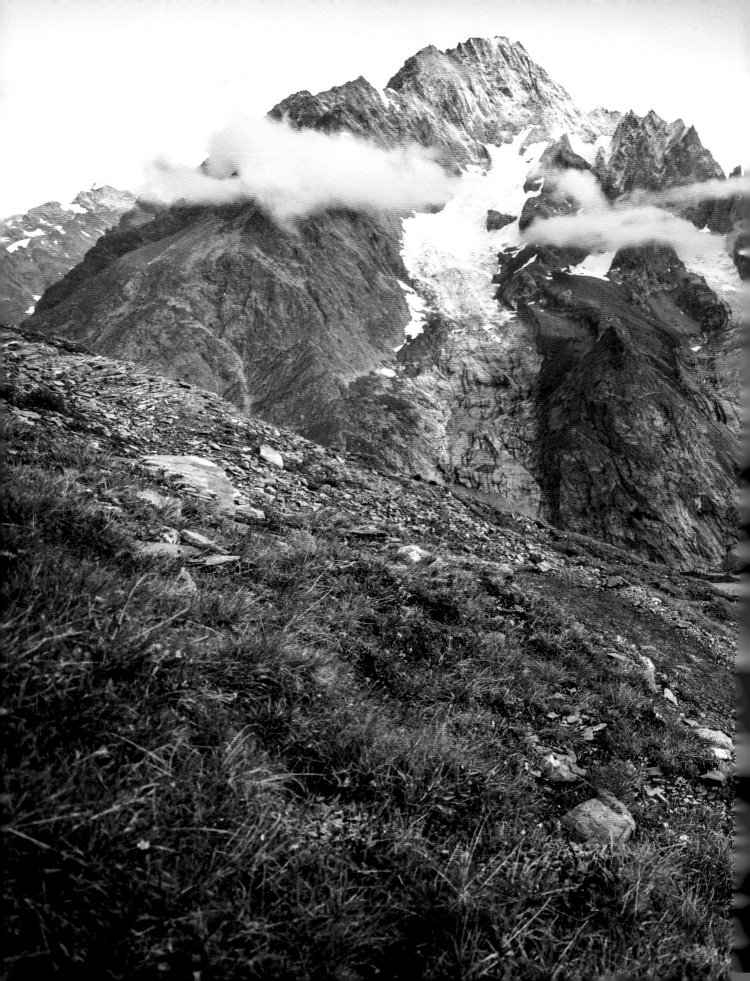

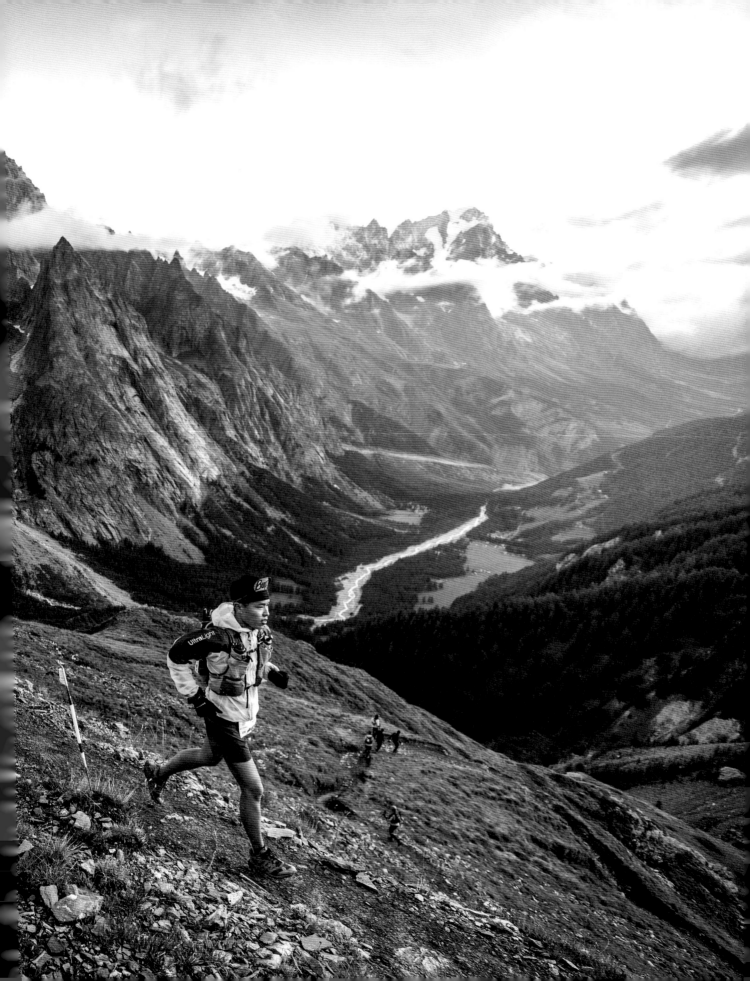

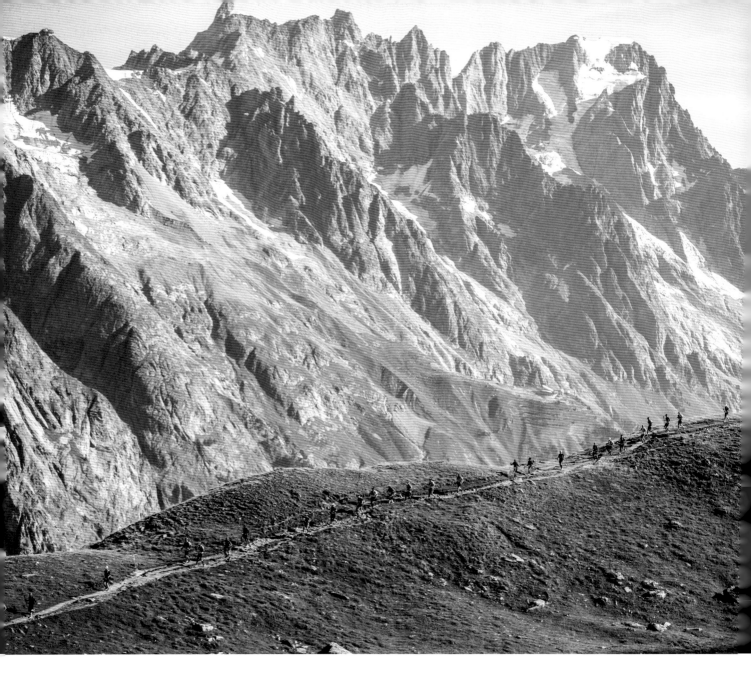

▶ run gives you much value for money. Sweeping green mountain-scapes, bright white snowcapped peaks, and brown scrambling trails are littered with more than 2,000 runners, all in awe of the mountains (and likely in pain). This is one of the most exhilarating events, made better by the finish line of all finish lines. Spectators fill the streets, balconies, and windows of the finish-arch area back in Chamonix. Surviving racers hear the clangs of cow bells and endless cheers for miles as they approach the town through the last twisting climb. The energy you thought you didn't have is ignited again briefly, as emotional and euphoric relief sets in—a moment every trail runner longs for. ∎

Length: 171 km (106 mi)

Location: Chamonix, France

Date: August/September

Type: trail/mountainous

Temperature Ø: 4–20 °C (39–68 °F)

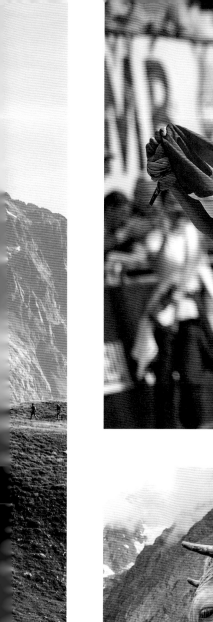

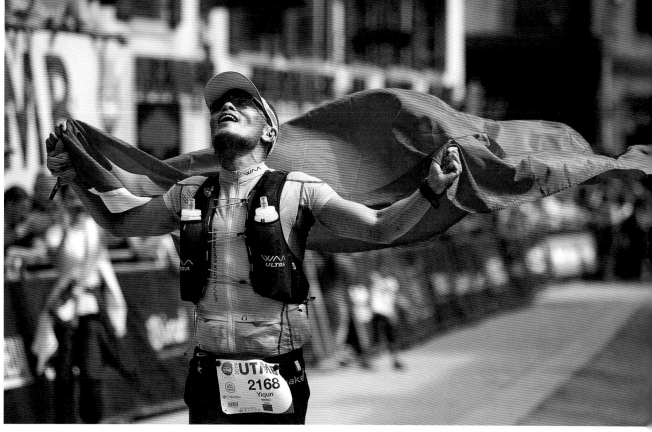

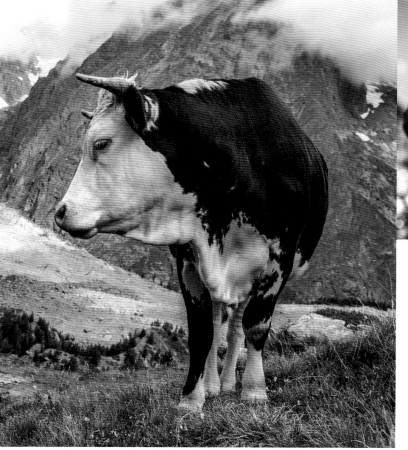

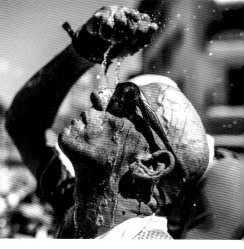

Top: the race starts and ends in Chamonix, on the French side of Mont-Blanc. Most runners will have had to run through two nights in order to complete the route in the specified time of 46 hours 30 minutes.

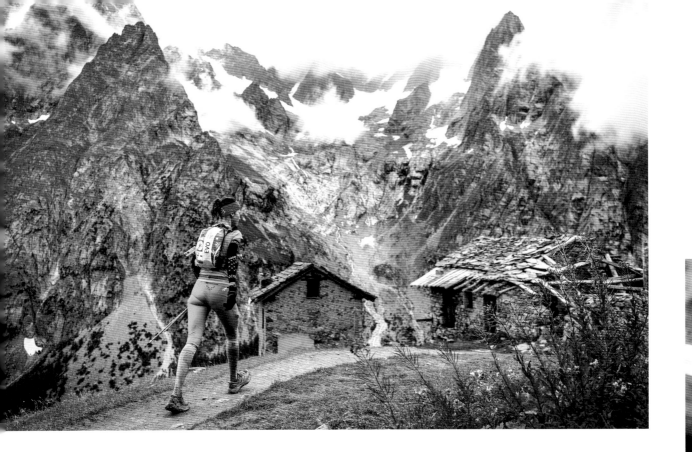

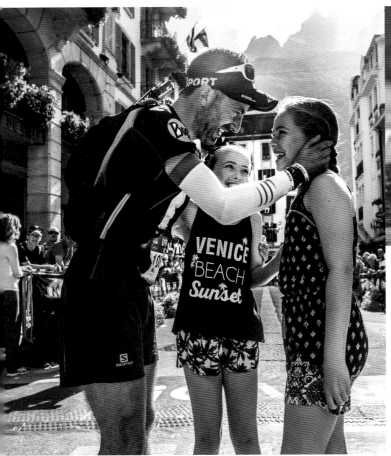

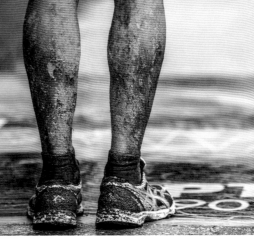

As the course unfolds, trail runners are pushed to their limits as they trek through valleys, over glaciers, and scale numerous peaks, the tallest of which is Col du Grand Ferret on the Swiss-Italian border.

There are aid stations and checkpoints along the way, but the race operates on a principle of "semi-autonomy," with runners expected to take responsibility for their own wellbeing and safety between these stations.

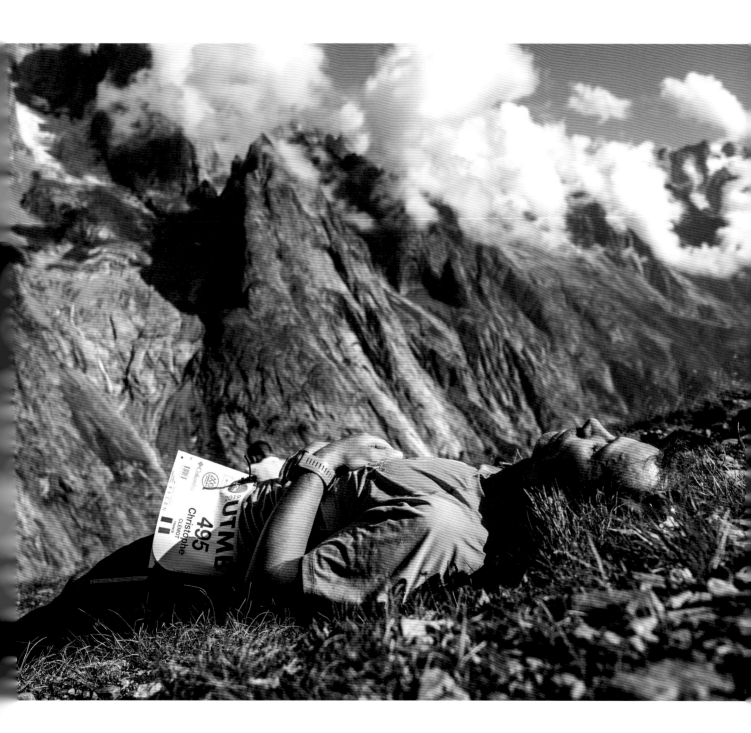

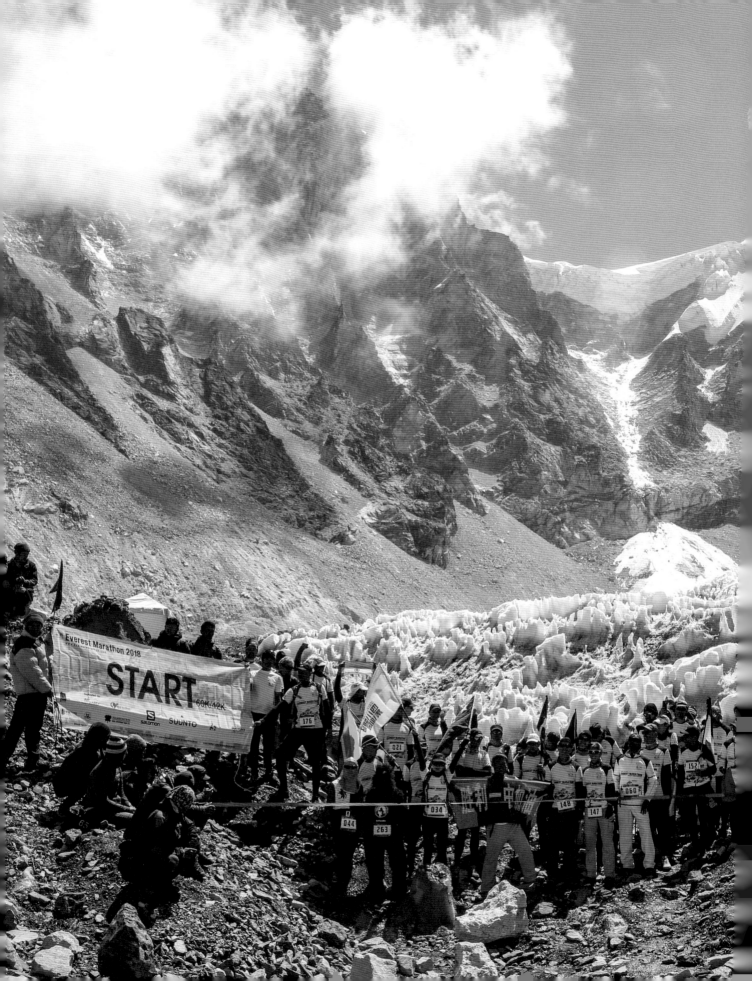

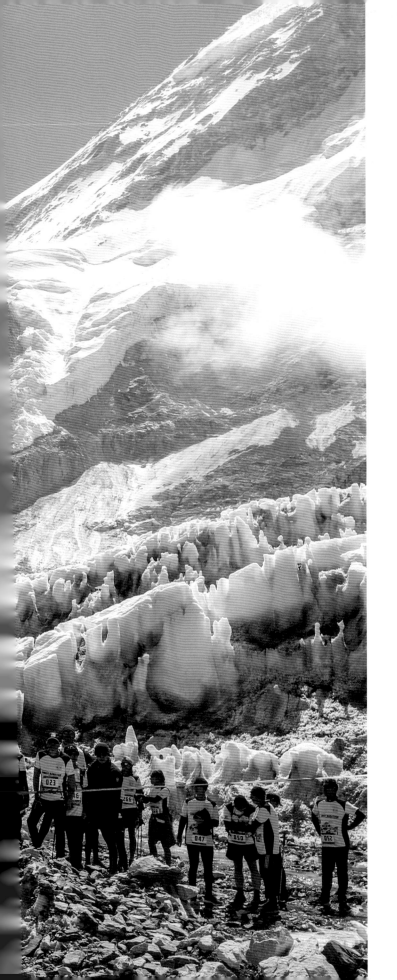

TENZING HILLARY EVEREST MARATHON

Welcome to the highest ultra marathon in the world. This race not only takes you through the high altitude of the Himalayas but offers an exclusive two-night stay at Everest Base Camp, where only climbers are normally allowed to stay. This is a must. It's Everest, for goodness' sake.

You will notice there's a fixed date for this event; that's because this marathon officially celebrates the ascent of Mount Everest made on May 29, 1953, by Edmund Hillary and Tenzing Norgay Sherpa, for whom the race is named. In honor of their historic adventure, runners from all over the world gather each year to race the trails of Khumbu valley in the Everest region, taking part in a high-altitude adventure. It is one of the biggest trail-running events in Nepal, and takes its status as a flagship race seriously.

There are three distances here, with the half-marathon recommended to novices (and only open to non-Nepal nationals)—it is described as "fun" and "fast," and is well supported. This is a far cry from the mass starts of a big-city race. It is in the marathon and ultra distances where things get really tough, although the ultra is really only for those with extreme endurance and a lust for adventure. ▶

Entrants get to spend two nights at Everest Base Camp, where normally only expedition climbers are allowed to stay. They start their respective races here, at an altitude of 5,356 meters (17,572 feet).

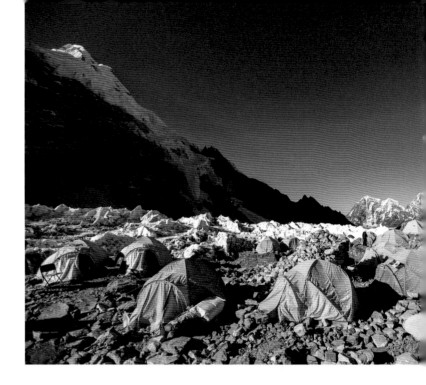

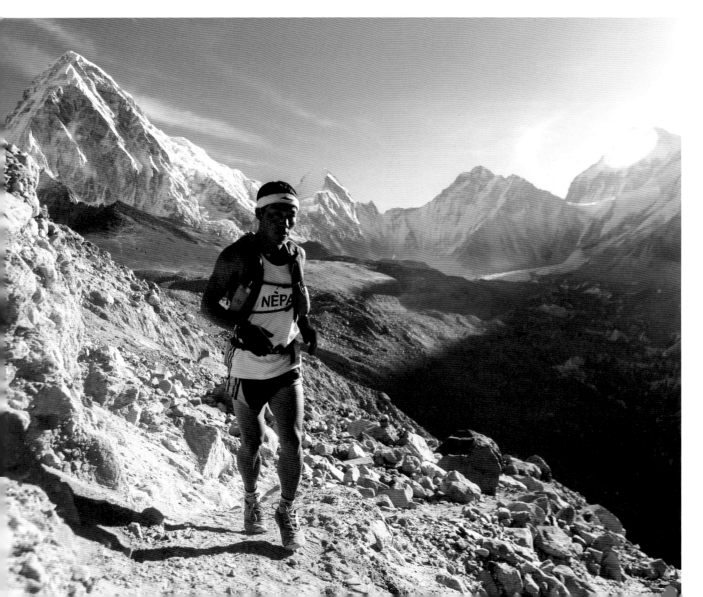

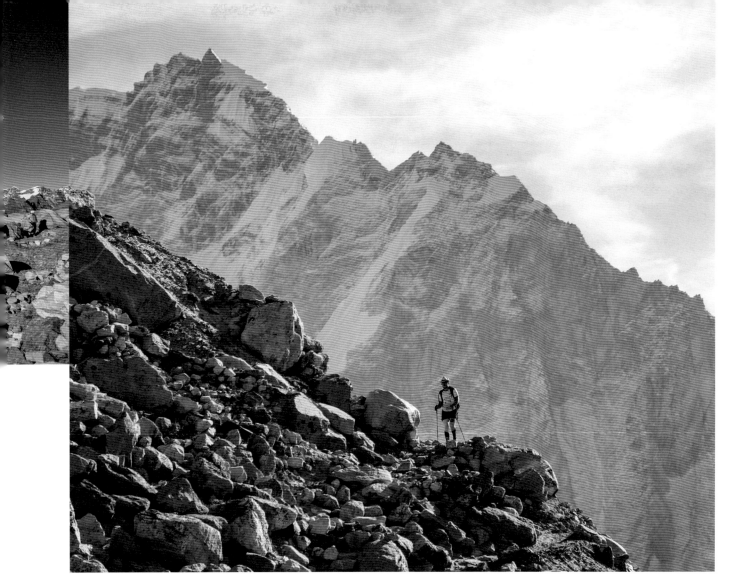

The marathon route is treacherous—almost all downhill on icy, uneven tracks; it is imperative that participants focus on their running. Thankfully, prior to racing, they climb Kala Patthar (5,6445 meters; 18,520 feet) for stunning views of Mounts Everest, Nuptse, and Lhotse.

▶ Entrants in both of these longer races get to spend two nights at Everest Base Camp, where normally only expedition climbers are allowed to stay. They start their respective races here, at an altitude of 5,356 meters (17,572 feet), beside the treacherous Khumbu Icefall. The end point for both races is the town of Namche Bazaar. For marathon runners, this route is mostly downhill, requiring caution and patience. Ultra runners, however, punctuate this course with a climb to the high mountain village of Machhermo, at 4,413 meters (14,478 feet), on a 20-kilometer (12.4-mile) "detour."

In case this doesn't sound extreme enough, remember this is the world's highest ultra-running event, with snow cover on many parts of the trail. In order to acclimate to the altitude and low oxygen levels, and avoid sickness, it's recommended that runners spend several days in the region prior to the race start. This is a prized destination for adventurers, however, and the race organizers also offer a number of packages that combine the race with hikes, climbs, and local accommodation. If you are looking for an extreme adventure holiday, look no further. ■

Length: 21.1, 42.2, or 60 km (13.1, 26.2, or 37.3 mi)

Location: Mount Everest Base Camp, Nepal

Date: May

Type: trail/mountainous

Temperature Ø: 5–20 °C (41–68 °F)

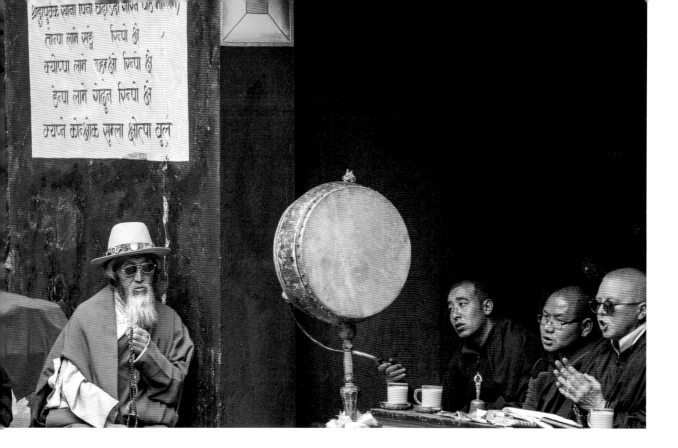

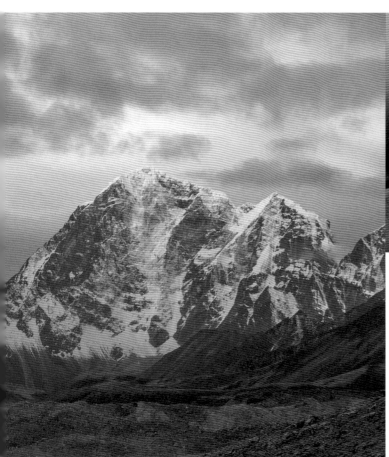

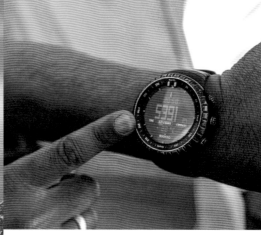

The marathon route crisscrosses the high Sherpa trails of the Khumbu valley before arriving at the finish line in Namche Bazaar. Referred to as the gateway to the high Himalayas, Namche is where many climbers spend time acclimating before attempting to ascend Mount Everest.

This is the world's highest ultra-running event, with snow cover on many parts of the trail. In order to acclimate to the altitude and low oxygen levels, it's recommended that runners spend several days in the region prior to the race start.

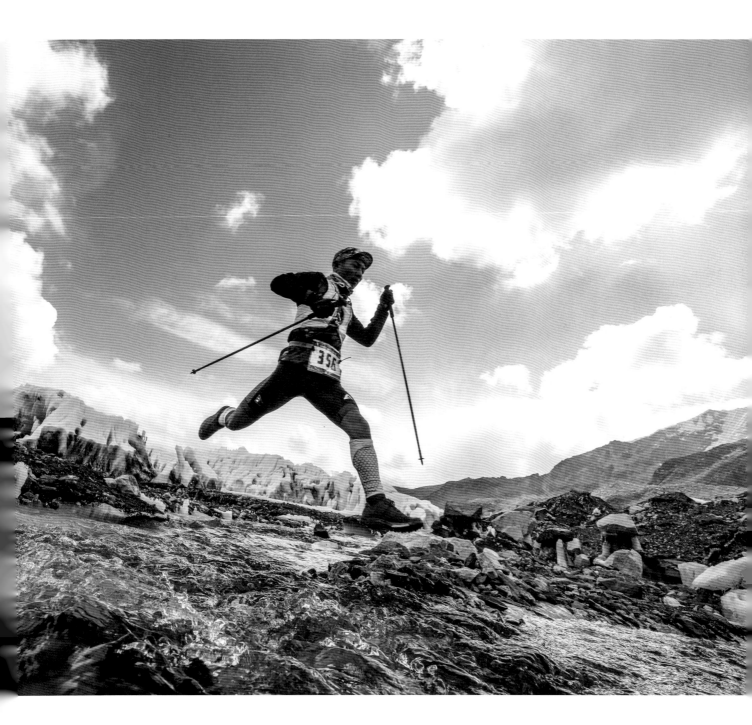

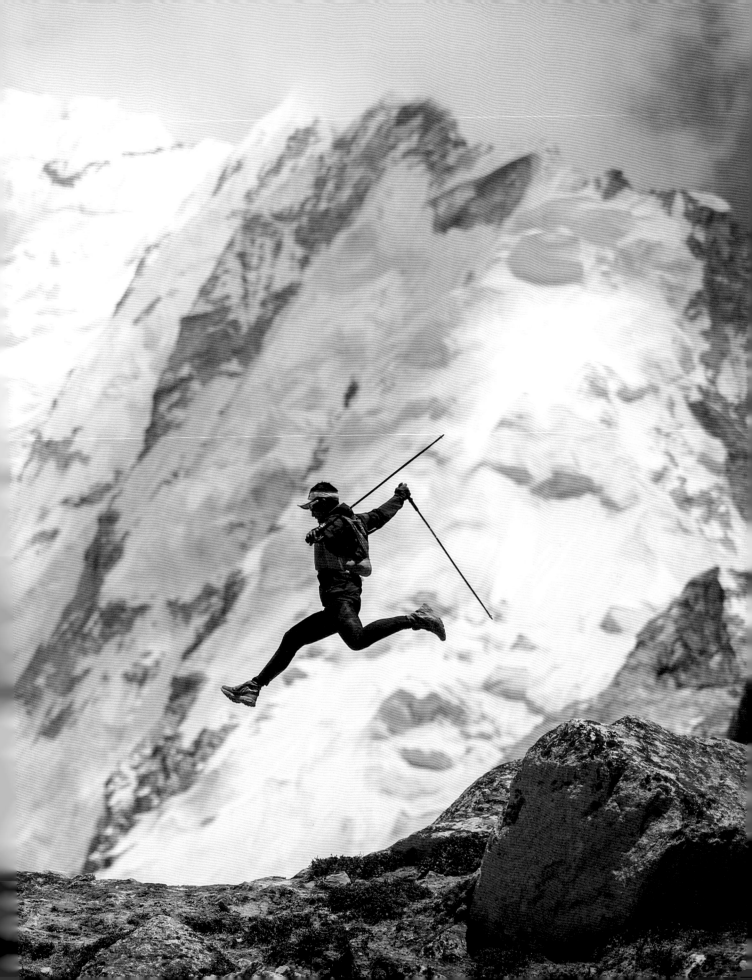

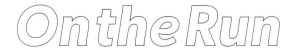

On the Run

Running Across the Globe

This book was conceived, edited, and designed by gestalten.

Edited by Robert Klanten and Lincoln Dexter
Contributing editor: Nicholas Butter

Text by Christian Näthler (pp. 5–19, 45–51, 81–82, 101–102, 175–176, 233–243)
Other texts by Nicholas Butter, edited by Faye Robson
Captions by Anna Southgate

Editorial Management by Adam Jackman and Anna Diekmann

Cover, design, and layout by Stefan Morgner

Photo Editors: Mario Udzenija and Madeline Dudley-Yates

Typeface: Gibson by Jamie Chang, Kevin King, Patrick Griffin, and Rod McDonald.

Cover image by João M. Faria for Madeira Island Ultra-Trail (MIUT)

Printed by Gutenberg Beuys Feindruckerei GmbH, Langenhagen
Made in Germany

Published by gestalten, Berlin 2021
ISBN 978-3-89955-864-7

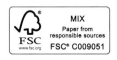

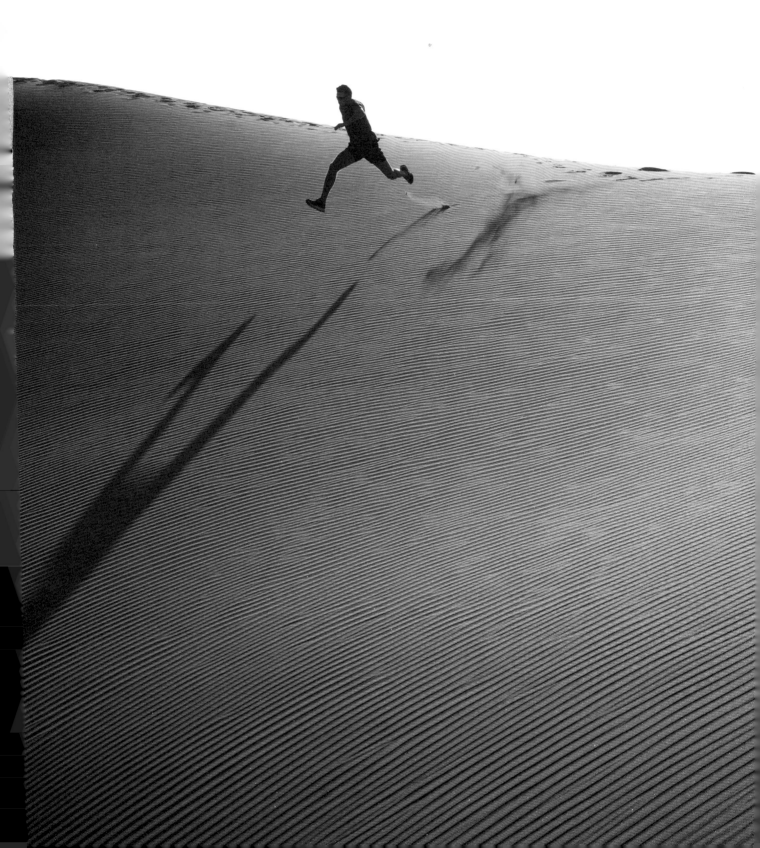

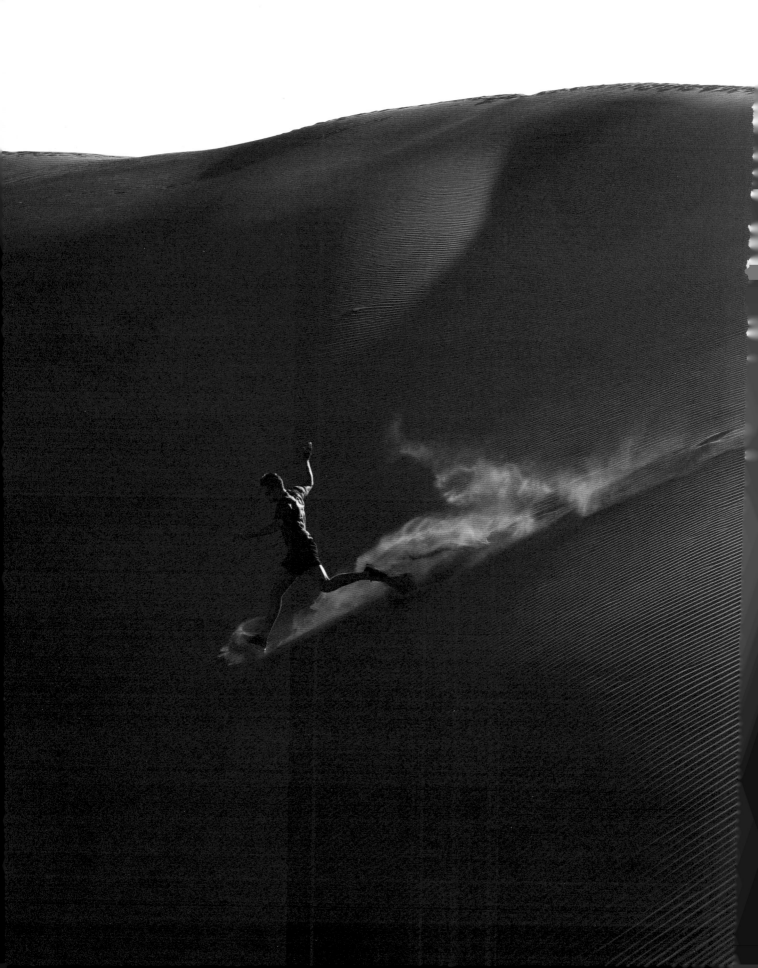